Secondary and Tertiary Arterial Reconstructions

Sachinder Singh Hans

Secondary and Tertiary Arterial Reconstructions

50 Clinical Cases

Springer

Sachinder Singh Hans
Vascular and Endovascular Services
Henry Ford Macomb Hospital
Clinton Township, MI, USA

ISBN 978-3-032-21213-9 ISBN 978-3-032-21214-6 (eBook)
https://doi.org/10.1007/978-3-032-21214-6

This Springer imprint is published by the registered company Springer Nature Switzerland AG
The registered company address is: Gewerbestrasse 11, 6330 Cham, Switzerland

This book is dedicated to my sister, Gurmit Kaur Dhillon, for her commitment, support, and dedication to enable my late brother, Dr. Jagjit Singh Hans, and me to pursue higher education and achieve our dreams.

Foreword

It is a pleasure to write an introduction for this vascular surgery book authored by Sachinder Hans, MD, from Henry Ford Health System in Michigan. All chapters deal with patients that he treated, although his associates participated in a few cases. Each chapter is clearly organized with an Introduction followed by key words, a case presentation, a discussion, photographs, three questions with answers relating to the case, and appropriate references.

The cases pertain to patients with commonly encountered vascular surgery pathology and issues. Dr. Sachinder's explanations of the cases, and particularly of the interventions, are very clear-cut and easy to follow. Not only is he clearly a master surgeon who has encountered a wide variety of vascular pathology, he is an expert dealing with a variety of complex and challenging cases. The reader will gain great insight into the management of each type of problem that he presents for your analysis. I particularly appreciate the inclusion of questions and answers after each case, which greatly enhance the learning experience. I wholeheartedly recommend this book to vascular surgery trainees and attending vascular surgeons.

Society for Vascular Surgery
Philadelphia, PA, USA

Keith Calligaro

Preface

Secondary and tertiary arterial reconstructions are often challenging even for an experienced Vascular surgeon. Besides technical difficulties, many patients requiring repeat arterial reconstruction are at high risk due to their advanced age and significant coexisting medical comorbidities. After a successful primary arterial reconstruction, some patients may require secondary procedures for management of recurrent disease, progression of distal disease, or late complications, such as anastomotic aneurysms, and occasionally a graft infection. Most textbooks in vascular surgery primarily emphasize primary reconstruction. A case-based book with a strong emphasis on secondary and tertiary arterial reconstruction was the impetus to publish this book for the benefit of vascular trainees, recent graduates of vascular surgery training programs, interventional radiologists, interventional cardiologists, primary care physicians, and emergency room physicians.

The 50 cases in this book are from the editor's clinical practice, except for a few cases by my colleagues at Henry Ford Medical Group vascular surgery. There were 25 patients who had two arterial reconstructions, 20 had three, and 13 had more than three arterial reconstructions. Two patients had primary arterial reconstruction but were included due to some interesting aspects in their care. Both satisfactory and suboptimal outcomes were included so that readers can learn from our unsatisfactory outcomes.

I would like to extend my sincere appreciation to Dr. Andi Peshkepija, Dr. Tamer Boules, Dr. Kate Rountree, Dr. Melissa Hetrick from Henry Ford, and Dr. Sean P. Lyden from the Cleveland Clinic, Cleveland, Ohio, and Dr. Muhammad Rishi from Soin Medical Center, Kettering, Ohio, for their participation in the care of two patients. I sincerely wish to thank Kristopher Spring, Executive Editor at Springer, for approval of this book project and his unrelenting support, Sharath Rangaraj, Production, Springer, and Melanie Bednarski, Librarian, Henry Ford Macomb Hospital, for their contributions in bringing this project to fruition.

Sincerely,
Sachinder Hans, MD

Clinton Township, MI, USA — Sachinder Singh Hans
8/15/2025

Contents

Rupture of Abdominal Aortic Aneurysm Due to Type IB Endoleak in a Patient with Prior Endovascular Repair for a Ruptured Abdominal Aortic Aneurysm

1

Presentation

An 84-year-old male presented to the emergency room of an out-of-state hospital with severe abdominal pain in December 2022. Medical comorbidities included controlled atrial fibrillation, hypertension, remote stroke with excellent recovery, and hyperlipidemia. In June 2016, the patient had undergone endovascular aneurysm repair for a ruptured abdominal aortic aneurysm (AAA) using the Endurant graft (Medtronic, Dublin, Ireland). The CTA abdomen and pelvis showed 9.4 × 9.1 cm AAA with right CIA 22 mm and left CIA 20 mm with periaortic hematoma (Fig. 1.1a, b). The main body (36 × 16 × 166 mm) was deployed from the right side. The contralateral limb (16 × 24 × 124 mm) and an ipsilateral limb (16 × 24 × 124 mm) were deployed. Completion aortogram showing satisfactory exclusion of the AAA (Fig. 1.2). A follow-up CTA abdomen and pelvis 1 month later showed that the size of the aneurysm sac was 9.6 × 9.2 cm. However, there appeared to be active extravasation of the contrast in the retroperitoneal hematoma associated with slight sac expansion. Patient underwent postoperative abdominal aortography, which did not show any evidence of endoleak and with satisfactory exclusion of the AAA (Fig. 1.3). Patient was followed by six monthly aortic-iliac duplex study, which showed a stable aneurysm sac without endoleak. In December 2022, he was admitted to an out-of-state hospital with severe abdominal pain. An emergency CTA of the abdomen and pelvis showed significant contrast enhancement outside the endograft in the arterial phase, compatible with a large endoleak. Arterial phase contrast enhancement extended into the lumen of the inferior vena cava, right common iliac vein, and right external iliac vein; findings suggestive of aortocaval fistula. The aneurysm sac measured 9.2 × 10.2 cm with infiltrate and attenuation surrounding the aneurysm sac, with fluid extension into the pelvis. The findings were suggestive of type IB endoleak with migration of the left limb proximally into the aneurysm sac. The patient was taken emergently to the operating room. A bilateral femoral artery access was obtained with ultrasound guidance and fluoroscopic assistance with the puncture site just inferior to the head of the femur using micro-puncture technique with placement of 7F sheaths on each side.

Two perclose devices were placed at "10 o'clock" and "2 o'clock" positions. The 7F sheath was upsized over a 0.035″ glidewire advantage, and Then using a glide catheter, an Amplatz super stiff wire was advanced into the proximal thoracic aorta, and 12F sheaths were advanced towards the main body of the graft from both sides. On the left side the tract had to be dilated to facilitate the passage of the sheath. Contrast injection via the left sheath confirmed a large type IB endoleak as a result of the retraction of the left iliac limb of the endograft

S. S. Hans, *Secondary and Tertiary Arterial Reconstructions*,
https://doi.org/10.1007/978-3-032-21214-6_1

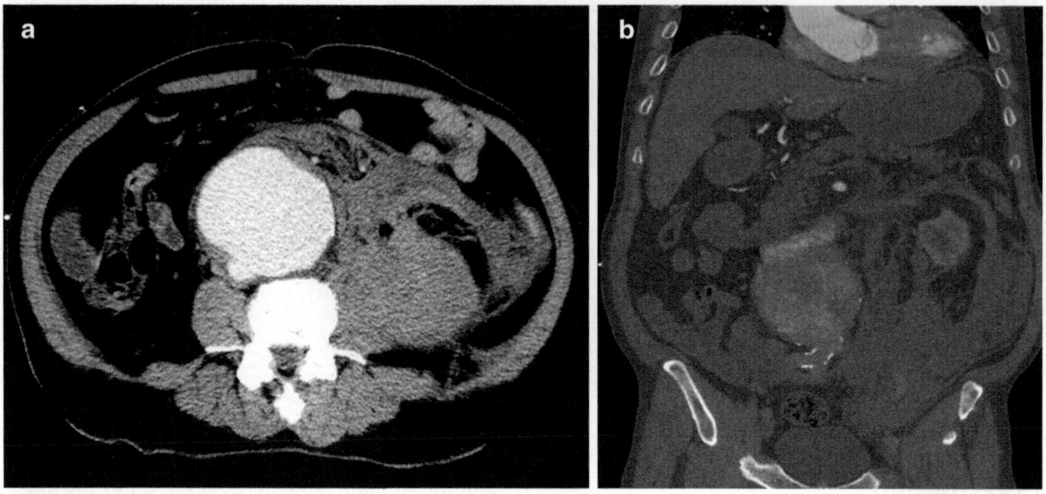

Fig. 1.1 (**a**) CTA is showing large AAA with retroperitoneal hematoma. (**b**) CTA is showing large AAA with retroperitoneal hematoma in coronal view

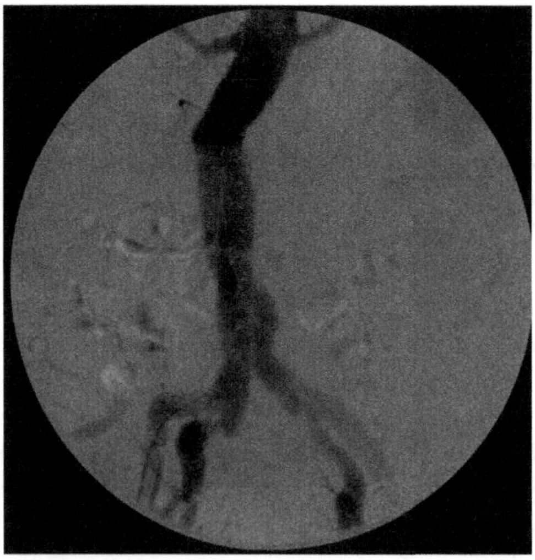

Fig. 1.2 Completion aortogram following EVAR

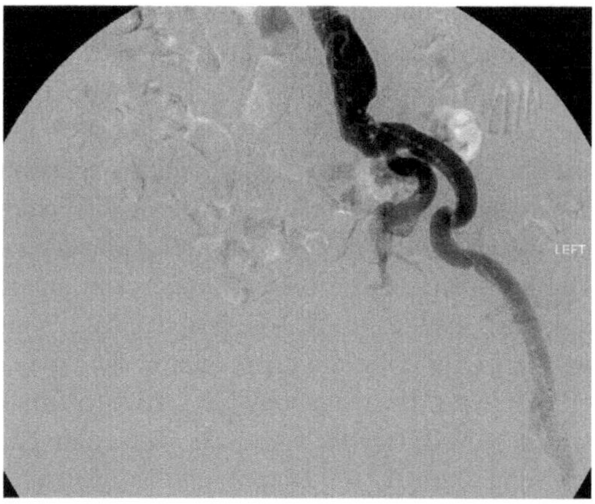

Fig. 1.3 Postoperative aortogram showing satisfactory deployment of the left iliac graft limb

into the dilated common iliac artery. The limb was realigned using a GORE EXCLUDER 16 × 14.5 × 140 mm limb extension from the gate to the proximal external iliac artery, followed by balloon angioplasty of the limb.

A very small type IB endoleak was still visualized. The left hypogastric artery was covered by a stent graft. The perclose device was deployed on the right side. On the left side, the left femoral artery was sutured with 4 "O" CV polypropylene (Ethicon, Cincinnati, OH) suture after performing a cutdown. A few months later, the patient underwent a coil embolization of the right hypogastric artery and deployment of a right iliac extension limb (Excluder) to the mid external iliac artery. Follow-up CTA of abdomen and pelvis showed satisfactory exclusion of the AAA with no evidence of endoleak (Figs. 1.4a, b and 1.5a, b). Patient was last seen on March 27, 2025, as he underwent a successful coil embolization for lower GI bleeding (cecal). A microcatheter was used to obtain access to the superior

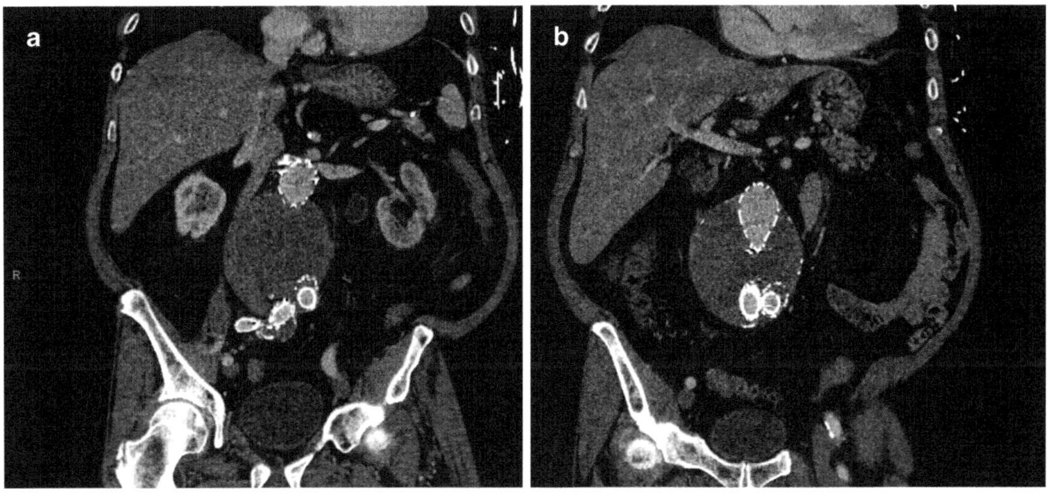

Fig. 1.4 (**a**, **b**) Postoperative CTA following EVAR for recurrent rupture of AAA due to Type IB endoleak with left iliac extension limb

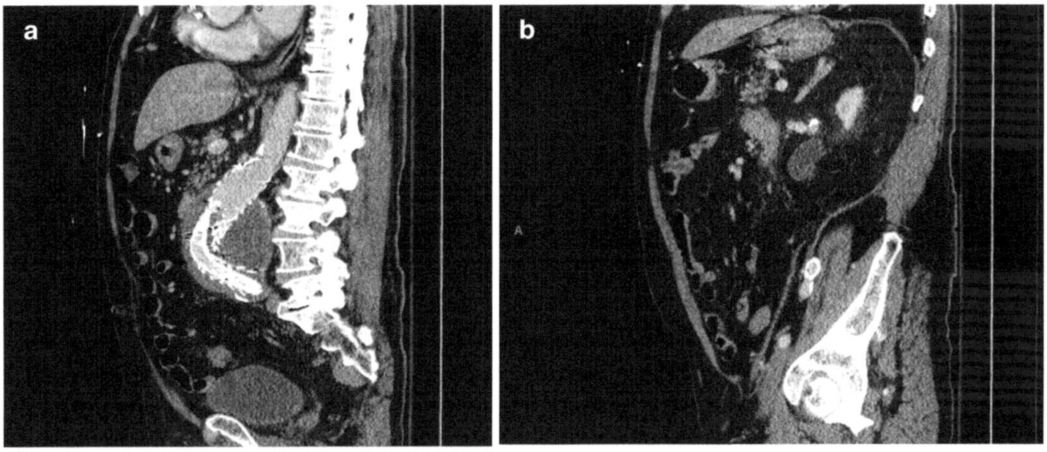

Fig. 1.5 (**a**, **b**) Sagittal view of CTA showing iliac extension limbs on both sides

mesenteric artery and into the branch of the ileocolic artery.

Discussion

From a scoping review of 27 articles Zuccon et al. reported a 0–8% incidence of type IB endoleak following EVAR [1]. Several anatomical factors, including a common iliac diameter of greater than 18 mm, a length of the common iliac artery landing zone of less than 20 mm, use of flared limbs (>20mm(greater than 20mm)), marked iliac artery, tortuosity, and large initial AAA size, increase the risk of type IB endoleak [1].

To decrease the incidence of type IB endoleak, a distal landing zone just proximal to the common iliac artery bifurcation should be attempted. In our patient, a large AAA (>9.0 cm) and dilated common iliac arteries increased the likelihood of the development of type IB endoleak. Most patients with type IB endoleak can be treated with endovascular techniques. This case also illustrates that in patients undergoing EVAR with large common iliac arteries, duplex imaging of the aortoiliac segment should be supplanted by CTA of the abdomen and pelvis for surveillance. In morbidly obese patients' accurate delineation of distal landing of the iliac limb may be difficult to obtain using aortoiliac duplex imaging. In patients with type IB endoleak, the size of the aneurysm sac may take longer to enlarge as compared to type IA endoleak.

Patients presenting with a ruptured AAA, with suitable anatomy for EVAR, have better outcomes with endovascular repair as compared to an open repair. Results of the IMPROVE trial, which randomized 613 patients with ruptured AAA, 316 to EVAR as the first strategy and 297 to open repair [2]. At 1 year, all-cause mortality was 41.5% for the endovascular repair group and 45.1% for the open repair group. There was no survival benefit for the EVAR group beyond 1 year, but it offered patients faster discharge and better quality of life [2]. The reintervention rate was similar in both groups [2]. Existing endograft provides neither acute nor one-year survival benefit after ruptured AAA repair. Doctors' evaluation reported 20% mortality in patients with prior endovascular repair and 38% with open repair ($p = 0.27$) in patients who had rupture of an AAA with prior endovascular repair [3].

Multiple Choice Questions

1. Results of the IMPROVE trial comparing EVAR to open repair for ruptured AAA demonstrated an all-cause mortality at 1 year of
   A. 60% for open repair, 50% for EVAR
   B. 50% for open repair, 45% for EVAR
   C. 45% for open repair, 41% for EVAR
   D. 50% for open repair, 60% for EVAR
2. From a scoping review of 27 articles, the incidence of type IB endoleak following EVAR is
   A. 0–8%
   B. 2–10%
   C. 4–12%
   D. Greater than 12%
3. The diameter of the common iliac artery at the time of EVAR predisposing to type IB endoleak following EVAR is
   A. 10–14 mm
   B. 14.1–16 mm
   C. 16.1–18 mm
   D. Greater than 18 mm

Answers: 1(C), 2(A), 3(D)

References

1. Zuccon G, D'Oria M, Gonçalves FB, et al. Incidence, risk factors, and prognostic impact of type IB endoleak following endovascular repair for abdominal aortic aneurysm: scoping review. Eur J Vasc Endovasc Surg. 2023;66(3):352–61. PMID:37356703.
2. Powell JT, Sweeting MJ, Thompson MM, et al. Endovascular or open repair strategy for ruptured abdominal aortic aneurysm: 30 day outcomes from IMPROVE randomized trial. BMJ. 2014;348:f7661. PMID:24418950.
3. Cho JS, Park T, Kim JY, Chaer RA, Rhee RY, Makaroun MS. Prior endovascular abdominal aortic aneurysm repair provides no survival benefits when the aneurysm ruptures. J Vasc Surg. 2010;52(5):1127–34. PMID:20674248.

2 Endovascular Repair of Hypogastric Artery Aneurysm Following Open Abdominal Aortic Aneurysm Repair

Presentation

An 85-year-old man was found to have a 5 cm (Tr/AP diameter) left Hypogastric artery aneurysm (HAA) detected by contrast enhanced CT scan abdominal and pelvis for back pain in January 2024 (Figs. 2.1 and 2.2). His comorbidities included Type II diabetes mellitus, CAD (Remote CABG), hypertension, pacemaker insertion, and chronic kidney disease. In June 2003, the patient underwent open repair of 5.5 cm infrarenal abdmonial aortic aneurysm (AAA) with interposition of an 18 mm aortic tube Gelsoft Dacron graft (Vascutek Ltd., Inchinnan, UK), with proximal anastomosis just inferior to the origin of renal arteries and distal anastomosis just above the aortic bifurcation.

On January 18, 2024, the patient underwent endovascular repair of the left HAA. Under ultrasound guidance, right femoral artery access was obtained using micro puncture technique. An abdominal aortogram using a 5F Omniflush catheter was obtained. It showed a large hypogastric aneurysm with satisfactory open repair with a tube graft (Fig. 2.3). The Omniflush catheter was removed. A Bentson 0.035″ wire (Cook Medical, Bloomington, IN) was used to place a 6F Pinnacle sheath on the right side. A 5F Cobra catheter was used to select the left hypogastric artery, which had a 50% stenosis at its origin. A 2.8F microcatheter was advanced through the Cobra catheter, and the aneurysmal anterior division of the HAA was selected with coil embolization using micro

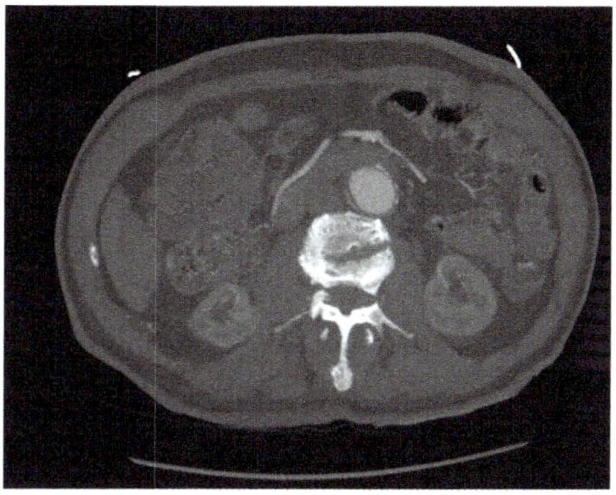

Fig. 2.1 CTA of abdomen showing previously placed aortic tube graft for the repair of AAA

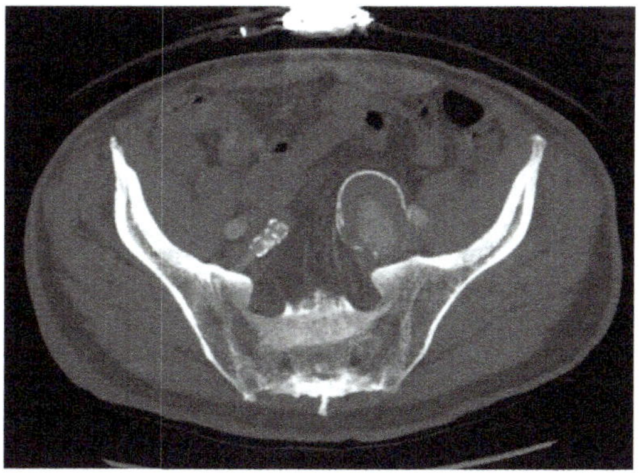

Fig. 2.2 CTA of pelvis showing a large hypogastric aneurysm

coils. Additional microcoils were placed through the microcatheter into the iliolumbar artery. Post embolization, fluoroscopic images did not demon-

S. S. Hans, *Secondary and Tertiary Arterial Reconstructions*,
https://doi.org/10.1007/978-3-032-21214-6_2

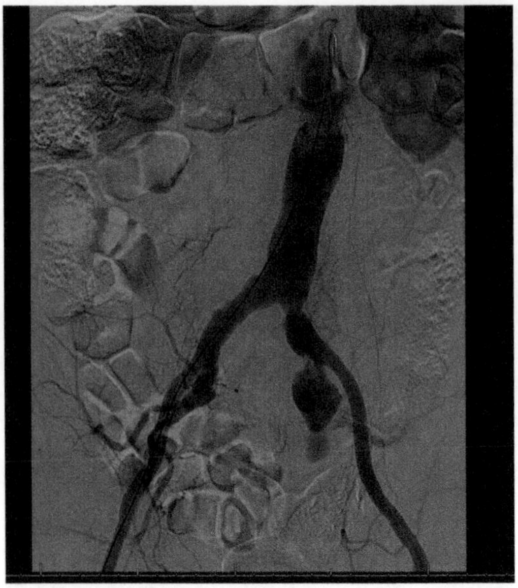

Fig. 2.3 Intraoperative Aortogram showing large left hypogastric aneurysm with prior open repair of AAA with a tube graft

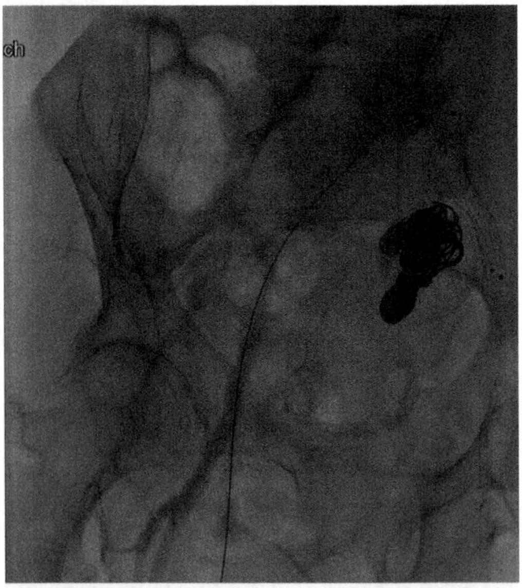

Fig. 2.4 Coil embolization of the left hypogastric artery using left femoral artery access

strate any flow into the iliolumbar artery, and there was no opacification of the HAA (Fig. 2.4).

Following coil embolization, left common femoral artery access was obtained using the

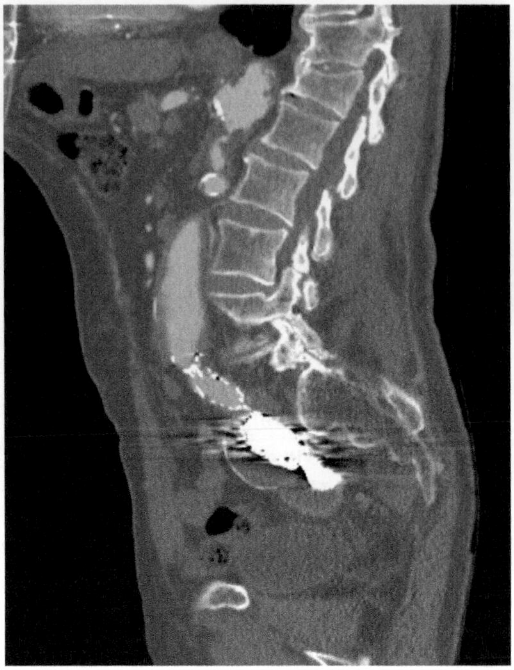

Fig. 2.5 Postoperative CTA showing successful thrombosis of left hypogastric artery aneurysm

micro-puncture technique under ultrasound image guidance, and a 7F sheath was advanced over a Bentson wire. The Bentson wire was exchanged for a 0.035″ exchange length Lunderquist wire (Cook Medical, Bloomington, IN). There was approximately 20% stenosis of the aorta at the proximal anastomosis and ectasia (15 mm) of the left common iliac artery. A 16 × 10 × 93 mm Endurant (Medtronic, Dublin, Ireland) was deployed from the proximal left CIA to the proximal left EIA, and a post-angioplasty using a Reliant balloon. A 14F Manta closure (Teleflex, Wayne, PA) device was used to close the puncture site in the left CFA. An angioseal device (Terumo, Somerset, NJ) was used to close the right CFA puncture site. Follow-up CTA of abdomen and pelvis 1 month later showed satisfactory exclusion of the left HA (Fig. 2.5). The Dacron graft replacement for AAA has shown gradual enlargement as expected. Postoperative CTA of the abdomen and pelvis showed complete thrombosis of the HA aneurysm (Fig. 2.5).

Discussion

Common iliac artery aneurysms are present in 10–20% of patients with AAA [1]. An isolated common iliac artery (CIA) and hypogastric artery aneurysm (HAA) are relatively uncommon, occurring in only 0.03% of the population, and are present in less than 2% and 0.4% of clinically noted aneurysmal disease, respectively. Common iliac and HAA are six times more common in men than in women [1]. Most HAA are degenerative and occasionally have a mycotic etiology. Most CIA and HAA with size >3.5 cm should be repaired in order to prevent rupture [1].

In contrast to the CIA aneurysm, the ability to preserve hypogastric artery flow is greatly reduced in patients presenting with large HA aneurysms, as adequate length of proximal and distal landing zones for repair with a stent graft is usually not feasible. Open procedures are generally not recommended because of the deep pelvic location of HAA, increased blood loss, and associated multiple comorbidities in elderly patients [1, 2].

Rupture may be the first presentation of HAA, manifesting as thigh, abdominal, or back pain with or without associated hypotension [1, 2]. Retroperitoneal rupture may be contained for a few hours, but intraperitoneal rupture leads to rapid exsanguination [3]. Rupture into the rectum, ureter, and urinary bladder has been reported [3]. Hypogastric artery aneurysms under 4 cm in Tr/AP diameter rarely rupture [3].

Multiple Choice Questions

1. Incidence of isolated Hypogastric artery aneurysm is
   A. 0.2%
   B. 0.4%
   C. 0.6%
   D. 0.8%
2. A 75-year-old man was found to have a 6 cm hypogastric aneurysm. He had a prior open AAA repair with a tube graft; the best management option is
   A. Place a covered stent across the opening of the Hypogastric artery
   B. Open repair
   C. Coil embolization of the anterior and posterior branches of the HA
   D. Coil embolization of the anterior and posterior branches and stent graft (covered stent) from the common iliac to the external iliac artery
3. Hypogastric artery aneurysm should be repaired when the aneurysm reaches the maximum diameter of
   A. 6 cm
   B. 5 cm
   C. 3.5–4 cm
   D. 3–3.5 cm

Answers: 1(B), 2(D), 3(C)

References

1. Hans SS. Endovascular repair of a large hypogastric aneurysm following open repair of abdominal aortic aneurysm. In: Challenging arterial reconstructions: 100 clinical cases. Cham: Springer; 2020. p. 327–8.
2. Murphy EW. Endovascular management of common and internal iliac artery aneurysms. Endoscopy Today, p. 76–81 (2012).
3. Laine MT, Björck M, Beiles CB, Szeberin Z, Thomson I, Altreuther M, et al. Few internal iliac artery aneurysms rupture under 4 cm. J Vasc Surg. 2017;65(1):76–81. PMID:28010870.

3 Endovascular Repair of Aortic Anastomotic Aneurysm Following Open Repair of AAA

Presentation

In January 1997, a 68-year-old man was admitted to the hospital via the emergency department with severe abdominal and back pain. He was found to have a 7.0 cm (AP/Tr diameter) infrarenal abdominal aortic aneurysm (AAA). Using a midline laparotomy incision, he underwent repair of a symptomatic AAA with a 16 mm gelsoft (Vascutek Inchinnan, UK) tube graft with reimplantation of the left lower pole accessory renal artery into the tube graft. Both femoral arteries were explored as the patient did not have Doppler flow in either foot at the completion of the operation. A limited common femoral endarterectomy with a vein patch taken from an accessory saphenous vein in the right groin and upper thigh was performed on both sides. Passage of a Fogarty catheter distally in each lower extremity did not retrieve any thromboembolic material. The patient had a satisfactory postoperative course and was followed yearly in the clinic.

In December 2013, the patient had a follow-up CTA scan of the abdomen and pelvis, which showed a 4.5 cm distal aortic anastomotic aneurysm and a 2.5 cm saccular proximal anastomotic aneurysm. He underwent an endovascular repair of both proximal and distal anastomotic aneurysms by groin cut-down access to the femoral arteries on each side. Groin dissection was challenging because of the prior exposure of the femoral arteries. The main body 32 × 16 × 150 mm of Endurant graft

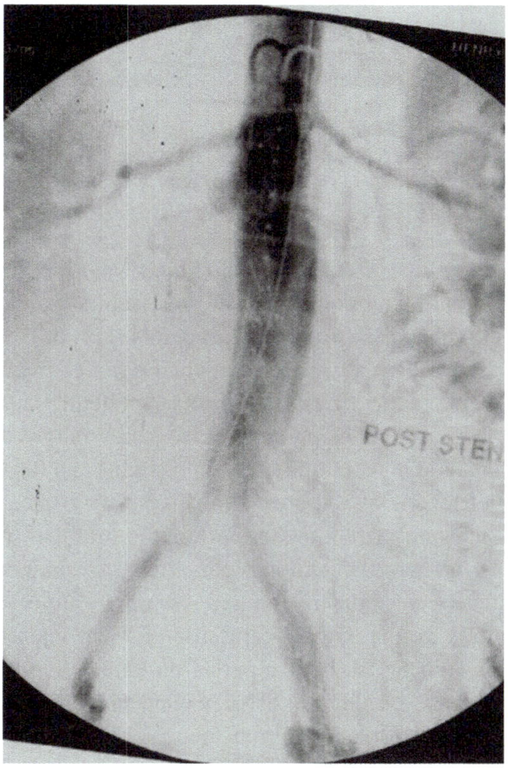

Fig. 3.1 Intraoperative completion aortogram showing exclusion of proximal and distal para-anastomotic aneurysm

(Medtronic, Dublin, Ireland) was deployed from the left side, and the contralateral right iliac limb 16 × 3 × 124 mm. Completion aortogram showed that both anastomotic aneurysms were successfully excluded (Fig. 3.1). A

S. S. Hans, *Secondary and Tertiary Arterial Reconstructions*,
https://doi.org/10.1007/978-3-032-21214-6_3

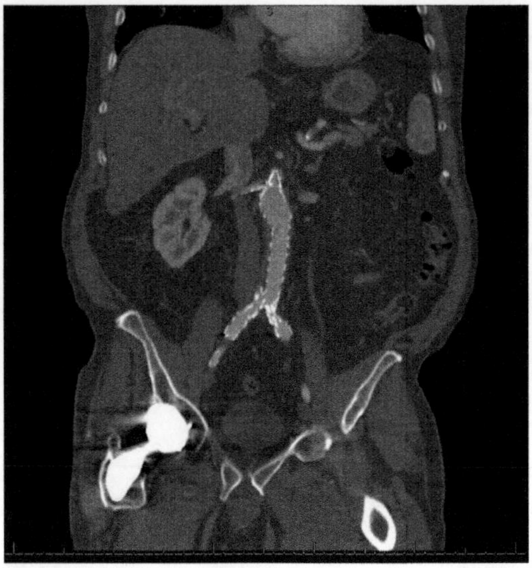

Fig. 3.2 Postoperative CTA of abdomen and pelvis showing successful exclusion of para-anastomotic aneurysm

follow-up CTA of the abdomen and pelvis 1 month later confirmed the satisfactory exclusion of the anastomotic aneurysms (Fig. 3.2).

In March 2023, the patient presented with symptomatic lifestyle-limiting bilateral calf claudication. Doppler arterial study showed an ankle brachial index of 0.46 (right) and 0.41 (left). CTA of abdomen and pelvis showed near occlusion of both common femoral arteries. In November 2023 and February 2024, the patient underwent bilateral staged common femoral artery and proximal deep femoral artery endarterectomy with bovine pericardial patch angioplasty. A vacuum-assisted wound closure was performed for each groin incision. The patient had marked improvement in his symptoms of intermittent claudication. Doppler arterial study in October 2024 showed ankle-brachial index 0.71 (right) and 0.78 (left).

Discussion

During the past 25 years, there has been an increasing number of reports describing successful endovascular repair of para-anastomotic aortic and iliac aneurysms with reduced morbidity and mortality as compared to open repair. The true incidence of para-aortic anastomotic aneurysms following open aortic reconstruction for aneurysmal and occlusive disease is unknown. The frequency of 2–2.9% has been reported. The exact incidence may be underestimated as a significant number of patients do not undergo imaging studies following open aortic reconstruction per SVS guidelines, and many are lost to follow-up.

The diagnosis of para-anastomotic aneurysms is usually made after 8–10 years of index repair. Paraaortic aneurysms following open aortic repair may represent a true progression of the disease or as result of an anastomotic disruption resulting in pseudoaneurysm formation. Hallett et al., reported that a proximal aortic para-anastomotic pseudoaneurysm developed in six patients (2.9%) from a retrospective study of 208 patients who survived open repair of AAA [1]. Conrad et al., reported a 15-year follow-up following open repair of AAA with 3.2% (26 patients) incidence of late complications, including anastomotic pseudoaneurysms in 23 and secondary aortoenteric fistula in the remaining three patients [2]. Following an open AAA repair, an anastomotic aneurysm or aneurysmal dilatation of the adjacent visceral segment or iliac arteries may occur in 1%, 5%, 20%, at 5, 10, 15 years, respectively [2]. Open repair of para-anastomotic aortic aneurysm is a challenging operation with a perioperative mortality of 17% in the elective setting and 24% in emergency cases. Perioperative mortality, including cardiac, pulmonary, neurologic, and infectious complications, is common. Sachdev et al., reported a 3.9% mortality of endovascular repair, and a 30-day complication rate, which included endoleak, was 23%. Overall mortality was 49% (mean follow-up of 18 months), and was significantly attributed to older age at the time of endovascular treatment (p=0.03) [3].

The Society for Vascular Surgery guidelines for management of abdominal aortic aneurysm recommend that the first CTA of the abdomen and pelvis should be obtained 5 years after open repair of AAA [4]. Most aortic and iliac anastomotic aneurysms remain asymptomatic. Large aortic and iliac anastomotic aneurysms can cause compression of surrounding structures like the ureter, lumbar plexus, and iliac vein, resulting in hydronephrosis, back or flank pain, and swelling of the lower extremity.

Multiple Choice Questions

1. According to SVS guidelines, the first CTA of the abdomen and pelvis following open repair of AAA should be obtained in
   A. 3 years
   B. 5 years
   C. 10 years
   D. 15 years
2. The incidence of para-anastomotic aneurysms following open repair of AAA is
   A. 1–2%
   B. 3–4%
   C. 5–7%
   D. >7%
3. Endovascular repair of para-anastomotic aneurysms, as compared to open repair, results in
   A. Reduced morbidity and mortality
   B. Reduced morbidity but similar mortality
   C. Increased morbidity but reduced mortality
   D. Reduced morbidity but increased mortality.

Answers: 1(B), 2(B), 3(A)

References

1. Hallett JW Jr, Marshall DM, Petterson TM, et al. Graft-related complications after abdominal aortic aneurysm repair: reassurance from a 36-year population-based experience. J Vasc Surg. 1997;25(2):277–84; discussion 285–286. PMID:9052562.
2. Conrad MF, Crawford RS, Pedraza JD, et al. Long-term durability of open abdominal aortic aneurysm repair. J Vasc Surg. 2007;46(4):669–75. PMID:17903647.
3. Sachdev U, Baril DT, Morrissey NJ, et al. Endovascular repair of para-anastomotic aortic aneurysms. J Vasc Surg. 2007;46(4):636–41. PMID:17764881.
4. Chaikof EL, Dalman RL, Eskandari MK, et al. The Society for Vascular Surgery practice guidelines on the care of patients with an abdominal aortic aneurysm. J Vasc Surg. 2018;67(1):2–77.e72. PMID:29268916.

4 Endovascular Aneurysm Repair (EVAR) in a Patient with Prior Iliac Covered Stent and Crossover Femoral–Femoral Graft

Presentation

In 2019, a 76-year-old man underwent left iliac covered stent placement and a crossover femoral-femoral graft at an outside hospital for right common iliac artery (CIA) and external iliac artery (EIA) occlusion and an inflow stenosis of the left CIA. He was seen in the vascular clinic in June 2022 with a complaint of constant back pain related to heavy lifting and with some relief from analgesics. He had a 60-pack-year smoking habit. He had been consuming 5–6 cans of beer daily for the past 55 years. His medical comorbidities included hyperlipidemia and chronic obstructive pulmonary disease. In July 2022, he was seen in the vascular clinic after having undergone a CTA of the abdomen and pelvis, which showed an enlargement of a known abdominal aortic aneurysm (AAA) from 5.2 cm to 5.5 cm (AP/Tr diameter). Because of multiple-associated comorbidities, surveillance with a follow-up CTA of the abdomen and pelvis in 6 months was planned. Aortoiliac duplex imaging in January 2023 showed that the AAA remained stable at 5.5 cm. However, aortoiliac duplex imaging in September of 2023 showed that the AAA had now enlarged and measured 5.9 cm in its greater AP/Tr diameter with a large amount of thrombus, with patency of the left common iliac artery stent. There was associated calcification of the left common and external iliac artery (Figs. 4.1 and 4.2a, b). In October 2023, the patient underwent digital subtraction arteriography (DSA) of abdomen, aorta, and pelvis as well as a runoff study using a percutaneous left brachial artery access as non-invasive arterial duplex imaging showed evidence of left iliac

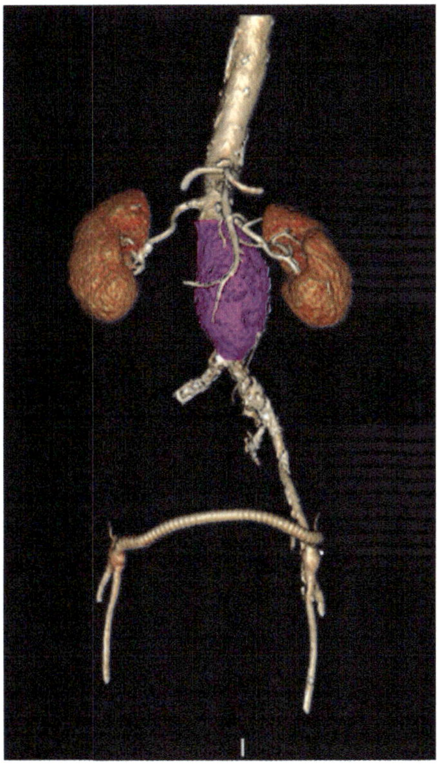

Fig. 4.1 CTA abdomen and pelvis showing infrarenal AAA with patent crossover femoral–femoral graft

S. S. Hans, *Secondary and Tertiary Arterial Reconstructions*,
https://doi.org/10.1007/978-3-032-21214-6_4

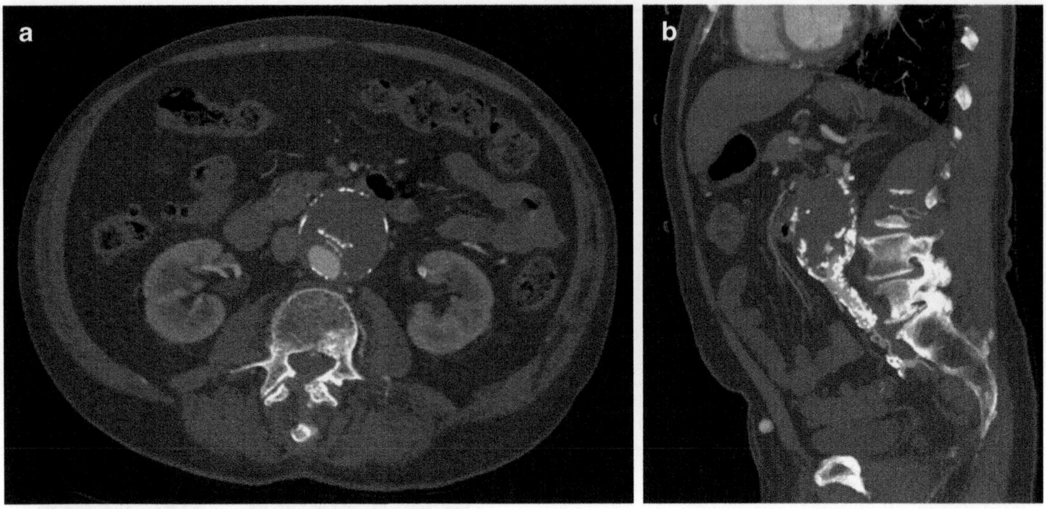

Fig. 4.2 (**a**) CTA Abdomen (axial image) showing 5.9 cm. AAA with large amount of thrombus. (**b**) CTA abdomen and pelvis (sagittal view) AAA: Left common iliac artery stent and calcification in the left iliac artery

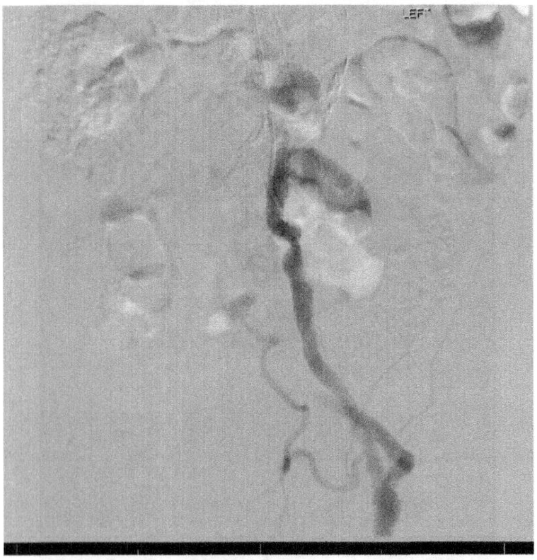

Fig. 4.3 Preoperative abdominal aortogram showed left iliac artery stenosis just distal to the previously placed stent

artery stenosis (Fig. 4.3). He underwent left iliac angioplasty for left iliac stenosis with an 8 mm × 4 cm Armada balloon (Abbott Medical, Chicago, IL).

Patient underwent EVAR with an aortouniliac (AUI) endograft on December 14, 2023. Left groin cutdown was performed. The crossover femoral–femoral graft was exposed. A moderate sized left femoral anastomotic aneurysm (3cm) was seen and mobilized. A simultaneous left brachial artery percutaneous access was obtained using ultrasound guidance. The left femoral artery was entered just inferior to the anastomotic aneurysm, and a 7F sheath was placed initially, a 0.035″ starter wire was exchanged for a Lunderquist wire, and its tip was placed in the proximal descending thoracic aorta using a Kumpe catheter (Angiodynamics, Latham, NY). An Omniflush catheter was placed in the suprarenal aorta via left brachial access. Because of the presence of left common iliac artery stenosis, the endograft delivery system could not be advanced. This necessitated the passage of an 18 mm Coons dilator followed by a 20 mm Coons dilator (Cook Medical, Bloomington, IN). Shockwave lithotripsy (Shock Wave Medical, Santa Clara, CA) and balloon angioplasty with an 8 × 60 mm Armada balloon (Abbott, Abbott Park, IL) were also performed. Following placement of a 20F Sentrant sheath (Medtronic, Dublin, Ireland) from just inferior to the presence of anastomotic aneurysm in the common femoral artery, the endograft delivery system could then be advanced just distal into abdominal aorta just proximal to AAA.

Both the SFA and the profunda femoris artery were controlled separately with silastic vascular loops. Aortouniiliac Endurant graft

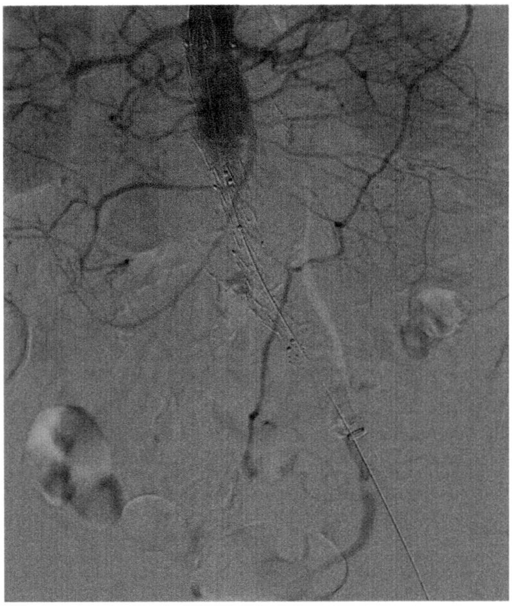

Fig. 4.4 Completion aortogram during EVAR showing encroachment of the left renal artery by the endograft

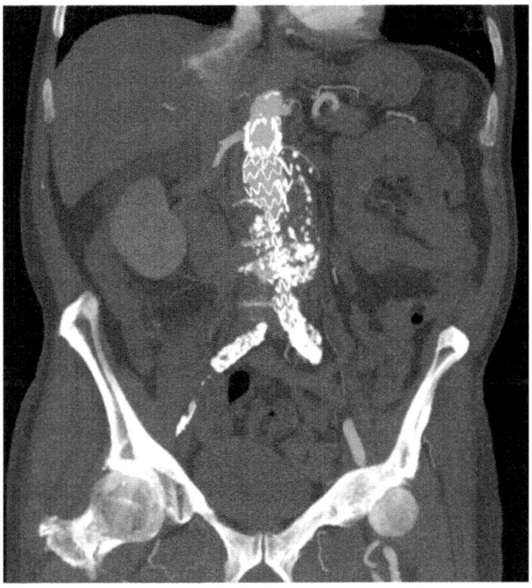

Fig. 4.5 Postoperative CTA abdomen and pelvis showing endograft with diminuitive left renal artery due to partial coverage by the stent graft

36 × 14 × 102 mm was deployed, followed by a left iliac limb extension (16 × 13 × 93 mm). A 10 × 39 mm left distal common iliac and proximal external iliac balloon expandable stent Omnilink (Abbott, Abbott Park, IL) was deployed distal to the iliac limb of the endograft. The left femoral anastomotic aneurysm was resected and repaired with a 5 cm, long 8 mm diameter interposition PTFE graft between the distal external iliac artery (using limited left lower quadrant retroperitoneal exposure) to the common femoral artery bifurcation. Crossover femoral graft was extended distally to the hood of the left external iliac and femoral interposition graft with another short 3 cm length of 8 mm PTFE graft.

Completion aortogram after endograft deployment showed slight encroachment of the fabric of the endograft into the orifice of the left renal artery (Fig. 4.4). A follow-up CTA of the abdomen and pelvis 1 month following EVAR showed that the proximal end of the endograft was encroaching upon the lumen of the left renal artery with poor flow in the left renal artery (Fig. 4.5). The patient was advised to undergo a left renal artery stent placement, but he refused to undergo the procedure. However, he did agree to the left renal stent placement 2 months later. An abdominal aortogram and pelvic arteriogram showed that the left renal artery had completely occluded in the interim with a patent crossover femoral-femoral graft following repair of the left femoral anastomotic aneurysm (Fig. 4.6a, b). His renal function remained satisfactory. The patient was subsequently admitted to the hospital with frequent falls, memory loss, and a T-12 compression fracture. The patient died in June 2024 from acute respiratory failure, superimposed on an advanced chronic obstructive pulmonary disease.

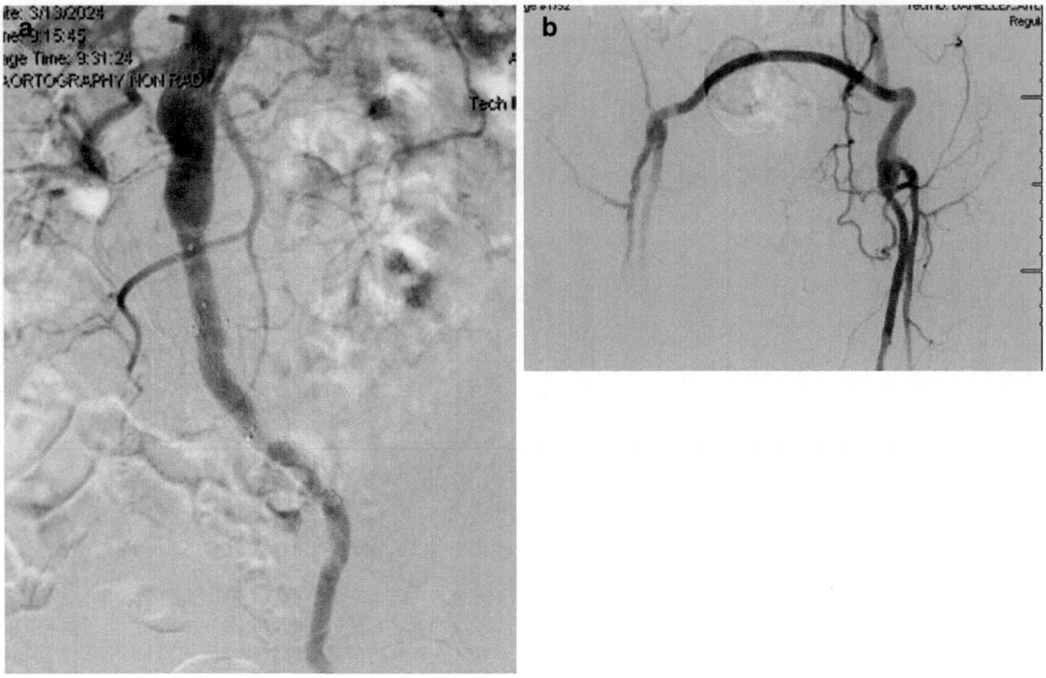

Fig. 4.6 (**a**) Postoperative aortography using brachial access shows left renal artery occlusion and exclusion of the AAA with aortouniliac graft. (**b**) Patient crossover femoral–femoral graft with repair of left femoral anastomotic aneurysm and interposition graft from distal EIA to CFA bifurcation

Discussion

Hinchcliffe et al. reported 231 patients (1994–2002) who underwent aorto-uniiliac stent graft and crossover femoral-femoral graft for repair of AAA. They reported an incidence of local wound complications in 11% of patients. In their series, the five-year patency of the femoral–femoral bypass graft was 83%. They concluded that when graft occlusion occurs it is due to inadequate inflow stenosis in the stent graft or intimal flap in the external iliac artery [1].

Dortch et al. reported 35 patients from 2002 to 2012 who underwent EVAR with commercially manufactured aorto-uniiliac endograpts with femoral–femoral bypass graft and reported a median follow-up of 40 months. In 26% of patients a secondary procedure was performed, and three patients underwent tertiary procedures. The authors concluded that in high-risk patients, aorto-uni-iliac graft is a potential alternative to open repair, as was the case in this report [2]. Hossain et al. studied contralateral hypogastric artery perfusion following aorto-uni-iliac device and crossover femoral–femoral grafting in 130 consecutive patients. With postoperative CTA imaging, they observed an incidence of 33% occlusion of the contralateral hypogastric artery and 24% incidence of stenosis of the contralateral hypogastric artery, with patients reporting buttock claudication in almost all patients when the hypogastric artery was occluded at follow-up [3].

Multiple Choice Questions

1. The incidence of renal dysfunction following EVAR is
   A. <1%
   B. 1–2%
   C. 2.1–3%
   D. 4.1–3.5%

2. A valuable aid in minimizing a "windsock effect" and an aid in precise deployment of the endograft in patients with challenging anatomy
   A. Placing the guidewire in the renal arteries using brachial artery access
   B. Parallax Correction
   C. Intraoperative hypotension
   D. All of the above
3. The complications of aortouniiliac stent graft and crossover femoral–femoral graft include
   A. Endoleaks
   B. Thrombosis of the limb and crossover femoral–femoral graft
   C. Stent migration
   D. All of the above
4. During EVAR, difficulty is encountered in advancing the endograft through the left iliac artery. The aids to be considered for successful passage of the endograft are
   A. Balloon angioplasty/covered stent deployment in the iliac artery
   B. Graduated Coons dilators
   C. Shockwave therapy
   D. All of the above

Answers: 1(C), 2(D), 3(D), 4(D)

References

1. Hinchcliffe RJ, Alrick P, Wenham PW, Hopkinson BR. Durability of femoral-femoral bypass grafting after aorto-uni-iliac endovascular aneurysm repair. J Vasc Surg. 2013;38:498–503.
2. Dortch JD, Oldenberg WA, Farres H, Rawal B, et al. Stent grafts for the endovascular repair of abdominal aortic aneurysm. Ann Vasc Surg. 2014;28(5):1258–65.
3. Hossain S, Steinmetz OK, Corrivean MM, Mackenzie KS. Patency of contralateral internal iliac artery in aorto-uni-iliac grafting. J Vasc Surg. 2016;60:974–82.

5 Physician Modified Endograft for Repair of Pararenal Anastomotic Aneurysm

Presentation

During surveillance with CTA abdomen and pelvis following open repair of a juxtarenal abdominal aortic aneurysm (AAA) in 2018, a 68-year-old man was found to have an asymptomatic perivisceral para-anastomotic AAA in May 2024 measuring 5.7 cm AP/Tr diameter (Figs. 5.1 and 5.2). Medical co-morbidities included chronic obstructive pulmonary disease (COPD), hypertension, hyperlipidemia, and atrial fibrillation. He was a current smoker witha history 65 pack-years. On September 11, 2024, the patient underwent a physician-modified endograft (PMEG) with four-vessel fenestration using bilateral percutaneous ultrasound-guided femoral artery access with placement of two Proglide sutures at the 10 and 2 o'clock position for closure of the arterial opening at the end of the graft deployment. A 32 mm × 142 mm Zenith T × 20 thoracic graft (Cook Medical, Bloomington, IN) was unsheathed on a back table to the level of the flow divider. A stencil was created on a sterile plastic sheet based on the centerline measurements of the celiac artery, superior mesenteric artery (SMA), and bilateral renal arteries for the endograft using a marking pen.

Fenestrations for the four vessels were created using a low-energy cautery. The fenestrations were outlined with a piece of ensnare wire sutured to the graft using a 5–0 EthibondZ suture. Two orientation markers were sewn to the graft to designate the anterior position. The diameter of the graft was then reduced by constraining each level of struts. The graft was then reintroduced into the device after shrinking the diameter with Rummel tourniquet and silk sutures in addition to the umbilical tape.

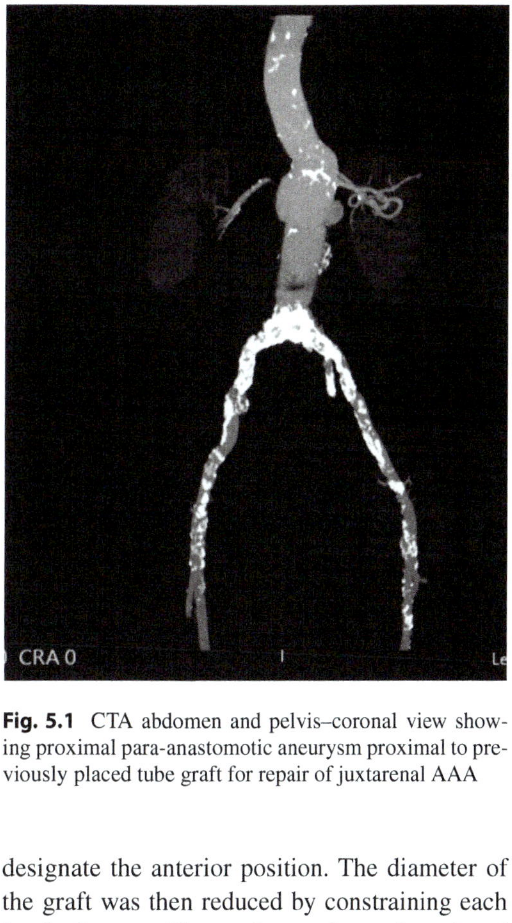

Fig. 5.1 CTA abdomen and pelvis–coronal view showing proximal para-anastomotic aneurysm proximal to previously placed tube graft for repair of juxtarenal AAA

S. S. Hans, *Secondary and Tertiary Arterial Reconstructions*,
https://doi.org/10.1007/978-3-032-21214-6_5

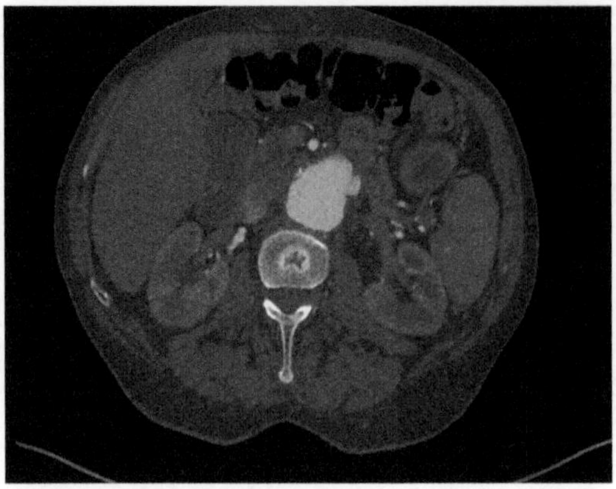

Fig. 5.2 CTA abdomen and pelvis–axial view showing proximal para-anastomotic aneurysm

This was followed by placement of an 8F sheath over the wire. A Lunderquist wire was advanced using a Kumpe catheter. Vessel navigation was available based on the previews of the CT scans and the 3D vessel navigator. Bilateral groin sites were dilated, and a 14F sheath was placed on the right side. The track was dilated to 22 mm, and the sheathed graft was advanced from the left side. The anteroposterior position of the endograft was confirmed based on its movement upon manipulation under fluoroscopy and the anterior position of the AP marker. The contralateral gate was accessed from the right side using a Kumpe catheter. The right femoral sheath was advanced into the gate and secured at the skin level with a silk suture.

A tour guide (Medtronic, Dublin, Ireland) was used from the right side over a glide wire advantage to access the left renal artery using the designated fenestration. The wire was advanced into the renal artery, followed by the passage of a Navicross catheter. The glide wire was then exchanged for a Rosen wire. An angiogram showed bleeding from the superior pole renal artery branch, which was coil embolized using 2 and 3 mm coils. Repeat arteriogram showed cessation of bleeding. Similar steps through the right sheath to gain access for the right renal, SMA, and celiac artery using a Rosen wire were under-

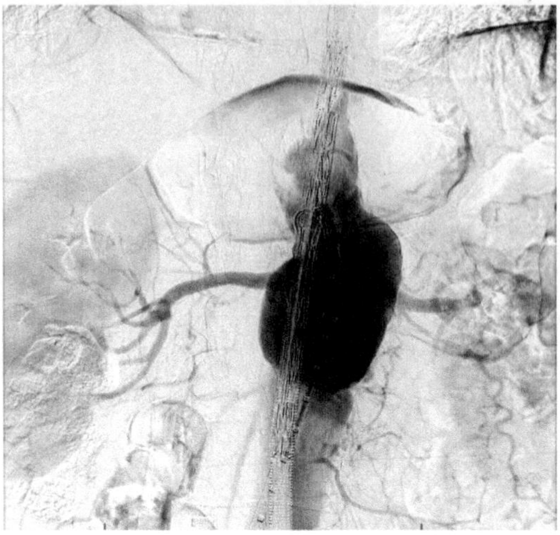

Fig. 5.3 Intraoperative aortogram during PMEG

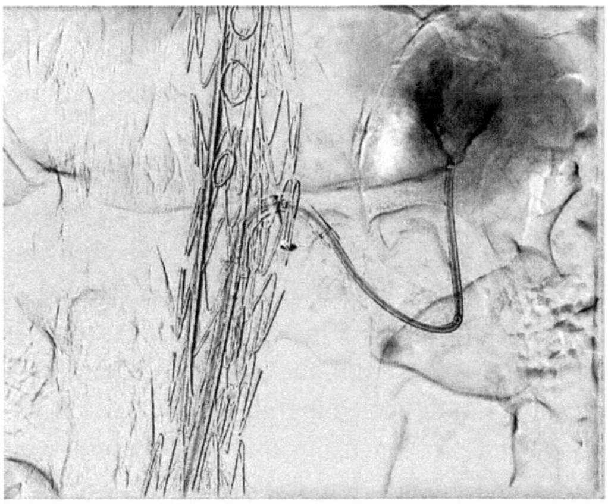

Fig. 5.4 Cannulation of the left renal artery

taken. A Coda balloon catheter was used to fully expand the graft by inflating and breaking the constraining sutures: 7 × 29 mm VBX stent—in the celiac artery (post dilation with 10 × 2 balloon); 8 × 29 VBX (post dilation and flaring with a $10\times^2$ mm balloon) and a 6 × 29 VBX stent was deployed in each renal artery and post dilated and flared with a 9 × 2 mm balloon (Figs. 5.3, 5.4, 5.5 and 5.6). A 10 × 80 mm Smart self-expanding stent (Cordis Johnson & Johnson, New Brunswick, NJ) was deployed to cover the right iliac artery dissection and was post-dilated

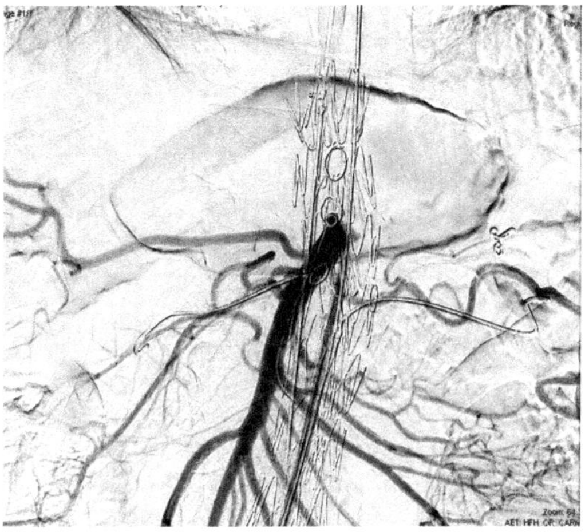

Fig. 5.5 Cannulation of SMA

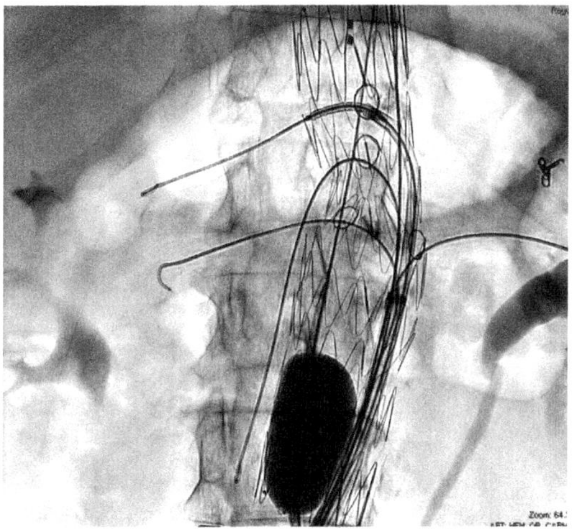

Fig. 5.6 Cannulation (wires) of Celiac, SMA, and SMA with Coda balloon in the endograft

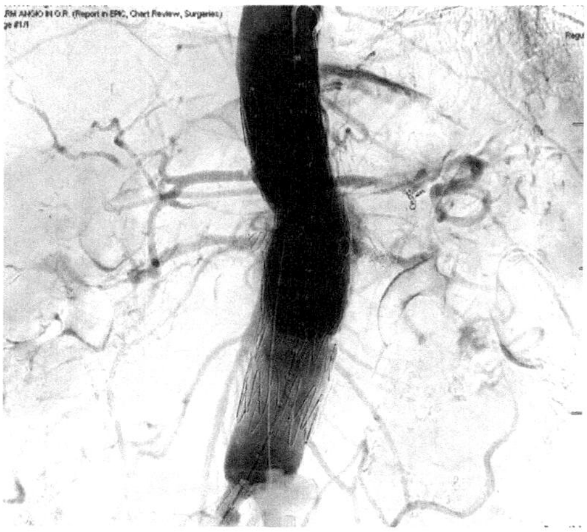

Fig. 5.7 Completion aortogram showing exclusion of para-anastomotic pararenal aneurysm

to 9 mm. Completion aortogram did not show any endoleak with successful exclusion of the aneurysm and patency of all four main branches of the abdominal aorta(celiac, SMA, and both renal arteries) (Fig. 5.7).

Postoperatively, the patient complained of left flank pain, which remained stable during the hospital stay. A CT scan showed a 9 × 14 × 19 cm left retroperitoneal hematoma, most likely the result of a guidewire perforation. The patient remained stable in the postoperative period as the hematoma did not show expansion. The patient was discharged on the ninth postoperative day. The 6-month follow-up CTA of the abdomen and pelvis showed satisfactory exclusion of the aneurysm without endoleak (Fig. 5.8a, b, c).

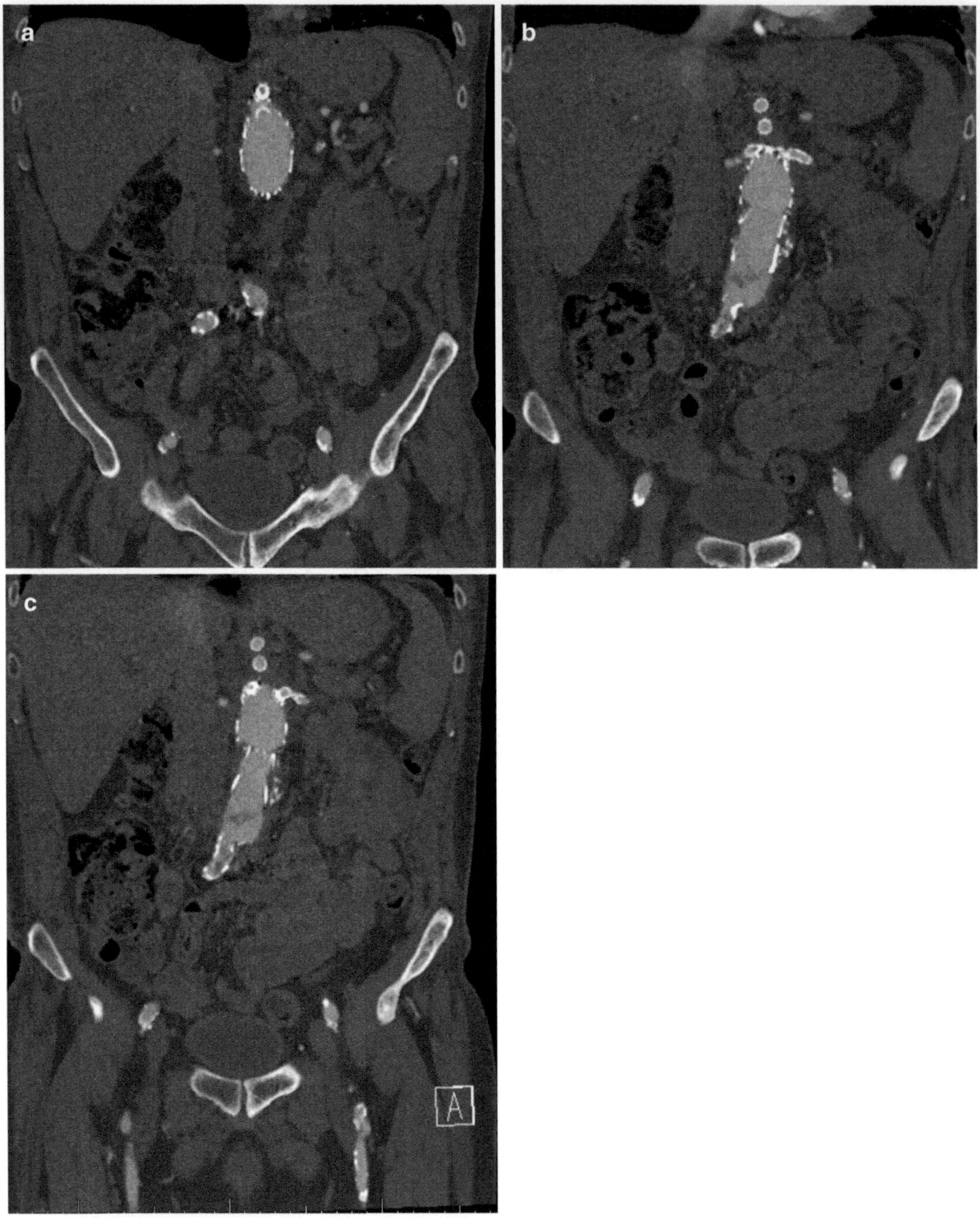

Fig. 5.8 (**a**) Follow-up CTA of the abdomen and pelvis showing patency of Celiac, SMA, and both renal arteries and exclusion of pararenal aneurysm without endoleak. (**b**) CTA showing patency of the Celiac, SMA, and both renal arteries and exclusion of aneurysm without endoleak. (**c**) CTA showing patency of the Celiac, SMA, and both renal arteries and exclusion of aneurysm without endoleak

Discussion

From an International multicenter single-arm cohort study analyzing the outcomes of PMEG's in complex abdominal aortic and thoracoabdominal aneurysms from 19 centers, reported the results in 1274 patients with a median age of 74; 75.7% were men, 45.7% had complex abdominal aortic aneurysms and 54.3% were thoracoabdominal aortic aneurysms, 65.5% patients presented electively, 24.6% were symptomatic and 9.9% were ruptured [1]. Most patients (83.1%) had fenestrated repair, and 3.6% had branched repair, and 13.4% had a combined fenestrated and branched repair. Most patients (85.8%) had ≥3 target vessels included. The overall technical success was 94%; 30-day mortality was 5.8% (4.1% in the elective setting, 7.6% in symptomatic, and 12.7 in ruptured aneurysms) [1]. Major adverse events occurred in 25.2% of cases. Freedom from intervention was 73.8%, 61.8%, and 51.4% at 1, 3, and 5 years, respectively. Overall survival and freedom from aortic-related mortality was 82.4%/92.9%, 69.9%/91.6%, and 55.0%/89.1% at 1, 3, and 5 years [1].

Starnes et al. reported long-term results of PMEGs for the treatment of elective, symptomatic, and ruptured juxtarenal abdominal aortic aneurysms in 228 patients over a 12-year study period. Of these patients, 59 patients completed the 5-year follow-up period [2]. A total of 575 fenestrations were created: 387 renal arteries, 181 superior mesenteric arteries, and 7 celiac arteries [2]. In 203 patients, 410 renal artery stents were deployed. There were no open conversions or device migrations and one occlusion [2]. Three ruptured (1.4%) occurred at late follow-up, with one presumed graft infection. The overall rate of major adverse events at 30 days was 15%. Technical success was 93.7; overall treatment success was 82.6%. According to the data, the authors concluded that PMEG is a safe and durable option for repair of juxtarenal aortic aneurysms [2].

Multiple Choice Questions

1. Reported 30-day mortality following PMEG is
   A. 2–3%
   B. 3.1–5%
   C. 5.1–6%
   D. >7%
2. The technical success of PMEG is
   A. 80%
   B. 85%
   C. 90%
   D. 93%
3. Overall survival and freedom from aortic mortality following PMEG at 5 years is
   A. 60%
   B. 55%
   C. 50%
   D. 45%

Answers: 1(C), 2(D), 3(B)

References

1. Tsilimparis N, Gouveia EMR, Tenorio ER, et al. Multicenter study on physician-modified endografts for thoracoabdominal and complex abdominal aortic aneurysm repair. Circulation. 2024;150(17):1327–42. PMID:38989565.
2. Starnes BW, Zettervall S, Larimore A, Singh N. Long-term results of physician-modified endografts for the treatment of elective, symptomatic, and ruptured juxtarenal abdominal aortic aneurysms. Ann Surg. 2024;280(4):633–9. PMID:38920026.

6 Endovascular Repair of an Abdominal Aortic Aneurysm in a Patient with Prior Iliac Stent Resulting in Graft Limb Occlusion

Presentation

A 75-year-old man underwent endovascular aneurysm repair (EVAR) using percutaneous access in August 2020 for a 5.5 cm (AP/Tr diameter) infrarenal AAA (Figs. 6.1 and 6.2). He had a prior history of bilateral common iliac artery stents with a right iliac stent (8 mm) projecting for a distance of about 2 cm into the lumen of the aneurysm sac. The main body of the Endurant™ graft (Medtronic, Dublin, Ireland), 36 × 14 × 103 mm, was deployed following a percutaneous puncture of the common femoral artery under ultrasound guidance.

The contralateral limb (16 × 10 × 124 mm) was deployed following percutaneous puncture of the right common femoral artery. The limbs were crossed, and the right limb of the endograft traversed through the iliac stent. An ipsilateral iliac extension limb (16 × 10 × 124 mm) was deployed (Fig. 6.3). Both hypogastric arteries were small in caliber, and previously placed iliac stents were partially covering the origin of the hypogastric arteries. Two kissing (9 × 59 Omnilink, Abbott, Chicago, IL) balloon--expandable stents were deployed in the main body extending into both iliac limbs. Closure of the femoral arteries was performed using the Manta closure device on both sides.

In the postoperative period, the patient developed occlusion of the right graft limb of the endograft. The right lower extremity remained viable due to collateral blood flow. Non-invasive Doppler arterial study showed an ABI right (0.32) left (0.89) showed right graft limb occlusion. An abdominal and pelvic arteriogram confirmed right graft limb occlusion and stenosis of the left common femoral artery (Fig. 6.4). The patient underwent a crossover femoral–femoral graft for symptoms of right calf claudication in May 2023, using an 8 mm Interring PTFE graft (W.L. Core, Newark, DE). The left common femoral artery had exuberant granulation tissue (Fig. 6.5) in the lumen of the artery, presumably as a reaction to the percutaneous closure device with associated thick posterior plaque. Left common femoral endarterectomy was per-

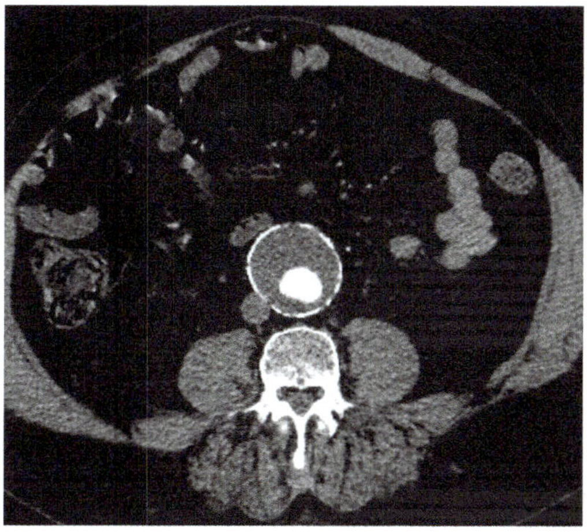

Fig. 6.1 CTA showing infrarenal AAA

S. S. Hans, *Secondary and Tertiary Arterial Reconstructions*,
https://doi.org/10.1007/978-3-032-21214-6_6

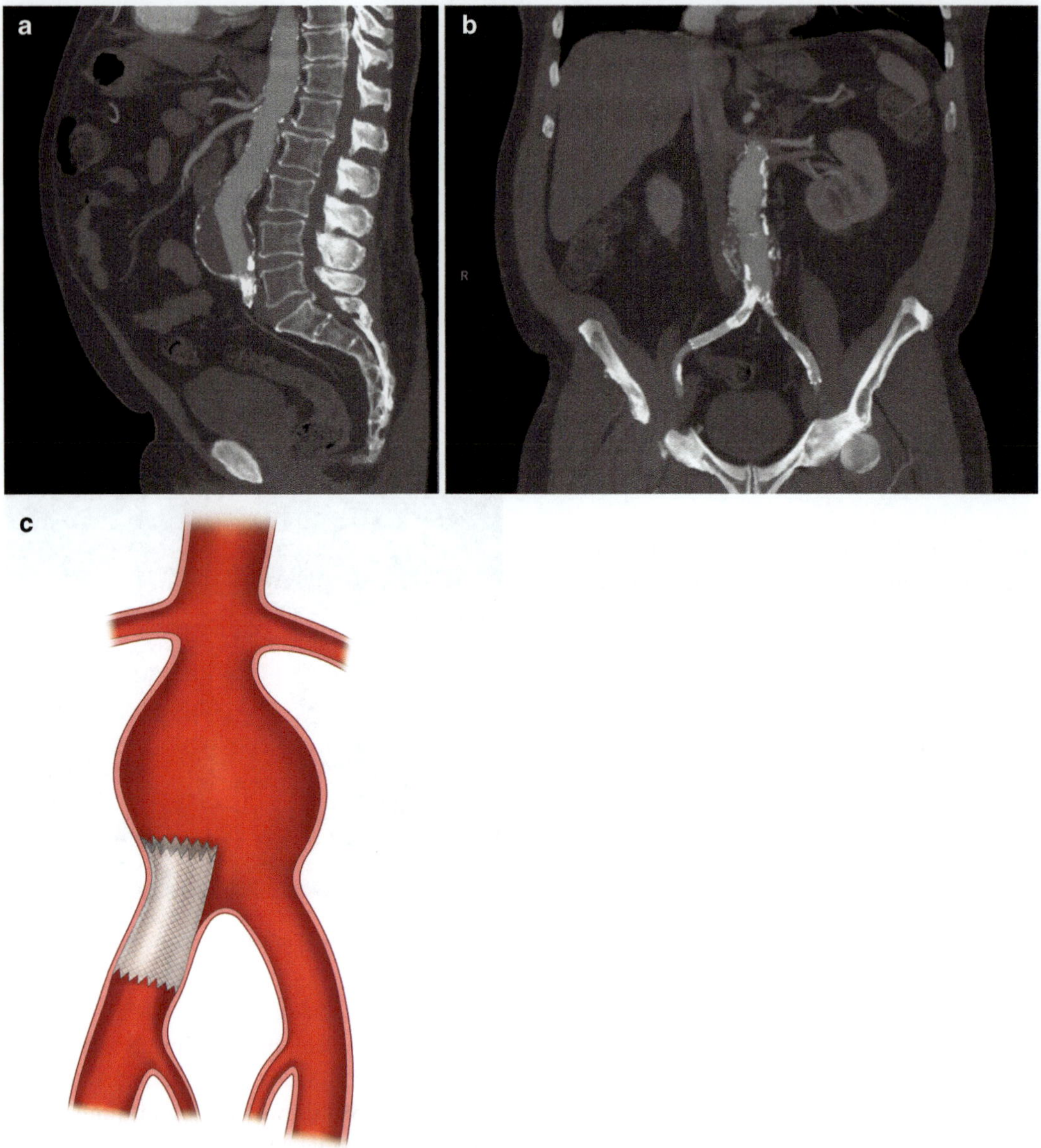

Fig. 6.2 (**a**) Sagittal view of CTA of abdomen and pelvis showing right common iliac stent projecting into the aneurysm sac. (**b**) Coronal view of CTA of abdomen and pelvis showing right common iliac stent projecting into the aneurysm sac. (**c**) Diagrammatic representation of right common iliac stent projecting into the aneurysm

formed with a bovine pericardial patch angioplasty, and the anastomosis of the origin of the crossover PTFE graft was performed at the middle of the pericardial patch. His postoperative course was uneventful. A follow-up Doppler arterial study in February 2024 showed ABI on the right (0.86) and (0.88) on the left side, with complete relief of the symptoms of intermittent claudication. He died in December 2024 from advanced carcinoma of the lung.

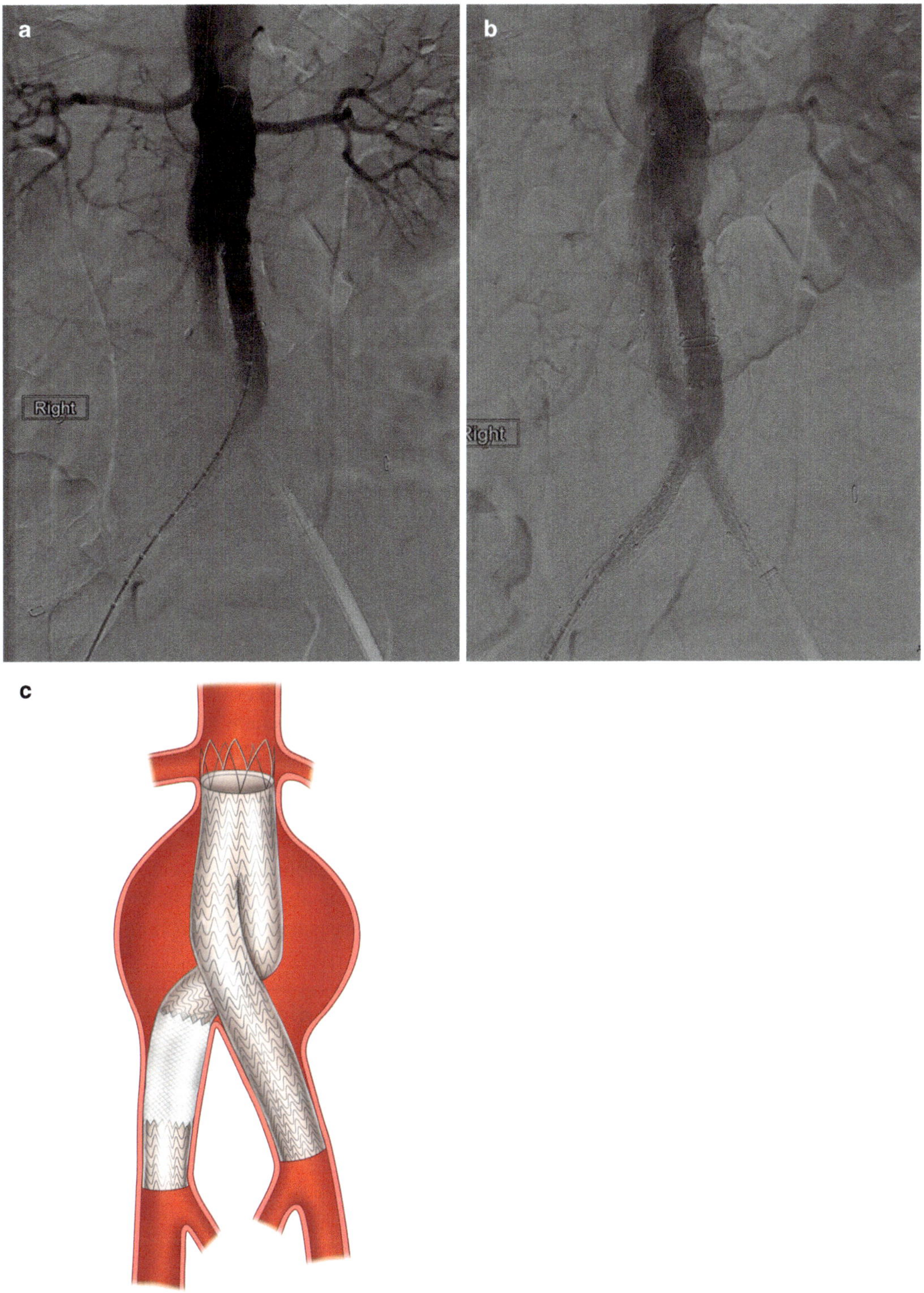

Fig. 6.3 (**a**) Completion aortogram showing crossing of the iliac limbs with angulation of the right iliac limb of the endograft. (**b**) Completion aortogram showing crossing of the iliac limbs with angulation of the right iliac limb of the endograft. (**c**) Diagrammatic representation of kinking of the right iliac limb as it traverses the protruding iliac stent in the aneurysm sac

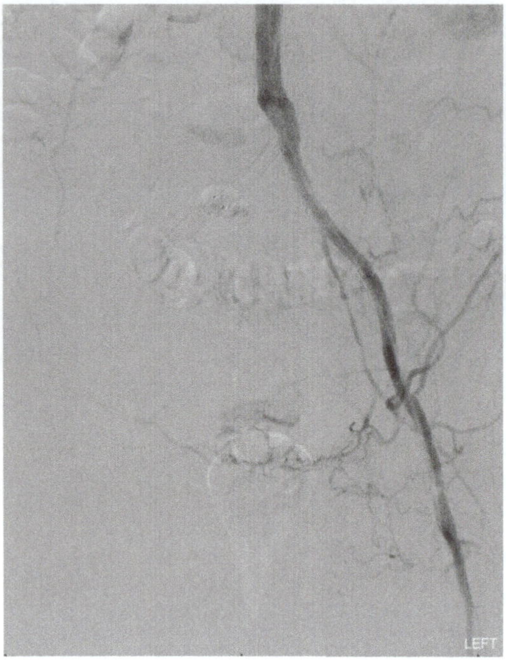

Fig. 6.4 Follow-up abdominal and pelvic aortogram, right, showing graft limb occlusion and stenosis of the left common femoral artery

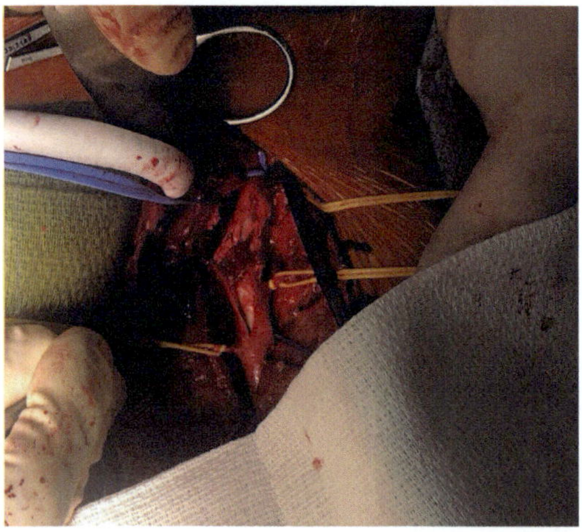

Fig. 6.5 Operative picture of the left common femoral artery showing marked intimal hyperplasia secondary to its closure with the Manta device

Discussion

From a meta-analysis of 13 studies comprising 5454 patients undergoing EVAR (1995–2014), iliac graft limb occlusion was reported in 5.6% of patients, with one-half of the patients presenting within 3 days of EVAR [1]. From another study, Mantas et al., reported 18 limb occlusions (4.1%) among 439 patients (2010–2013) [2]. The significant predictors of graft limb occlusion were the presence of calcification and angulation of the iliac arteries, as well as excessive limb oversizing. Faure et al., reported 42 graft limb occlusions in 39 patients (3.4%) from the Endurant stent graft Natural Selection Global Post Market Registry (ENGAGE) [3]. Three important predictors for limb occlusions were distal landing zone in the external iliac artery (EIA), EIA diameter of less than 10 mm and kinking and tortuosity of the CIA [3]. Chacko et al., reported GLO in 23 limbs among 319 patients (7.2%) available for analysis following EVAR, and found that a small diameter EIA, graft limb extension into the EIA, and the presence of prior iliac stent were the main factors leading to graft limb occlusion [4]. Early graft limb occlusion can be managed by thrombectomy with the aid of thrombectomy devices with or without TPA. In some cases, the patient may need extension of the graft to the EIA. Patients with late graft limb occlusion may present with symptoms of mild claudication and may not need arterial reconstruction. In a patient with symptoms of disabling claudication, a crossover femoral–femoral graft is a suitable option to be considered in most instances with late graft limb occlusions.

Multiple Choice Questions

1. The incidence of graft limb occlusion following EVAR is
   A. >8%
   B. 7.3–8%
   C. 3.4–7.2%
   D. <3.4%
2. The important predictors of graft limb occlusion
   A. Small diameter EIA(<10 mm)
   B. Distal landing zone of the iliac limb into the external iliac artery

   C. Kinking and tortuosity and heavy calcification of the common iliac artery
   D. All of the above
3. Early GLO is best managed by
   A. Conversion to open repair
   B. Crossover femoral-femoral graft
   C. Pharmacomechanical thrombectomy
   D. Anticoagulation

Answers: 1(C), 2(D), 3(C)

References

1. Hammond A, Hansrani V, Lowe C, et al. Meta--analysis and meta-regression analysis of iliac limb occlusion after endovascular aneurysm repair. J Vasc Surg. 2018;68(6):1916–24.e1917. PMID:30366653.
2. Mantas GK, Antonopoulos CN, Sfyroeras GS, Moulakakis KG, Kakisis JD, Mylonas SN, Liapis CD. Factors predisposing to endograft limb occlusion after endovascular aortic repair. Eur J Vasc Endovasc Surg. 2015;49(1):39–44. PMID:25453234.
3. Faure EM, Becquemin JP, Cochennec F. Predictive factors for limb occlusions after endovascular aneurysm repair. J Vasc Surg. 2015;61(5):1138–45.e1132. PMID:25656594.
4. Chacko P, Hans SS, Nahirniak P, Morton K. Clinical patterns, predictors, and results of graft limb occlusion following endovascular aneurysm repair. Ann Vasc Surg. 2023;94:341–6. PMID:36918093.

7 Explantation of Aortic Endograft Due to Recurrent Type IA Endoleak

Presentation

A 75-year-old woman was seen in October 2010 with a 6.0 cm (Ap/Tr diameter) infrarenal AAA, with a horseshoe kidney (Fig. 7.1a, b). Medical co-morbidities included hypertension, hyperlipidemia, and obesity (BMI 42). She underwent EVAR using an AneuRx graft (Medtronic, Dublin, Ireland). The main body of the endograft (26 × 15 × 135 mm) was deployed using the right femoral artery access, which was obtained by using a left groin cut-down. The contralateral iliac limb (15 × 15 × 115 mm) was deployed from the left femoral artery access obtained by a groin or cut-down. The right iliac extension limb (15 × 15 × 85 mm) was deployed with a landing zone in the distal CIA. Following Reliant™ (Metronic, Dublin, Ireland) balloon angioplasty of the aortic neck, patient became hypotensive, and contrast injection showed extravasation at the aortic neck (Fig. 7.2). Immediately the aortic balloon was inflated in the suprarenal aorta and a 26 × 26 × 40 mm AneuRx aortic cuff was deployed just inferior to the origin of the left renal artery with satisfactory control of the leak from aortic neck.

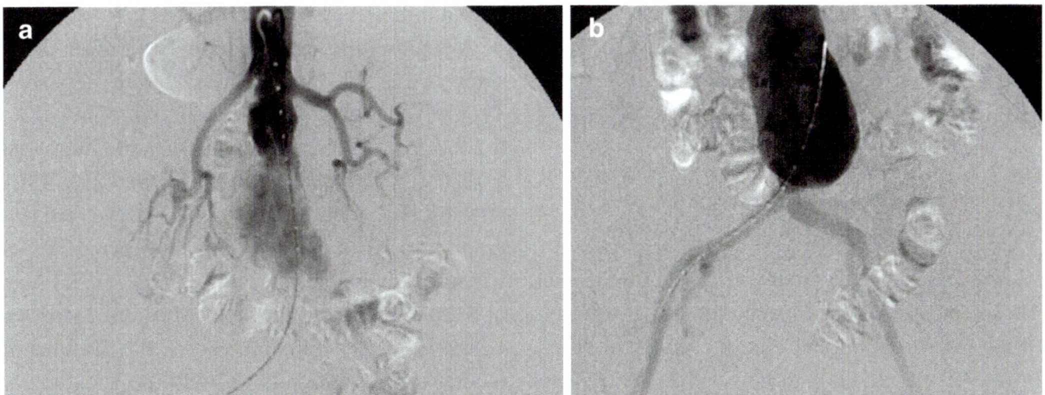

Fig. 7.1 (**a**) Aortogram of abdominal and pelvis showing infrarenal AAA. (**b**) Aortogram showing infrarenal AAA

S. S. Hans, *Secondary and Tertiary Arterial Reconstructions*,
https://doi.org/10.1007/978-3-032-21214-6_7

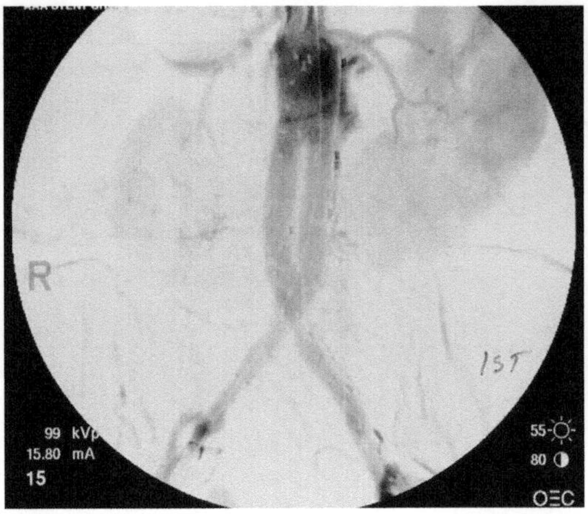

Fig. 7.2 Aortogram showing extravasation of contrast at the aortic neck following endograft deployment

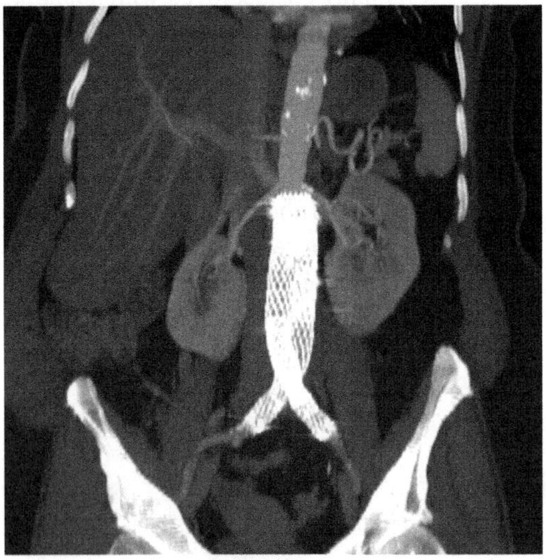

Fig. 7.3 Postoperative CTA after EVAR with an aortic cuff, with satisfactory exclusion of the AAA

A CTA scan of the abdomen and the pelvis on the second postoperative day showed resolution of the extravasation with minimal residual blood in the left periaortic area (Fig. 7.3). The patient was followed with aortic duplex imaging and CTA of the abdomen and pelvis. In July 2012, the aneurysm sac measured 3.5 × 3.8 cm. In July 2015, the CTA showed an enlargement of the residual aneurysm sac (5.3 × 5.9 cm), with distal migration of the endograft, with a Type II endoleak most likely resulting from an accessory renal artery supplying the isthmus of the kidney. There

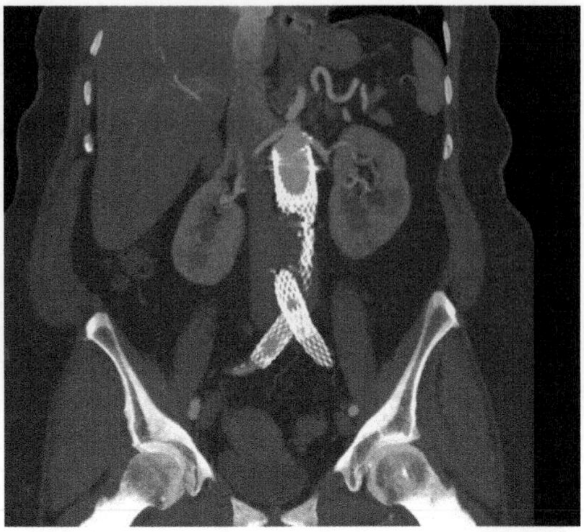

Fig. 7.4 CTA showing distal migration of the endograft resulting in Type IA endoleak

was also a strong suspicion of a Type IA endoleak (Fig. 7.4). In August 2018, using a right femoral artery access with a groin cut down and a left brachial artery percutaneous access, coil embolization of the proximal false aneurysm sac was performed. An iCAST™ (Atrium, Charlotte, NC) 6 × 38 mm stent and an Endurant™ (Medtronic, Dublin, Ireland) cuff were deployed simultaneously using a snorkel technique to gain additional length for the proximal attachment seal zone of the Endurant™ cuff (Fig. 7.5a, b, c).

A follow-up CTA scan in September 2018 showed a stable aneurysm sac with persistent Type II endoleak. As the aneurysm enlarged to 6.2 × 5.8 cm (Sept. 2019), the patient underwent a repeat abdominal aortogram, selective SMA arteriogram, and bilateral hypogastric arteriogram, which did not show any evidence of Types I, II, or III endoleaks (January 2021). A CTA scan of the abdomen and pelvis in April 2022 showed a large Type IA endoleak (Fig. 7.6). Because of recurrent Type IA endoleak with no satisfactory endovascular option available for management of a Type IA endoleak, she underwent explant of the endograft in June 2022 under general anesthesia.

The patient was placed in a right lateral decubitus position. A thoracoabdominal incision was made through the left ninth intercostal space. The crus of the diaphragm was divided. There was dense inflammation along the lateral side of the

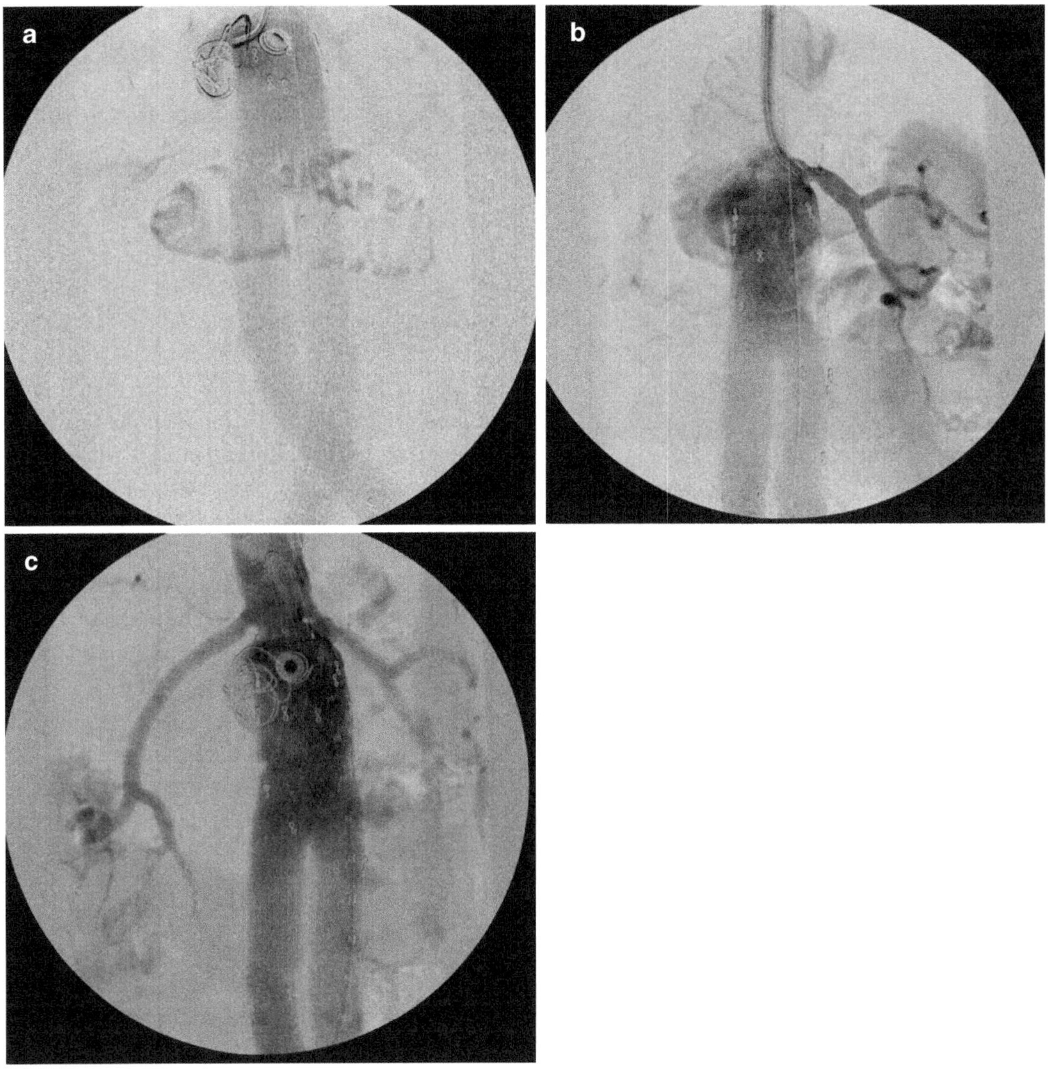

Fig. 7.5 (**a**) Coil embolization of the periaortic sac. (**b**) Snorkeling with the sheath (using left brachial access) in the left renal artery. (**c**) Deployment of Left Iliac ICAST stent with Snorkeling

aorta near the horseshoe kidney. The supraceliac aorta was exposed and mobilized. There were two lumbar arteries in the vicinity needing ligation and division. There was dense inflammation surrounding the iliac arteries, left gonadal vein, and several draining veins from the horseshoe kidney in the pelvis were ligated and divided. The lumbar branch of the left renal vein was ligated and divided. Mannitol infusion was started by the anesthesia team. Intravenous Heparin was administered to keep ACT in the therapeutic range (close to 300 s). The left renal artery was dissected with its proximal division into two main branches with a covered stent in the renal artery. Both common iliac arteries were clamped with a vascular clamp, with simultaneous clamping of the limbs of the AneuRx graft. The supraceliac aorta was clamped. The aneurysm was opened just proximal to the origin of the celiac artery posterolaterally. The aorta was transected flush at the origin of the right renal artery, and the left renal artery was implanted as a carrell patch. Cold heparinized saline solution was injected into the orifice of the right renal artery. The Endurant™ cuff and covered stent

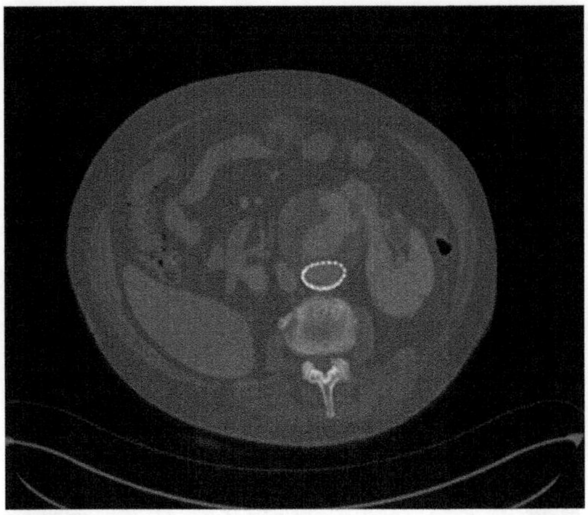

Fig. 7.6 Recurrent Type IA endoleak

from the left renal artery were removed. The AneuRx device was transected and partially removed, leaving the iliac limbs. An endarterectomy of the left renal artery was performed to a satisfactory endpoint. An 18 × 9 mm Hemashield gold Dacron graft (Maquet, Rastatt, Germany) was sutured to the suprarenal aorta flush at the level of the right renal, celiac, and superior mesenteric artery with 26 min of visceral ischemic time. The graft was then clamped distal to the proximal anastomosis using an aortic Satinsky clamp. A graftotomy was made in the anterolateral wall of the graft with removal of a portion of the Dacron graft and reimplantation of the left renal artery into the Dacron graft as a carrel patch with a continuous 5′0″ cardiovascular polypropylene suture (Ethicon, Raritan, NJ). The left renal ischemia time was 35 min. Iliac limbs of the Dacron graft were sutured to the divided common iliac arteries with limbs of the AneuRx™ graft and anastomosed to both common iliac arteries.

After restoration of flow to both lower extremities, heparin was reversed with protamine sulfate. Platelets, fresh frozen plasma, and cryoprecipitate were administered to reverse the coagulopathy once hemostasis was achieved. A 28 F chest tube was placed, and the incision was closed in the layers, including the diaphragm. The patient was discharged on the eighth postoperative day. Patient was last seen in March 2025 with follow-up CTA of the abdomen and pelvis showing patent repair with post-surgical changes.

Discussion

The explant of an aortic endograft is required in only 1–5% of cases following EVAR. It is associated with significant morbidity and mortality. From a single-center retrospective study of 32 patients (2002–2017) who underwent explantation, with a majority undergoing complete removal of the endograft (59%). The reported failure was due to endoleak in 91% (Type I 38%, Type II 32%, Type III 13%, Type IV 13%) [1]. The mortality was 6.3% (3.8% elective, 16.7% ruptured) with major complications at 31%. Feldman et al., reported 52 patients who underwent explantation of endovascular aortic repair devices, including 32 who underwent partial explant [2]. Partial explant was performed in sicker patients and those with acute presentation, and had similar outcomes as complete explantation. A complete explantation is required in all patients with an endograft infection.

Three approaches are used for complete excision. One technique involves pouring ice-cold saline onto nitinol stents with thermal memory to ease removal from the aortic neck by decreasing device diameters close to the pre-deployment state. Another technique described by Koning and collaborators uses a sterile 20 mL syringe that is prepared by removing the plunger, cutting the end of the barrel with a saw, and rounding the edges of the cylinder with a file [3]. After the iliac limbs are disconnected from the main body, the syringe barrel is slid proximally over the main body, and a Kelly clamp or an umbilical tape is used to grasp the main body at the inferior end of the syringe. The syringe is advanced superiorly over the main body with downward tension on the clamp or the tape. Once the hooks are detached, downward tension on the Kelly clamp brings the main body out of the aortic neck. This approach works with Zenith® Flex (Cook Medical Inc., Bloomington, IN) and Talent (Medtronic, Dublin, Ireland) stent graft, but not with the newer Endurant™ II AAA stent graft system. This graft has reverse barbs on its suprarenal stent, making en bloc removal with this technique impossible. In this situation, suprarenal struts should be cut from the infrarenal portion of the main body of graft with sterile wire cutters and removed piecemeal from the Para-visceral aorta, with a vertical aortotomy extending above the renal arteries. Following complete excision of an Endurant™ II AAA stent graft system, aortic reconstruction usually requires a beveled anastomosis, incorporating suprarenal aortotomy, and may also require reimplantation of the left renal artery. The extent of endograft excision often depends on the pre-existing device seal, the presence or absence of suprarenal fixation struts. In the absence of infection, the fabric of a well--incorporated endograft is included with native aortic tissue in the anastomosis.

The incidence of late open conversion following EVAR is usually less than 5% [4–6]. The indications for graft explantation include Type IA endoleak despite unsuccessful secondary interventions to correct the endoleak, graft infection, and refractory graft occlusion [4–6]. The type of the endograft used at the index operation has no relation to the incidence of explant. Endograft failure within 1 year is most commonly the result of failure to achieve a satisfactory proximal seal at the index operation and underscores the need to understand the device limitations if used outside the instructions for use (IFU) [6]. Late failures most commonly are the result of aneurysmal degeneration at the seal zones, device material failure, and may occur even after a decade of successful EVAR repair [4–6]. Emergent repair is most often required for rupture or infection [6]. Both retroperitoneal and transabdominal approaches can be used for endograft explant, and suprarenal clamping is required in most cases [6]. Aortoiliac reconstruction is the most common type of reconstruction following endograft explant. In an elective setting, mortality should be less than 5%, and in an emergent explant, 40%. For graft infection, complete removal of the endograft is required. Partial graft excision can be judiciously employed in patients with sac expansion and rupture secondary to endoleak.

The EUROSTAR registry reported on 2464 patients (1996–2000) with a mean follow-up of 12.19 months, with a confirmed rupture in 14 patients [7]. The cumulative risk of rupture was 1% per year. Forty-one patients underwent late conversion to open repair. The cumulative risk of late conversion was approximately 2.1% per year. In this report, the first generative endograft for EVAR was first deployed. With improvement in graft technology, with use of newer generation of endograft, and better patient selection, the incidence in contemporary practice should be lower.

Multiple Choice Questions

1. Late open conversion following EVAR occurs in
   A. <1% of patients
   B. 1–5% of patients
   C. 5–10% of patients
   D. 11–12% of patients
2. The best strategy to facilitate the complete removal of suprarenal stents during the explant of an aortograft is
   A. Use of a 20-cc syringe as a sheath to encircle and collapse the suprarenal stents and struts.
   B. Release of barbs from the main body with a circumferential wire cutter.
   C. Use of ice-cold saline on the nitinol element to collapse the metal.
   D. Release of barbs with a wire cutter and ice saline in a syringe to collapse the suprarenal segments.
3. Which of the following statements best reflects the incidence of late conversion and risk of delayed rupture following EVAR?
   A. Overall incidence of late conversion is 2.1%, and the delayed risk of rupture is 1% per year.
   B. Overall incidence of late conversion is 5%, and the delayed risk of rupture is 2% per year.
   C. Overall incidence of late conversion is 5%, and a delayed risk of rupture is 3% per year.
   D. Overall incidence of late conversion is 1%, and a delayed risk of rupture is 0.5% per year.

Answers: 1(B), 2(C), 3(A)

References

1. Arnaoutakis DJ, Sharma G, Blackwood S, Shah SK, Menard M, Ozaki CK, Belkin M. Strategies and outcomes for aortic endograft explantation. J Vasc Surg. 2019;69(1):80–5. PMID:29914836.
2. Feldman ZM, Kim D, Roddy C, Sumpio BJ, DeCarlo CS, Kwolek CJ, et al. Partial and complete explantation of aortic endografts in the modern era. J Vasc Surg. 2023;77(1):97–105. PMID:35868421.
3. Koning OH, Hinnen JW, van Baalen JM. Technique for safe removal of an aortic endograft with suprarenal fixation. J Vasc Surg. 2006;43(4):855–7. PMID:16616252.
4. Chaar CI, Eid R, Park T, Rhee RY, Abu-Hamad G, Tzeng E, et al. Delayed open conversions after endovascular abdominal aortic aneurysm repair. J Vasc Surg. 2012;55(6):1562–9.e1561. PMID:22503183.
5. Kelso RL, Lyden SP, Butler B, Greenberg RK, Eagleton MJ, Clair DG. Late conversion of aortic stent grafts. J Vasc Surg. 2009;49(3):589–95. PMID:19135829.
6. Turney EJ, Steenberge SP, Lyden SP, Eagleton MJ, Srivastava SD, Sarac TP, et al. Late graft explants in endovascular aneurysm repair. J Vasc Surg. 2014;59(4):886–93. PMID:24377945.
7. Harris PL, Vallabhaneni SR, Desgranges P, Becquemin JP, van Marrewijk C, Laheij RJ. Incidence and risk factors of late rupture, conversion, and death after endovascular repair of infrarenal aortic aneurysms: the EUROSTAR experience. European collaborators on stent/graft techniques for aortic aneurysm repair. J Vasc Surg. 2000;32(4):739–49. PMID:11013038.

8 Repair of Type Ib Endoleak Following EVAR

Presentation

A 77-year-old man underwent EVAR for a 5.3 cm (AP/Tr diameter) infrarenal abdonimal aortic aneurysm (AAA) that had increased in size by 5 mm in the preceding 6 months (Fig. 8.1a). CTA of the abdomen and pelvis showed infrarenal AAA of the long neck and a non-flow limiting dissection flap of the middle portion of the right common iliac artery (CIA) (Fig. 8.1b). Percutaneous EVAR using a Manta (Teleflex, Wayne, PA) closure device was performed. The main body of the Endurant™ graft, measuring 28 × 14 × 103 mm, contralateral limb 16 × 16 × 93 mm, and ipsilateral extension limb 16 × 16 × 93 mm, was deployed (February 2023). Bilateral balloon expandable 10 x 29 mm Omnilink stents (Abbott Medical, Abbott Park, IL) were deployed in the distal aorta extending into the common iliac arteries.

At the 1-month follow-up, CTA of the abdomen and pelvis showed a Type Ib endoleak (Fig. 8.2). The patient was taken to hybrid operating room and a right iliac arteriogram performed by contrast injection via the right femoral sheath which showed incomplete apposition of the right iliac limb of the endograft to the medial wall of the common iliac artery. A deployment of an 11 × 39 mm VBX balloon expandable covered stent (W.L. Gore, Newark, DE) at the site of the

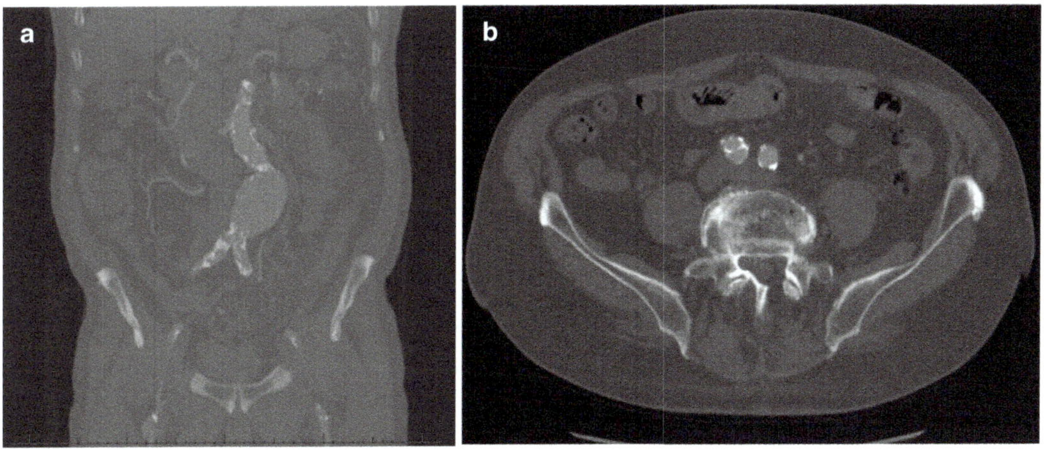

Fig. 8.1 (**a**) CTA (Coronal view) showing infrarenal AAA. (**b**) CTA of abdomen and pelvis (Axial view) showing dissection flap in the right common iliac artery

S. S. Hans, *Secondary and Tertiary Arterial Reconstructions*,
https://doi.org/10.1007/978-3-032-21214-6_8

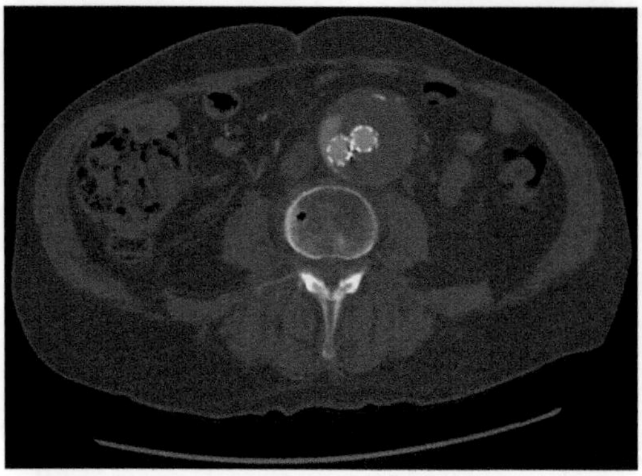

Fig. 8.2 CTA showing Type Ib endoleak

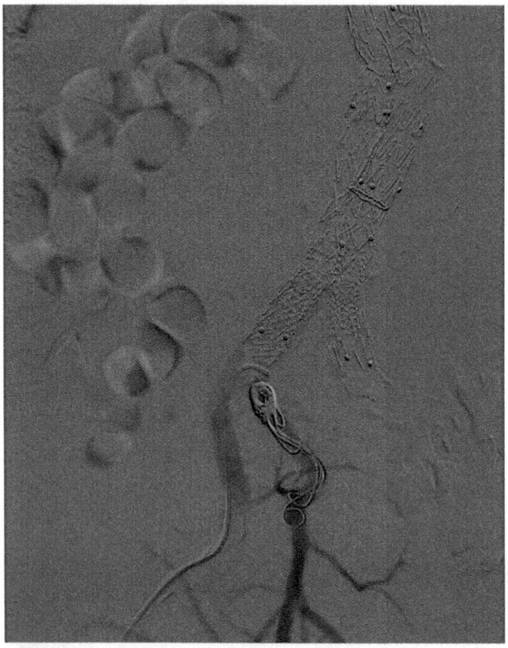

Fig. 8.3 Arteriogram showing coil embolization of the right hypogastric artery

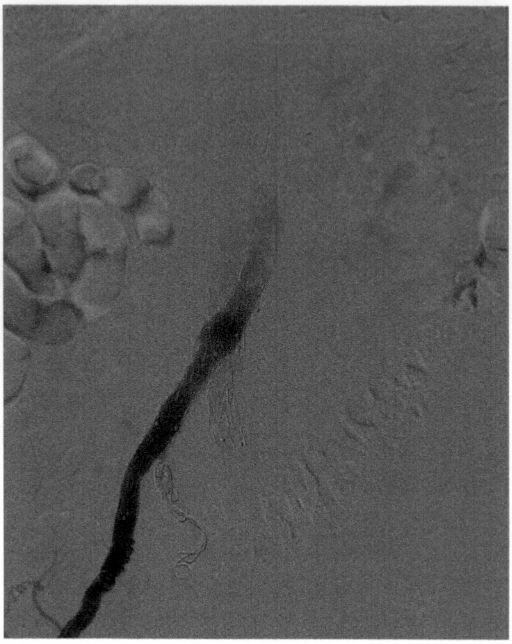

Fig. 8.4 Completion arteriogram showing occlusion of right hypogastric artery and extension of the iliac limb into the external iliac artery

endoleak did not result in the resolution of the Type Ib endoleak. Therefore, a coil embolization of the branches of the right hypogastric artery using AZUR coils was performed (Terumo, Tustin, CA) (Fig. 8.3) An iliac limb extension into the external iliac artery using a 16 × 10 × 124 mm Endurant™ limb (Fig. 8.4) was performed. A follow-up CTA of the abdomen and pelvis 1 month later showed resolution of the Type Ib endoleak. The patient was last seen in the clinic in August 2024, with aortoiliac duplex imaging showing satisfactory exclusion of the AAA with a stable residual aneurysm sac (5.3 cm) with no evidence of endoleak.

Discussion

A dissection flap with slight aneurysmal dilatation of the right CIA prevented an adequate seal of the right limb of the iliac endograft. In such situations, a completion arteriogram via the right femoral sheath, balloon angioplasty, and deployment of a balloon-expandable covered stent at the time of index repair AAA, might have prevented a Type Ib endoleak.

From a scoping review of 27 articles comprising 7197 patients, Zuccon et al., reported an incidence of 0–8% of Type Ib endoleak [1]. The anatomical features that could increase the risk of Type Ib endoleak included CIA diameter of greater than 718 mm, or requiring the use of flared limbs of 720 mm, length of CIA landing zone of <20 mm, marked iliac tortuosity, and a large initial diameter AAA. According to the review, most Type Ib endoleaks can be corrected by endovascular means with an immediate technical success of 100% [1].

Multiple Choice Questions

1. The incidence of Type Ib endoleak following EVAR is
   A. 0–4%
   B. 0–6%
   C. 0–8%
   D. 0–10%
2. What minimum length of common iliac artery landing zone causes to increased incidence of Type Ib endoleak is
   A. <26 mm
   B. <24 mm
   C. <22 mm
   D. <20 mm
3. The technical success for the repair of Type Ib endoleak with endovascular techniques approaches
   A. 70%
   B. 80%
   C. 90%
   D. 100%

Answers: 1(C), 2(D), 3(D)

Reference

1. Zuccon G, D'Oria M, Gonçalves FB, Fernandez-Prendes C, Mani K, Caldeira D, et al. Incidence, risk factors, and prognostic impact of Type Ib endoleak following endovascular repair for abdominal aortic aneurysm: scoping review. Eur J Vasc Endovasc Surg. 2023;66(3):352–61. PMID:37356703

9 Endovascular Repair of Symptomatic Recurrent Infrarenal AAA Following Remote Open Repair of AAA

Presentation

A 74-year-old woman was seen in the ER with abdominal pain in August 2011. She had an open repair of AAA with a tube graft in 1991 at an outside hospital using a midline laparotomy. The details of the operation and the type of graft used were not available. Medical comorbidities included advanced chronic obstructive pulmonary disease (COPD) and hypertension. CTA of the abdomen and pelvis showed a 6.0 cm AAA just above the aortic bifurcation (Fig. 9.1a). It was not clear whether the aneurysm was a true aneurysm distal to the previously placed distal anastomosis or a para-anastomotic aneurysm. Both iliac arteries were calcified and small in caliber (Fig. 9.1b). In August 2011, she underwent endovascular repair of AAA using bilateral transverse groin incisions. The main body of the Endurant™ graft 23 × 13 × 124 mm (Medtronic, Dublin, Ireland) was advanced from the right side after 14 mm and 16 mm Coon dilators (Cook Medical, Bloomington, IN) were passed. A contralateral iliac limb 16 × 10 × 93 mm, and an ipsi-

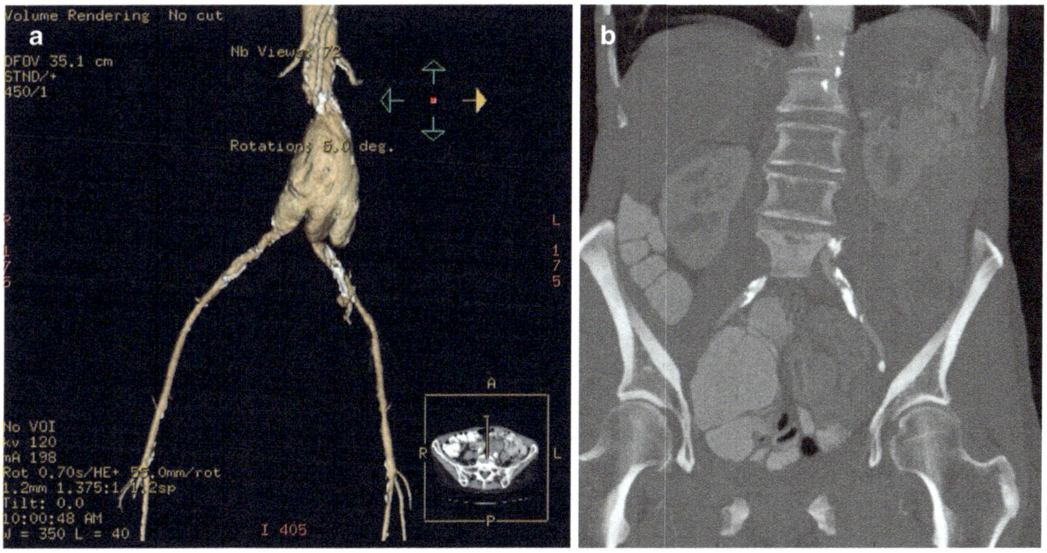

Fig. 9.1 (**a**) CTA showing large recurrent distal saccular AAA (**b**) CTA showing small diameter calcified iliac arteries

S. S. Hans, *Secondary and Tertiary Arterial Reconstructions*,
https://doi.org/10.1007/978-3-032-21214-6_9

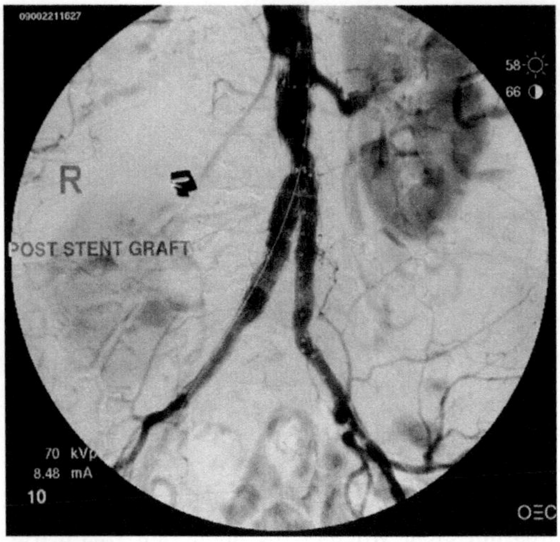

Fig. 9.2 Completion aortogram showing satisfactory endovascular repair. Right kidney is located in the right hemi-pelvis

lateral extension limb of 13 × 13 × 82 mm were also deployed to completely exclude the aneurysm. A completion aortogram showed satisfactory exclusion of the recurrent AAA (Fig. 9.2).

Right common and proximal SFA endarterectomy was performed with bovine pericardial patch grafting. The patient was discharged on the third post-operative day in satisfactory condition. A follow-up CTA 6 weeks later showed satisfactory exclusion of the AAA without endoleak. The patient died in January 2013 from progressive respiratory failure secondary to chronic obstructive disease.

Discussion

True aortic aneurysms proximal and distal to the open repair of AAA, as well as para-anastomotic aneurysms, occur following open repair of aortic aneurysms and can be diagnosed with follow-up imaging studies. In many instances, the native aorta continues to enlarge due to inherent weakness (degeneration) of the aortic wall. The results of the repair of these aneurysms have improved due to the availability of endovascular options. Open repair of recurrent aortic aneurysm is associated with a significantly higher morbidity and mortality and should be avoided unless there are no endovascular options available, and the patient is an acceptable risk for an open repair.

With the increasing use of physician-modified endografts (PMEGs), para-anastomotic aortic aneurysms can now be treated in centers specializing in advanced aortic pathology. From an international multicenter single-arm cohort study analyzing the outcomes of PMEGs in the treatment of elective, symptomatic, and ruptured complex abdominal aortic aneurysms and thoracoabdominal aortic aneurysms of 1274 patients from 19 centers, the median age was 74 years (IQR 68–79) and 75.7% were men with 45.7% were complex abdominal aortic aneurysms, and 54.3% were thoracoabdominal aortic aneurysms; 65.5% patients presented electively, 24.6% were symptomatic, and 9.9% were ruptured. [1] Most patients had a fenestrated repair, 3.6% branched repair, and 13.4% a combined fenestrated and branched repair. Most patients (85.8%) had ≥3 target vessels included. The overall technical success was 94%. Thirty-day mortality was 5.8% (4.1% in elective, 7.6% in symptomatic, and 12.7% in ruptured aneurysms). Major adverse events occurred in 25.2% of cases. Median follow-up was 21 months (5.6–50.6). Freedom from reintervention was 73.8%, 61.8%, and 51.4% at 1, 3, and 5 years; primary target vessel patency was 96.9%, 93.6%, and 90.3%. Overall survival and freedom from aortic-related mortality were 82.4%/92.9%, 69.9%/91.6%, and 55.0%/89.1% at 1, 3, and 5 years, respectively [1]. The study authors concluded that PMEGs are a safe and effective treatment for elective, symptomatic, and thoracoabdominal aneurysms, but recommend that future comparative studies with other established techniques are needed in both the elective and urgent setting.

Multiple Choice Questions

1. The overall technical success of PMEGs is
   A. 80%
   B. 84%
   C. 90%
   D. 94%

2. The 30-day mortality of PMEGs is
   A. 5.8%
   B. 6.5%
   C. 7%
   D. >7%
3. Freedom from reintervention at 5 years following PMEGs is
   A. 65%
   B. 60%
   C. 55%
   D. 50%

Answers: 1(D), 2(A), 3(C)

Reference

1. Tsilimparis, N., Gouveia, E. M. R., Tenorio, E. R., Scali, S., Mendes, B., Han, S., . . . Oderich, G. S. (2024). Multicenter study on physician-modified endografts for thoracoabdominal and complex abdominal aortic aneurysm repair. Circulation, 150(17), 1327–1342. PMID:38989565.

10 Repair of Saccular Aneurysm of Infrarenal Aorta with Iliac and Femoral Artery Occlusive Disease

Presentation

A 69-year-old woman was seen in the clinic with a 5.2 cm saccular infrarenal AAA in January 2017. The distal aorta just inferior to the aneurysm was small in caliber (12 mm diameter). Abdominal aortography showed infrarenal AAA with a long neck and small-diameter iliac arteries (Fig. 10.1a, b). She had a history of a right common iliac artery stent and left CIA angioplasty for symptomatic iliac artery disease. The patient had a history of hypertension, hyperlipidemia, and hyperthyroidism. The patient was a current smoker and consumed six beers daily. In April 2017, she underwent endovascular aneurysm repair (EVAR) with the deployment of the main body from the left femoral artery access obtained by a groin cutdown. The main body 23 × 14 × 103 mm of Endurant ™ graft (Medtronic, Dublin, Ireland) was deployed from the right side. The contralateral limb, 16 × 10 × 82 mm, was deployed using left femoral access via a left groin cutdown. An ipsilateral extension limb (16 × 10 × 93 mm) and two balloon expandable (10 mm × 59 mm) Omnilink stents (Abbott, Abbott Park, IL) were deployed. She developed a surgical site infection (SSI) in the right groin, which was treated with local wound care and antibiotics.

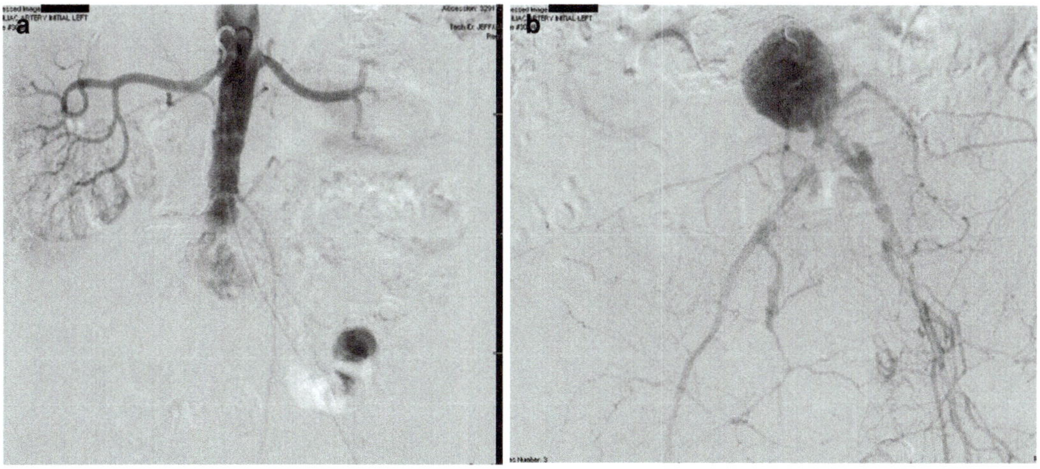

Fig. 10.1 (**a**) Abdominal aortography showing infrarenal AAA with a long neck and small diameter iliac arteries (**b**) Abdominal aortography showing infrarenal AAA and small diameter iliac arteries

S. S. Hans, *Secondary and Tertiary Arterial Reconstructions*,
https://doi.org/10.1007/978-3-032-21214-6_10

A follow-up CTA scan of the abdomen and pelvis 5 weeks after EVAR revealed a marked decrease in the size of the aneurysm sac. She was lost to follow-up for 2 years. A CT angiogram of the abdomen and pelvis for bladder cancer was obtained by a urologist in October 2019, which showed diffuse thickening of the wall of the urinary bladder and an incidental finding of stenosis in the distal end of the right iliac limb, with the narrowing of the right iliac diameter to a patent lumen of 2 mm.

At a follow-up clinic visit in February 2022, the aneurysm sac had regressed to 3.3 × 3.0 cm with no evidence of endoleak by Duplex ultrasound of the aorta. A non-invasive arterial doppler study showed an ABI (0.57- right) and (0.62- left). In February 2023, the patient had worsening symptoms of intermittent claudication (IC) with progression to ischemic rest pain. CTA of abdomen and pelvis showed occlusion of the right limb of the EVAR (Fig. 10.2a, b). She underwent open right femoral artery exposure following a challenging dissection in the right groin as a result of previous groin exposure and a subsequent SSI. A 7F introducer sheath was placed in the right CFA. The Shockwave 8 mm balloon angioplasty catheter was used to cross the known segment of narrow calcified plaque. On the left side, an ultrasound-guided puncture of the left common femoral artery was performed with two Perclose closure devices (Abbott Vascular, Redwood City, CA) with the introduction of a 12F sheath, and a 14 mm 4 cm long balloon was inflated in the left iliac limb to prevent distal embolization. Mechanical thrombectomy of the occluded right limb was performed using the Rotarex™ Atherectomy system (Becton Dickinson Franklin Lakes, NJ). The right iliac limb was then relined with three covered stents starting distally and extending up to the flow divider using (8 × 39 mm, 9 × 39 mm 10 × 39 mm) covered stents (VBX, W.L. Gore, Newark, DE) (Fig. 10.3a, b).

Completion aortogram performed via the left femoral access (12F sheath) demonstrated a plug of thrombus just proximal to the newly placed covered stents. Therefore, it was decided to raise the flow divider to exclude the thrombus by deploying two 16 × 10 × 93 mm Endurant™ iliac graft limbs. A completion aortogram demonstrated a dissection flap in the right external iliac artery (EIA). A 7 mm × 10 cm long Viabahn self--expanding covered stent graft (E.L. Gore, Newark, DE) was deployed distal to the origin of the hypogastric artery, extending into the junction of the EIA and the CFA, with post-

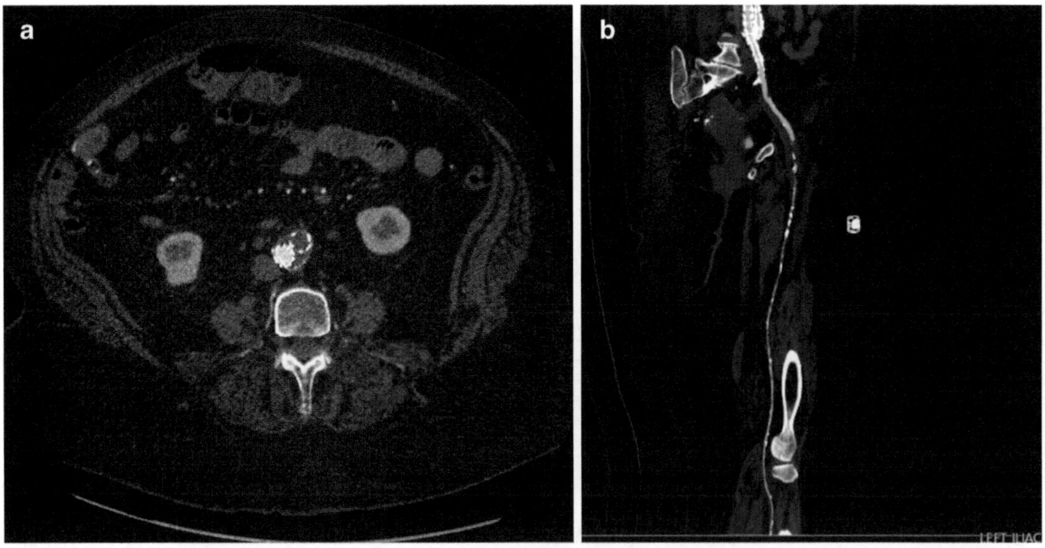

Fig. 10.2 (**a**) CTA of the abdomen and pelvis showing occlusion of the right graft limb (**b**) Abdominal CTA (MIP images) and runoff showing right graft limb occlusion

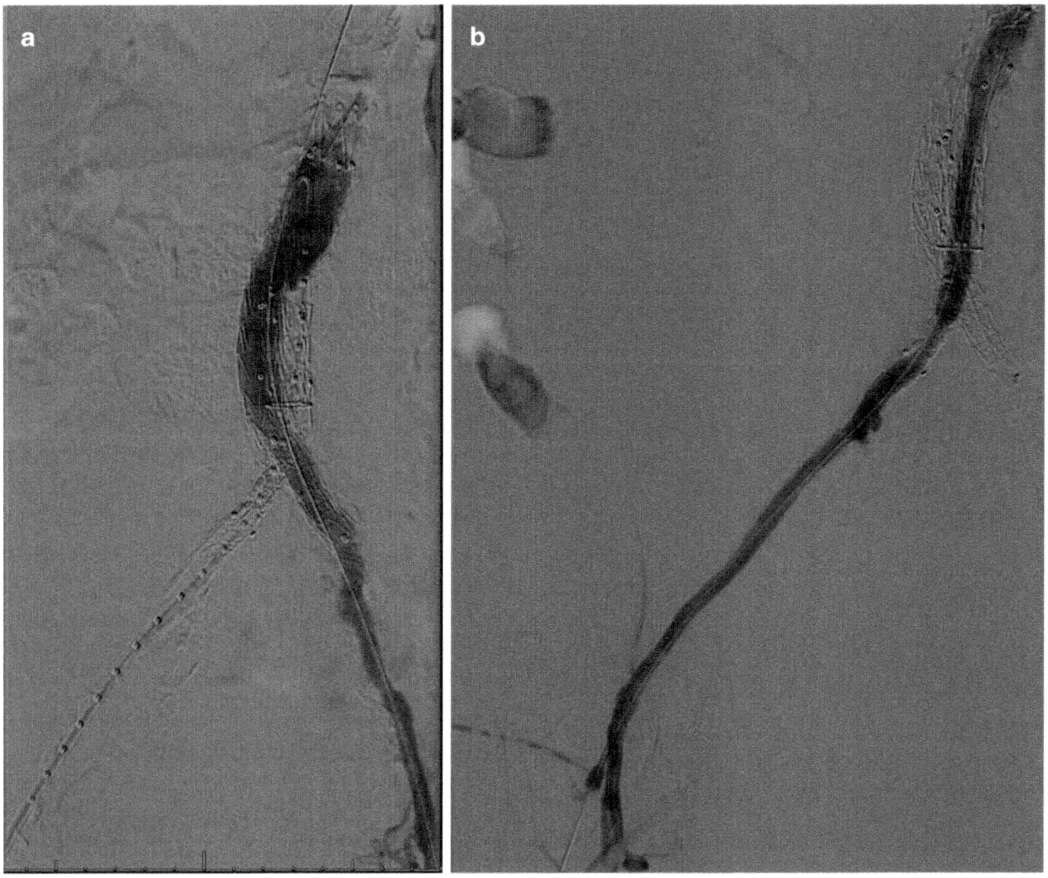

Fig. 10.3 (**a**) Intraoperative aortogram showing occlusion of right graft limb (**b**) Aortogram showing partial recanalization of right iliac limb following mechanical thrombectomy

angioplasty using a 6 mm × 10 cm. Armada balloon (Abbott Medical, Abbott Park, IL) (Fig. 10.4).

An arteriotomy incision in the right CFA was sutured using a continuous 5′0″ cardiovascular polypropylene suture. On the left side, two Perclose devices were deployed as the 12F sheath was removed with its dilator. A third Perclose device at the "12 o'clock" position was also deployed to obtain complete hemostasis on the left side. During the evening of the operation, the patient developed ischemic left lower extremity (LE), and CTA of the abdomen and pelvis demonstrated an occlusion of the left CFA at the origin of the profunda femoris artery. The patient was taken back to the OR and underwent re-exploration of the left groin. The ProGlide sutures were removed. Proximal control of the distal EIA was obtained, and left CFA endarterectomy, including the orifice of the profunda, was per-

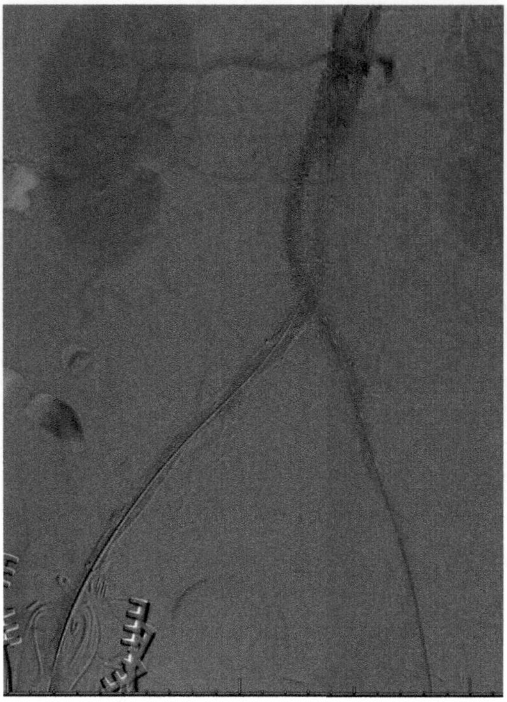

Fig. 10.4 Completion Aortogram showing satisfactory endovascular repair with proximalization of flow divider by deployment of covered stents extending proximally in each iliac endograft

formed with application of a pericardial patch with restoration of satisfactory blood flow to the LLE.

Discussion

The ProGlide® vascular closure device (Abbott Vascular, Abbott Park, IL) is approved for the closure of arterial puncture (5–26F) sheaths with a maximum diameter of 26F. A failure rate of 2–8% is reported [1]. Chen et al., from a retrospective study of 458 patients with the use of ProGlide® vascular closure devise reported failure in 7.6% of cases [1]. Factors contributed to failure included a history of peripheral arterial disease ($p < 0.001$), the presence of common femoral artery calcification ($p < 0.001$), and the depth of the skin puncture site ≥33 mm ($p < 0.001$). Body mass index of ≥28.7 kg/m^2 ($p < 0.001$) and use of sheath size of ≥19F ($p < 0.001$) [1]. Careful patient and closure device selection are important factors to prevent failure of the vascular closure device.

Graft limb occlusion (GLO) following EVAR was reported in 5–6% of the patients from a meta-analysis of 13 studies comparing 5454 patients [2]. Mantas et al., reported 18 grafts (4%) among 439 patients (from 2010 to 2013) [3]. Factors contributing to GLO were angulation and tortuosity of the iliac artery, iliac artery calcification, and excessive limb oversizing. Faure et al., reported 42 GLOS's in 39 patients (3.4%) from the Endurant™ stent graft natural selection [4]. Global post-market registry (ENGAGE), the strongest independent predictors for limb occlusions were the distal landing zone in the EIA. EIA diameter <10 mm and the kinking and tortuosity of the iliac arteries [4]. Chacko et al., reported 5.9% incidence of GLO; predictors of GLO were a small diameter EIA, prior CIA stenting and graft limb extension to the EIA [5].

Multiple Choice Questions

1. The incidence of GLO following EVAR is
   A. 4–6%
   B. 7–8%
   C. 9–10%
   D. >10%
2. From the ENGAGE post-market registry, the strongest predictor of GLO of Endurant™ graft was
   A. Oversizing of the graft by greater than 20%
   B. Iliac artery tortuosity and calcification
   C. Short landing zone in CIA
   D. Distal landing zone in EIA
3. In sheaths greater than 16F, access site closure failure with the use of Proglide sutures occurs in
   A. 5.6% of patients
   B. 6.6% of patients
   C. 7.6% of patients
   D. 8.6% of patients

Answers: 1(A), 2(D), 3(C)

References

1. Chen IM, Lee TH, Chen PL, Shih CC, Chang HH. Factors in ProGlide® vascular closure failure in sheath Arteriotomies greater than 16 French. Eur J Vasc Endovasc Surg. 2019;58(4):615–22. PMID:31500989
2. Hammond A, Hansrani V, Lowe C, Asghar I, Antoniou SA, Antoniou GA. Meta-analysis and meta-regression analysis of iliac limb occlusion after endovascular aneurysm repair. J Vasc Surg. 2018;68(6):1916–1924.e1917. PMID:30366653
3. Mantas GK, Antonopoulos CN, Sfyroeras GS, Moulakakis KG, Kakisis JD, Mylonas SN, Liapis CD. Factors predisposing to endograft limb occlusion after endovascular aortic repair. Eur J Vasc Endovasc Surg. 2015;49(1):39–44. PMID:25453234
4. Faure EM, Becquemin JP, Cochennec F. Predictive factors for limb occlusions after endovascular aneurysm repair. J Vasc Surg. 2015;61(5):1138–14.
5. Chacko P, Hans SS, Nahirniak P, Morton K. Clinical patterns, predictors, and results of graft limb occlusion following endovascular aneurysm repair. Ann Vasc Surg. 2023;94:341–6. PMID:36918093 5.e1132. PMID:25656594

11 Chyle Leak Following Carotid Subclavian Artery Bypass and Thoracic Endovascular Aortic Repair (TEVAR)

Presentation

A 69-year-old woman underwent a left carotid subclavian artery bypass and thoracic endovascular aortic repair (TEVAR) (Figs. 11.1 and 11.2). She had an open repair of thoracic aortic coarctation at the Children's Hospital of Michigan during her childhood. The exact details of the operation were not available. Approximately 1 week after TEVAR and carotid-subclavian artery bypass, she presented to the emergency room with swelling in the left neck with drainage of chylous fluid and Horner's syndrome. Medical comorbidities included hypertension, atrial fibrillation, hyperlipidemia. She was started on a fat-free diet supplemented with medium chain trigylcerides and Octreotide (Sandostatin) 100 mg/daily. However, she did not respond to conservative treatment and therefore, underwent foam sclerotherapy with injection of contrast medium in the sinus tract. Foam solution (Sotradeclol 3% and air) with manual compression of the neck was performed for 10 min. However, chylous leak persisted with daily output of 1000–1400 ml. Negative pressure wound therapy was applied. A CT scan of the neck showed a 7 × 8.5 × 8 cm soft tissue fluid collection in the left side of the neck (Figs. 11.3 and 11.4).

In June 2015, the patient underwent lymphangiography of the pelvis and abdomen (bilateral) under ultrasound guidance, lymph nodes in both groins were accessed sequentially. Once each lymph node was assessed, a small amount of iodinated contrast was injected under fluoroscopy to confirm the position of the needle in the lymph node. A slow injection of Lipiodol was started. A total of approximately 20 mL of Lipiodol was injected into both right and left inguinal lymph nodes. Prominent lymphatics were noted on both sides of the pelvis and there

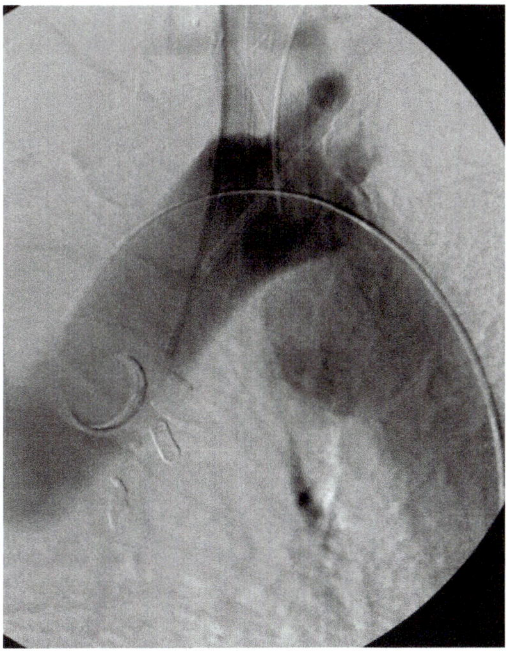

Fig. 11.1 Thoracic aortogram showing thoracic aortic aneurysm at the site of coarctation repair

S. S. Hans, *Secondary and Tertiary Arterial Reconstructions*,
https://doi.org/10.1007/978-3-032-21214-6_11

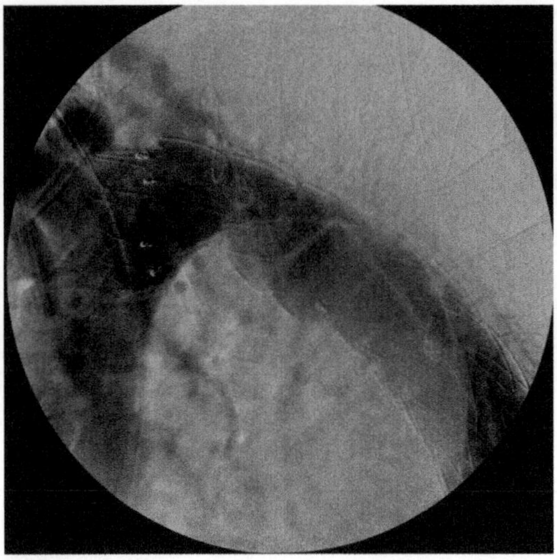

Fig. 11.2 Deployment of thoracic aortic stent graft

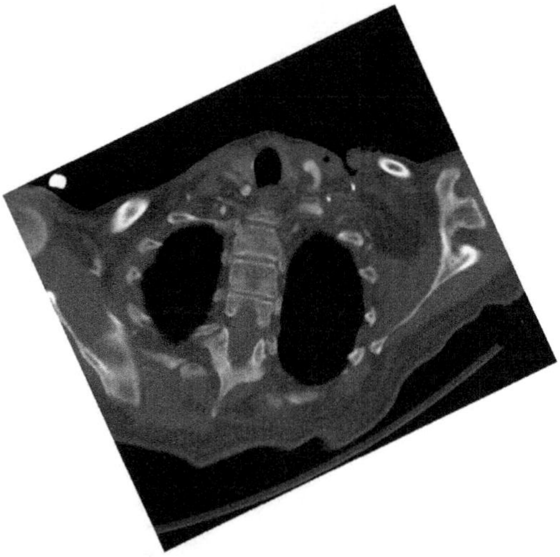

Fig. 11.3 CT of the soft tissue of the neck showing patent carotid subclavian bypass with evidence of fluid collection and gas in soft tissues of the neck with overlying skin breakdown

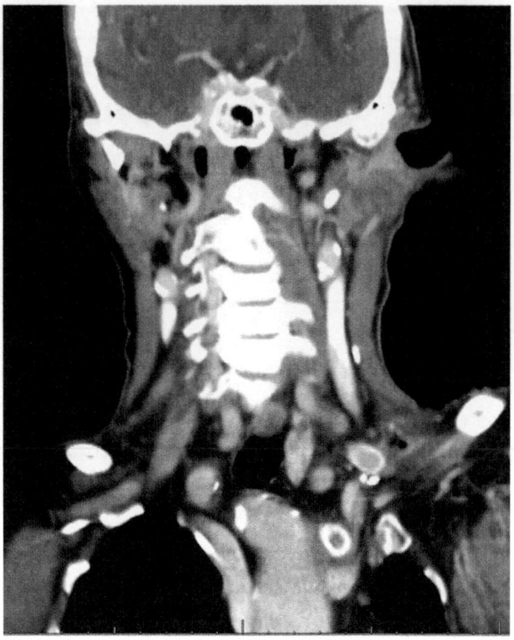

Fig. 11.4 Coronal view—CT of the soft tissue of the neck showing patent carotid-subclavian artery bypass evidence of fluid collection and gas in soft tissues of the neck and skin breakdown

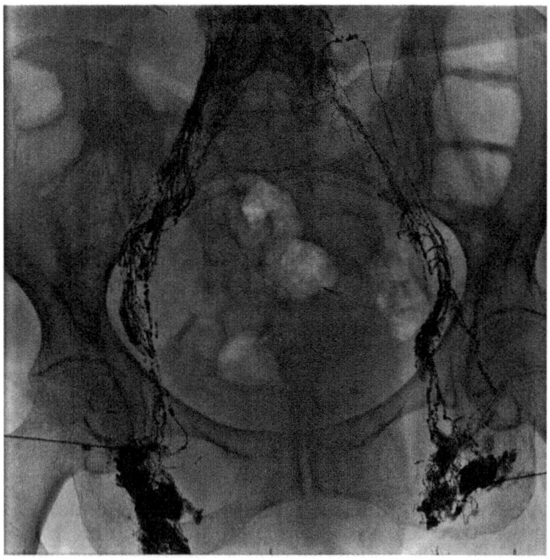

Fig. 11.5 Lymphangiography of abdomen and pelvis showing inguinal, pelvic, and lower abdominal lymphatics

was rapid filling of the lymphatics at the level of the lumbar spine (Fig. 11.5). Further fluoroscopic imaging showed continued filling of the lymphatics, eventually reaching the mid and upper abdomen and finally transitioning to fill the thoracic duct in the thorax (Fig. 11.6). In the neck, adjacent to surgical clips there was extravasation of lipiodol from the open left neck wound (Fig. 11.4). Three dimensional CT scan was performed to delineate the location of the lymphatics in the upper abdomen. There were two lymphatic channels in the upper abdomen on the right lateral side of the aorta. Under fluoroscopic guidance, one of these lymphatic channels was

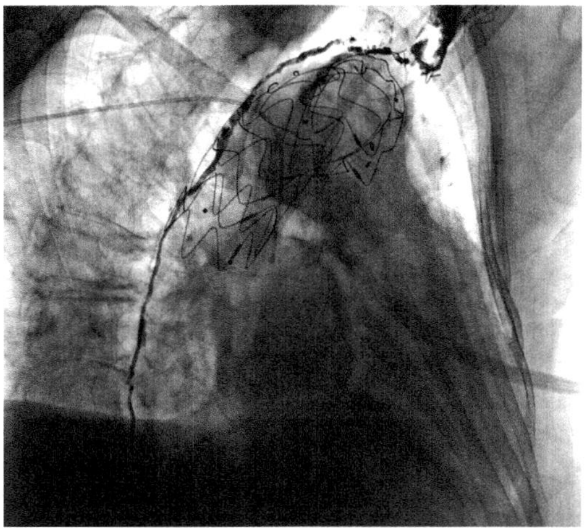

Fig. 11.6 Lymphangiography showing visualization of thoracic duct with extravasation of lipiodol in the left neck

punctured percutaneously using an anterior approach with a 20-gauge spinal needle. A nitinol cope wire (Cook Medical, Bloomington, IN) was advanced proximally in the thoracic duct through the needle access. Once the wire was in a satisfactory position, an Aprima set (Cook Medical, Bloomington, IN) micro-puncture introducer and the distal end of the severed microcatheter was successful and advanced to the site of the chyle leak. The short nitinol wire was exchanged for a 150 cm V18 wire. The severed segment of the microcatheter was removed, and a new microcatheter was advanced to the site of the chyle leak. Multiple Tornado coils were deployed at the site of the chyle leak, and contrast injection showed occlusion at the site of the coils. The remaining segment of the thoracic duct was occluded with a mixture of glue and lipiodol mixed at a ratio of 1:4. The microcatheter was withdrawn.

The patient developed abdominal pain and signs of peritonitis following the procedure. A CT scan of the abdomen showed free fluid but without the presence of free air. There was a concern for a perforated viscus. The patient underwent attempted laparoscopy, but because of the presence of adhesions, and with the findgings of a significant amount of bile surrounding the liver and a hematoma within the omental adhesions, it was converted to a laparotomy. There was no evidence of gastrointestinal perforation. A 19F Blake drain was inserted within the lesser sac. The patient developed atrial fibrillation with a rapid ventricular response. She died 3 weeks later from multiple organ failure.

Discussion

Protack et al., reported a 0.7% (2 patients) incidence of lymphatic leak following subclavian artery revascularization in patients undergoing TEVAR [1]. Following thyroidectomy, the reported incidence of chylous leak is 0.5–1.4%, and the incidence increases to 8.1% following neck dissections. Accumulation of chylous fluid in the neck leads to local irritation, delayed wound healing, wound dehiscence, electrolyte imbalance, malnutrition, and immunosuppression. Chylous leak is the result of iatrogenic injury to the thoracic duct or one of its tributaries in the lower neck. Patients may present with a palpable fluid collection in the surgical bed, as increased outputs from the surgical drain increase following resumption of the oral diet. The fluid is creamy with an increased level of triglycerides (more than 110 mg/dl).

Initially, patients should be placed on a low-fat diet, medium-chain triglycerides, and high-protein content. Patients who are non-responsive to dietary manipulation should be started on total dietary parental nutrition with medium-chain triglycerides. Somatostatin or its analogue Octreotide, with a longer half-life in a dosage of 100 mcg once daily subcutaneously, helps reduce the lymph flow.

For patients not responding to conservative means, thoracic duct embolization (TDE) should be considered. Catheter embolization of the thoracic duct is safe, feasible, and successful in eliminating high-output chyle leak in 71% of patients [2]. Transgression of the needle through visceral organs, arteries, and vessels can result in bile leakage, bleeding, and peritonitis. Long-term complications include chronic lower extremity edema, chronic diarrhea, and abdominal ascites. Transabdominal embolization may not always be feasible (e.g., when lymph vessels are less than 2–3 mm in diameter). As an alternative, retrograde cannulation of thoracic duct, using a transvenous approach or through a cannulation via a lymphocele [3]. Direct percutaneous cervical access to the thoracic duct with retrograde embolization in a high-output cervical fistula has also been reported [4].

Multiple Choice Questions

1. The incidence of lymphatic leak following carotid subclavian artery bypass in patients undergoing TEVAR is
   A. 0.2%
   B. 0.5%
   C. 0.7%
   D. 1%
2. The triglyceride content of chylous fluid is
   A. <50 mg/dL
   B. 50–75 mg/dL
   C. 76–109 mg/dL
   D. >110 mg/dL
3. The success rate of thoracic duct embolization for chylous leak in patients unresponsive to conservative treatment is
   A. 90%
   B. 80–89%
   C. 72–79%
   D. Approximately 70%

Answers: 1(C), 2(D), 3(D)

References

1. Protack CD, Smith A, Moennich LA, Hardy D, Lyden SP, Farivar BS. Midterm outcomes of subclavian artery revascularization in the setting of thoracic endovascular aortic repair. J Vasc Surg. 2020;72(4):1222–8. PMID:32093914
2. Chen E, Itkin M. Thoracic duct embolization for chylous leaks. Semin Intervent Radiol. 2011;28(1):63–74. PMID:22379277
3. Moussa AM, Maybody M, Gonzalez-Aguirre AJ, Buicko JL, Shaha AR, Santos E. Thoracic duct embolization in post-neck dissection Chylous leakage: a case series of six patients and review of the literature. Cardiovasc Intervent Radiol. 2020;43(6):931–7. PMID:32342160
4. Pieper CC, Schild HH. Direct cervical puncture for retrograde thoracic duct embolization in a postoperative cervical lymphatic fistula. J Vasc Interv Radiol. 2015;26(9):1405–8. PMID:26314650

12 Cervical Chyloma Following Left Common Carotid Artery (CCA) to Subclavian Artery Bypass Performed in Conjunction with Thoracic Endovascular Aortic Repair (TEVAR) for Aortic Dissection

Presentation

A 74-year-old woman was emergently admitted to the hospital with a near-syncopal episode. She had a history of recurrent dizziness. Carotid duplex imaging showed left subclavian artery occlusive disease with retrograde flow in the left vertebral artery. CTA of the head and neck showed a near occlusion of the first portion of the left subclavian artery with retrograde flow in the left vertebral artery (Fig. 12.1). A left subclavian artery angioplasty/stenting using left brachial artery access was attempted, but the procedure was terminated as the lesion could not be crossed by the guidewire. Arteriogram at the end of the attempted subclavian intervention showed a non-flow-limiting dissection at the junction of the transverse and descending thoracic aorta (Fig. 12.2). She complained of upper thoracic back pain after the procedure. A follow-up CTA of the neck and chest showed chronic type B thoracic aortic dissection. In May 2024, she underwent a left common carotid artery (CCA) to the subclavian artery bypass as a staged procedure, a day prior to endovascular repair of thoracic aortic dissection (TEVAR). A left supraclavicular incision starting from the medial border of the sternocleidomastoid (SCM), a few centimeters above the clavicle and extending towards the shoulder for a distance of approximately 6 cms was made. The clavicular head of the SCM was divided, and the carotid sheath was opened. The anterior scalene fat pad was mobilized, preserving the phrenic nerve. The insertion of the scalene anticus was also divided exposing the second portion of the subclavian artery. A small pleural rent was repaired with a 2′0′ Vicryl suture. An 8 mm externally supported ringed PTFE graft (W.L. Gore, Newark, DE) was selected and anastomosed to the posterolateral wall of the CCA in an end-to-side fashion. The graft was brought behind the internal jugular vein (IJV) and anastomosed to the subclavian artery in an end-to-side fashion in its third portion.

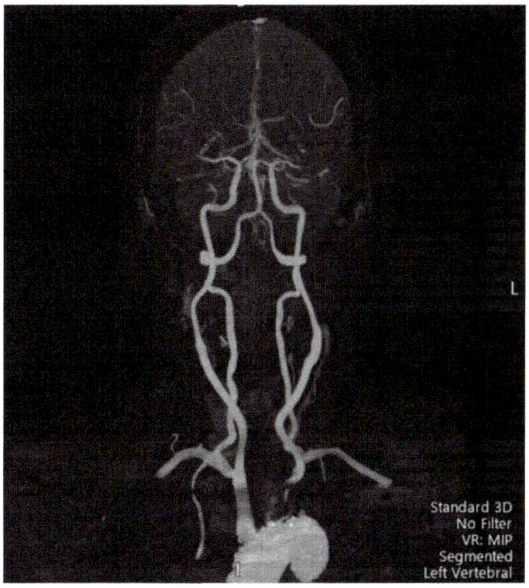

Fig. 12.1 CTA of the head and neck (MIP images) showing near occlusion of the left subclavian artery

S. S. Hans, *Secondary and Tertiary Arterial Reconstructions*,
https://doi.org/10.1007/978-3-032-21214-6_12

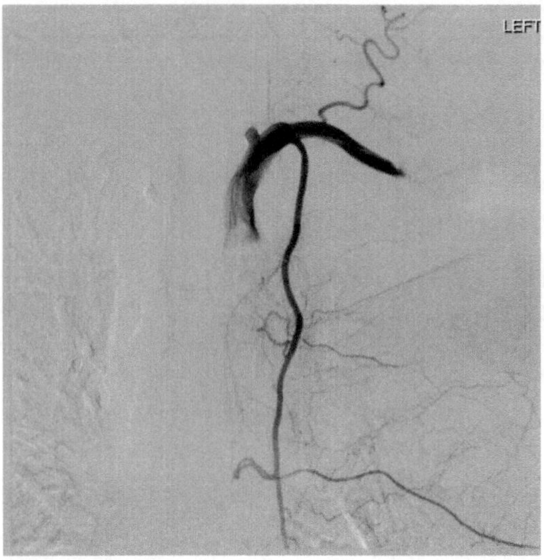

Fig. 12.2 Left upper extremity arteriogram using brachial access showing non-flow-limiting subclavian artery dissection

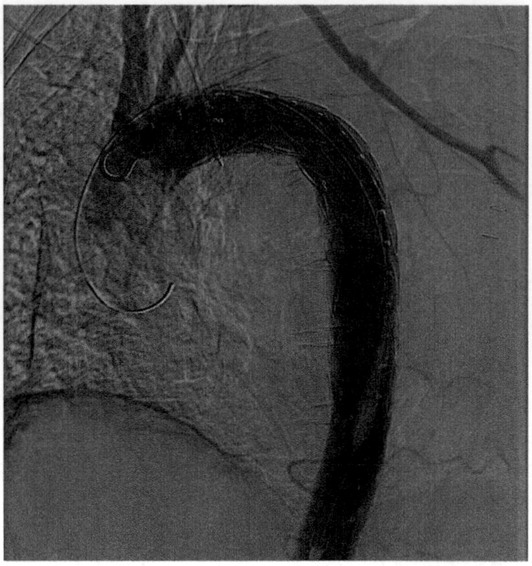

Fig. 12.3 Repair of thoracic aortic dissection with endograft

The following day, she underwent TEVAR using bilateral percutaneous femoral artery access under ultrasound guidance with the passage of a 7F sheath in each common femoral artery (CFA). Intra-arterial lithotripsy balloons were introduced over 0.014″ glidewire advantage wire and positioned just above the aortic bifurcation. The intra-arterial balloon impulses were delivered for a total of 300 impulses across the distal abdominal aorta, aorta bifurcation, and the common and external iliac arteries. A 90 cms. long Omniflush sizing catheter (AngioDynamics, Latham, NY) was introduced through the right femoral access sheath and parked in the descending thoracic aorta. Two ProGlide (Abbott Medical, Chicago, IL) were deployed in the left groin. On the left side, a 0.035″ Storq wire (Cordis, Dublin, OH) was exchanged for a Lunderquist (Cook Medical, Bloomington, IN) wire using a glide catheter. A 30 mm × 150 mm Captiva thoracic endograft (Medtronic, Dublin, Ireland) was advanced from the left side. The graft was deployed covering the left subclavian artery and the area of dissection. Completion aortogram demonstrated satisfactory deployment of the thoracic endograft (Fig. 12.3). There were no abnormalities in the abdominal aorta, common iliac, and external iliac arteries. ProGlide-mediated suture closure was performed for the left femoral artery access. A Star close device was used for closure of the right femoral artery access.

She presented to the clinic three months later with swelling in the left neck (Fig. 12.4). A CTA of the neck demonstrated a 5.8 cms. fluid collection consistent with a chyloma (Fig. 12.5). She subsequently sought two opinions at two different outside facilities for the management of the chyloma, which remained asymptomatic. Post-op CTA demonstrated patent carotid-subclavian bypass (Fig. 12.6) and satisfactory thoracic endograft without any evidence of endoleak. An MRI of the neck demonstrated a 6 cm chyloma in the left supraclavicular area. The patient has been reluctant to undergo excision of the cervical chyloma. She was seen in the clinic in June 2025 with significant decrease in the size of the swelling in the neck (Fig. 12.7).

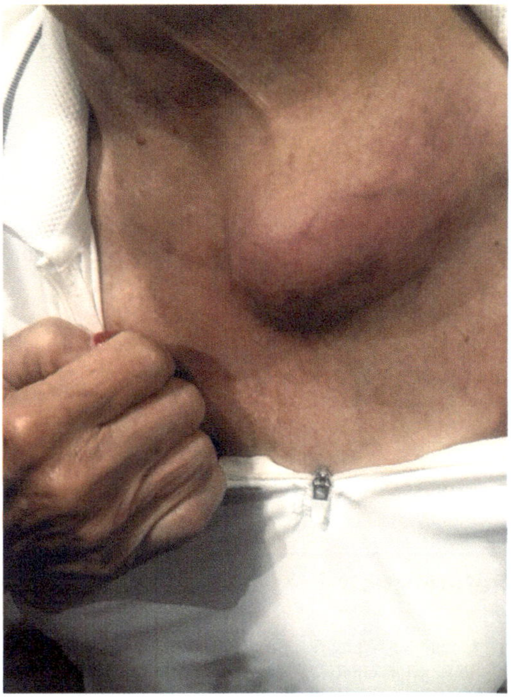

Fig. 12.4 Cervical chyloma left neck 3 months after common carotid to left subclavian artery bypass and TEVAR

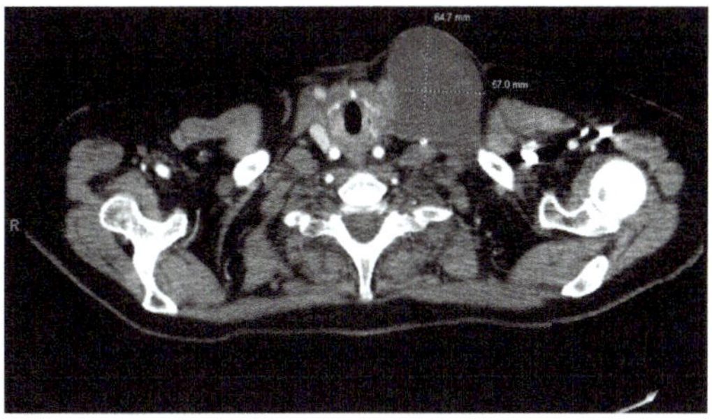

Fig. 12.5 Follow-up CTA neck showing Chyloma in the left neck

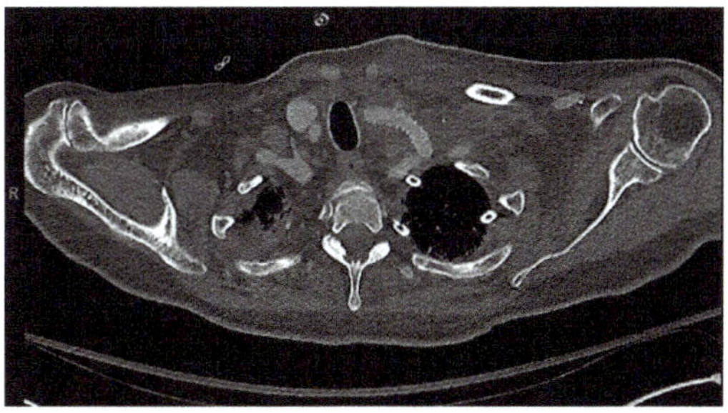

Fig. 12.6 Follow-up CTA neck and chest shows patent left carotid-subclavian bypass with fluid collection in the left neck

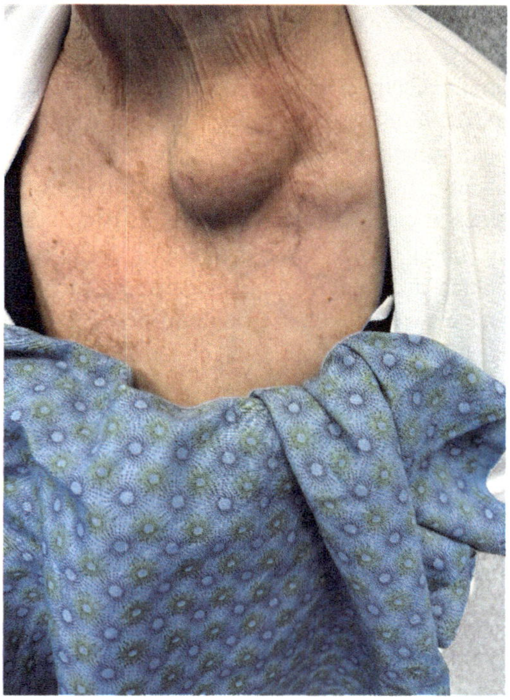

Fig. 12.7 Decrease in the size of Cervical Chyloma 14 months after the carotid subclavian bypass and TEVAR

Discussion

The results of a meta-analysis of 32 studies by Chen et al., assessing the outcomes of revascularization after intentional coverage of the left subclavian artery (LSA) for thoracic endovascular repair, showed a decreased risk of cerebrovascular accident and spinal cord ischemia, but at the cost of higher local complications such as possible vocal cord paresis, other nerve injuries, and chyle leak [1]. The 30-day mortality rates after TEVAR were not significantly different between the LSA revascularization and non-revascularization groups. According to the Society for Vascular Surgery guidelines, routine preoperative revascularization is recommended in selected patients with anatomy that compromises the perfusion to the brain, spinal cord, heart, and left arm [2]. The timing of LSA revascularization done synchronously with TEVAR or just prior to TEVAR does not affect the incidence of perioperative stroke.

Other complications following carotid-subclavian artery bypass include vocal cord paralysis, vagus nerve injury, phrenic nerve injury, thoracic duct injury, and Horner syndrome. Chylous leak, Chyloma, or Chylothorax are the result of thoracic duct injury or one of its main tributaries. In patients undergoing cervical node dissection, chyle leak occurs in 1–6% of cases. It can also result from trauma to the neck and chest, thyroid surgery, complications of lymphoma, and superior vena cava obstruction. Most patients will require excision of the chyloma and identification with ligation of the feeding thoracic duct or its major branch.

Multiple Choice Questions

1. Intentional coverage of the left subclavian artery with TEVAR
   A. Increase in local complications but decrease in incidence of perioperative stroke
   B. Decrease in local complications and decrease in incidence of perioperative stroke
   C. Increase in incidence of both local complications and perioperative stroke
   D. Similar incidence of stroke and local complications with or without coverage of the left subclavian artery
2. According to SVS guidelines, routine preoperative revascularization is recommended for anatomy that compromises perfusion to
   A. Brain
   B. Spinal cord
   C. Left arm
   D. Brain, spinal cord, left arm
3. Incidence of chylocele in the neck (Chyloma) after cervical node dissection is
   A. 0–0.25%
   B. 0.25–0.95%
   C. 1–6%
   D. 7–10%

Answers: 1(A), 2(D), 3(C)

References

1. Chen X, Wang J, Premaratne S, Zhao J, Zhang WW. Meta-analysis of the outcomes of revascularization after intentional coverage of the left subclavian artery for thoracic endovascular aortic repair. J Vasc Surg. 2019;70(4):1330–40. PMID:31176636
2. Matsumura JS, Lee WA, Mitchell RS, Farber MA, Murad MH, Lumsden AB, et al. The Society for Vascular Surgery Practice Guidelines: management of the left subclavian artery with thoracic endovascular aortic repair. J Vasc Surg. 2009;50(5):1155–8. PMID:19878791

13 Management of Type Ia Endoleak Following Endovascular Aneurysm Repair with First-Generation Aortic Endograft

Presentation

An 83-year-old woman was scheduled to undergo transaortic valve replacement (TAVR) and was found to have Type Ia endoleak following endovascular aneurysm repair for abdominal aortic aneurysm (EVAR). It was detected by a CTA of the abdomen and pelvis in January 2023 (Figs. 13.1 and 13.2). She had undergone EVAR in 2008 with a first-generation aortic endograft (AneuRx, Medtronic, Dublin, Ireland). Type Ia endoleak was associated with angulation of the aortic neck (approximately 60 degrees) with distal migration of the endograft. Review of the medical records indicated that the bilateral femoral artery cutdowns were performed for deployment of an aortic endograft in 2008. The patient had her last post-EVAR follow-up at the primary hospital in 2015 and did not have any subsequent follow-up. In January 2023, the patient underwent deployment of an Endurant aortic cuff (32 × 32 × 49 mm). A repeat left femoral cutdown and a left brachial artery access were obtained by a cutdown with insertion of a 5F sheath. An Omniflush catheter (Angiodynamios, Latham, NY) was advanced over an exchange length (260 cm) 0.035 glide wire (Terumo, Somerset, NJ). The common femoral artery was significantly calcified, and Coon's dilators (Cook Medical, Bloomington, IN) were used to help advance the endograft (aortic cuff). After deployment of the aortic cuff, Heli-Fx Endoanchors (Medtronic, Dublin, Ireland) were deployed. A completion aortogram following deployment of the aortic cuff and endoanchors showed a satisfactory resolution of the Type Ia endoleak (Fig. 13.3). Because of the severe left common femoral artery occlusive disease, left common femoral endarterectomy was performed, and a bovine pericardial patch was sutured at the site of endarterectomy. The patient underwent TAVR in March 2023 using a 26 mm Edwards TAVR (Lifesciences, Irvine, CA) and right percutaneous femoral artery access, with closure using two ProGlide sutures. In May 2023, the patient underwent right common femoral endarterectomy

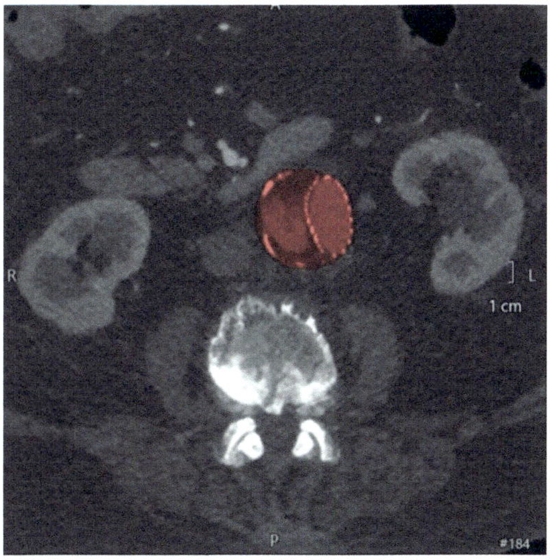

Fig. 13.1 CTA Abdomen and pelvis (axial image) show a large Type Ia endoleak at the proximal endograft site

S. S. Hans, *Secondary and Tertiary Arterial Reconstructions*,
https://doi.org/10.1007/978-3-032-21214-6_13

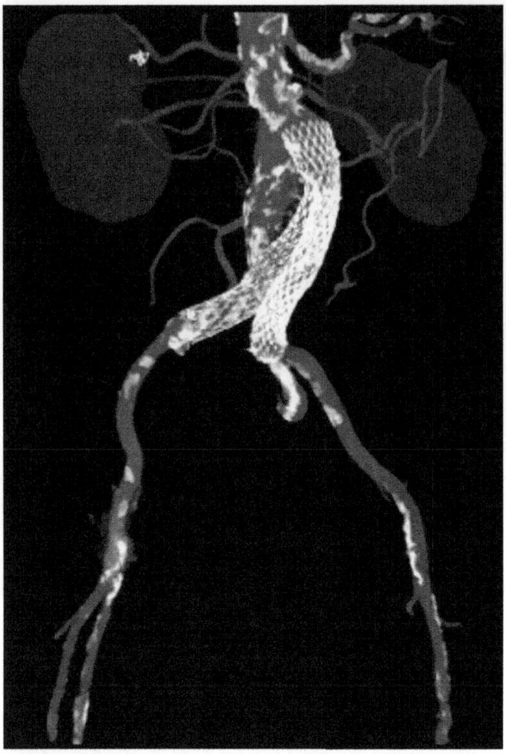

Fig. 13.2 CTA abdomen and pelvis MIP images show significant caudal migration of the AnuRx endograft

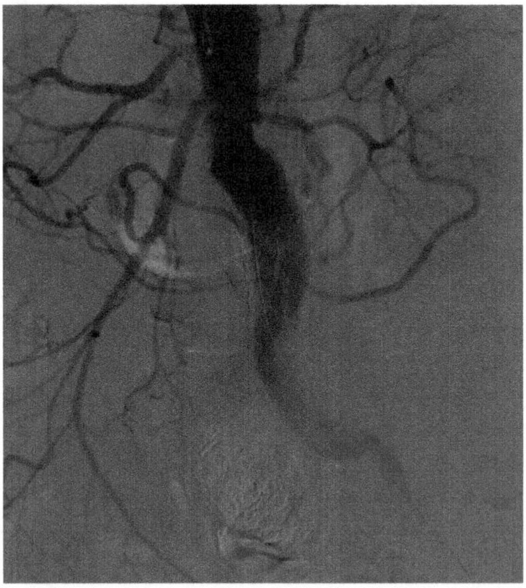

Fig. 13.3 Completion aortogram via Omniflush catheter from brachial access shows resolution of endoleak and a large mesenteric collateral following deployment of aortic cuff

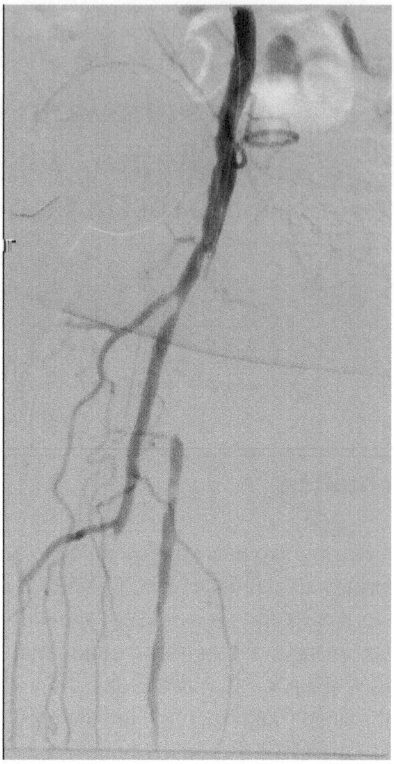

Fig. 13.4 Arteriogram shows proximal right SFA occlusion and mid-segment stenosis of the SFA. The profunda femoris artery shows moderate stenosis 3 cm beyond its origin, with distal occlusion of profunda femoris.

and a bovine pericardial patch angioplasty for near occlusion of the right common femoral artery with critical ischemia in the right lower extremity.

In January 2024, the patient presented with pre-gangrene of the toes and non-healing ulceration of the right heel. The profunda femoris artery demonstrated distal occlusion and a 50% stenosis in it's proximal 3cm. There was occlusion of the proximal superficial femoral artery (SFA) with segmental distal stenosis. (Fig. 13.4). She underwent proximal and mid-superficial femoral artery angioplasty and deployment of a self-expanding SMART stent (6 cm × 8 cm) (Cordis, Cardinal Health, Dublin, OH) (Fig. 13.5). There was gradual healing of the ulcer at an extended care facility. The patient was last seen in the clinic in November 2024 in a stable condition.

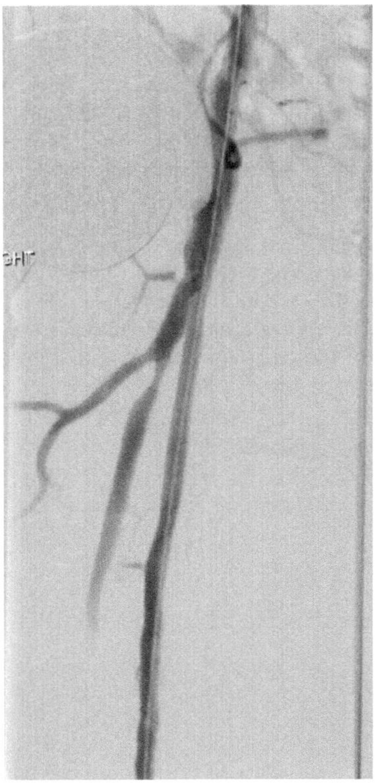

Fig. 13.5 Arteriogram following angioplasty and stenting of the SFA

Discussion

The development of Type Ia delayed endoleak is caused by the aortic neck degeneration resulting in its dilatation aortic neck, excessive graft oversizing greater than 30%, loss of proximal seal in patients due to angulation of the aortic neck, and the use of first-generation endografts without proximal fixation. In patients with persistent Type Ia endoleak, explantation of the endograft may have to be considered if repeated endovascular methods fail to resolve the endoleak.

Major et al., reported an incidence of 8.2% (n = 32) of the Type Ia endoleak among 389 patients undergoing EVAR. [1] This was associated with increased all-cause and aneurysm-related mortality. In their series, Type Ia endoleak presented at a median time of 52 months after EVAR. [1] Patients who had a successful intervention did not show any significant difference in median survival compared with the remaining EVAR cohort (140 months vs 120 months, p = 80) [1]. Those with persistent intraoperative Type Ia endoleak had a higher risk of postoperative Type Ia endoleak as compared with the EVAR overall cohort and had decreased median survival without increased aneurysm-related mortality [1]. Patients undergoing EVAR outside the IFU for the device have been reported to have an increased incidence of Type Ia endoleak.

Delayed Type Ia endoleak (>1 yr) after EVAR is associated with aneurysm sac growth. Occasionally, early Type Ia endoleak after EVAR may resolve spontaneously without any secondary intervention. O'Donnell et al., reported an incidence of 8% of Type Ia endoleak among 1484 EVARs from 1998 to 2015 in a single institution following completion arteriography following graft deployment [2]. They observed that persistent Type Ia endoleak was not independently associated with an increase in sac size on surveillance imaging [2]. Aneurysm rupture secondary to persistent Type Ia endoleak is rare. Extensive neck calcification is the only independent predictor of persistent Type Ia endoleak. They concluded that in select patients, early persistent Type Ia endoleak can be safely observed. [2]

Multiple Choice Questions

1. The incidence of postoperative Type Ia endoleak in patients undergoing EVAR is
   A. 5–6%
   B. 6.1–7%
   C. 7.1–8%
   D. 8.2%
2. Delayed Type Ia endoleak following EVAR occurs at a median time of
   A. 52 months
   B. 48 months
   C. 44 months
   D. 40 months

3. Development of Type Ia endoleak following EVAR is associated with
   A. Increased all-cause mortality
   B. Increased aneurysm-related mortality
   C. Increased all-cause mortality and aneurysm-related mortality
   D. No difference in all-cause mortality or aneurysm-related mortality

Answers: 1(D), 2(A), 3(C)

References

1. Major M, Long GW, Eden CL, Studzinski DM, Callahan RE, Brown OW. Long-term outcomes and interventions of postoperative type 1a endoleak following elective endovascular aortic aneurysm repair. J Vasc Surg. 2022;75(1):136–143.e131. PMID:34324969
2. O'Donnell, T. F. X., Corey, M. R., Deery, S. E., Tsougranis, G., Maruthi, R., Clouse, W. D., . . . Conrad, M. F. (2018). Select early type IA endoleaks after endovascular aneurysm repair will resolve without secondary intervention. J Vasc Surg, 67(1), 119–125. PMID:29268912.

Graft Limb Occlusion of Thoracic Aorta to Femoral Bypass Graft

14

Presentation

A 60-year-old woman presented to the hospital in May 2011 with history of shortness of breath. She was diagnosed with community acquired pneumonia and was treated with appropriate antibiotics. She was found to have ischemic ulceration on the outer aspect of the left foot with ischemic rest pain in May 2011. She had undergone a thoracic aorta to bilateral femoral artery bypass 5 years prior at an outside hospital. The details of the operation could not be obtained. A non-invasive arterial Doppler at this admission showed ABI on the right was 0.42 and 0.17 on the left. She underwent an abdominal aortogram and run-off study using right femoral artery access, which showed occlusion of the left limb of the thoracic aorta to femoral artery bypass and mild stenosis of the right limb. (Figs. 14.1, 14.2, 14.3 and 14.4). Medical comorbidities included hypertension, Type II diabetes mellitus, COPD (current smoker-45 pack years), hyperlipidemia, and morbid obesity. Because of the history of chest discomfort and equivocal cardiolite study (myocardial perfusion imaging), a coronary angiography was performed using right brachial artery percutaneous access, which showed 60% mid-segment stenosis of the right coronary artery with minor plaquing in the left main and left anterior descending artery. She was scheduled for crossover femoral–femoral artery graft reconstruction. However, she developed a sudden onset of rapid atrial fibrillation the day of the operation, and the surgery was postponed. She underwent a crossover femoral–femoral graft with an 8 mm PTFE Interring graft (WL Gore Inc., Newark, DE) 3 weeks later, after her cardiopulmonary condition had stabilized. Ischemic lesions in the left foot eventually

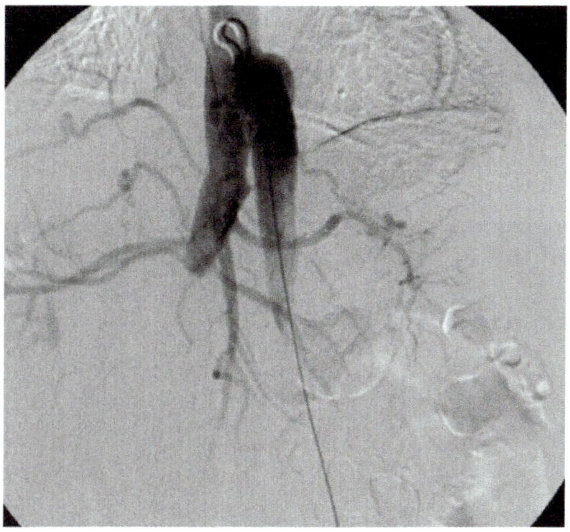

Fig. 14.1 Abdominal aortogram showing patent main body of thoracofemoral bypass and occlusion of abdominal aorta below the origin of the inferior mesenteric artery

S. S. Hans, *Secondary and Tertiary Arterial Reconstructions*,
https://doi.org/10.1007/978-3-032-21214-6_14

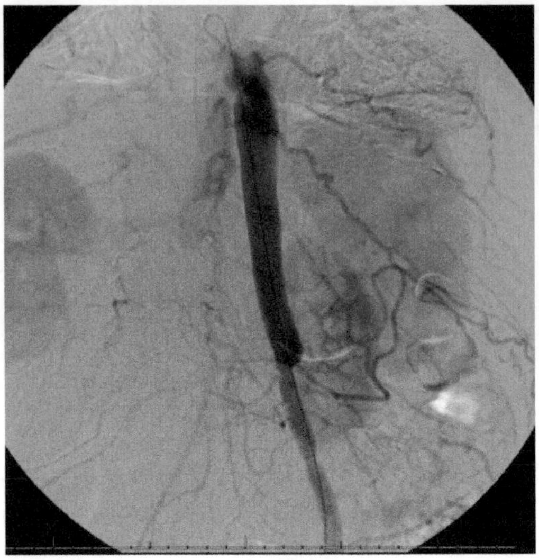

Fig. 14.2 Abdominal aortogram showing occlusion of one limb of the thoracofemoral bypass graft

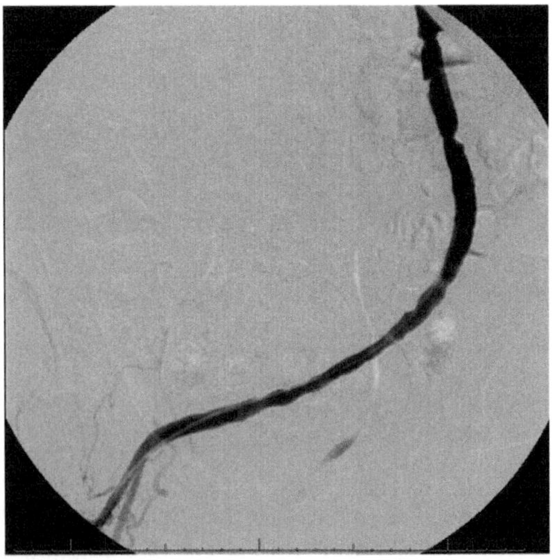

Fig. 14.3 Aortogram showing patent right limb of the thoracofemoral bypass and mild stenosis and occlusion of the left limb

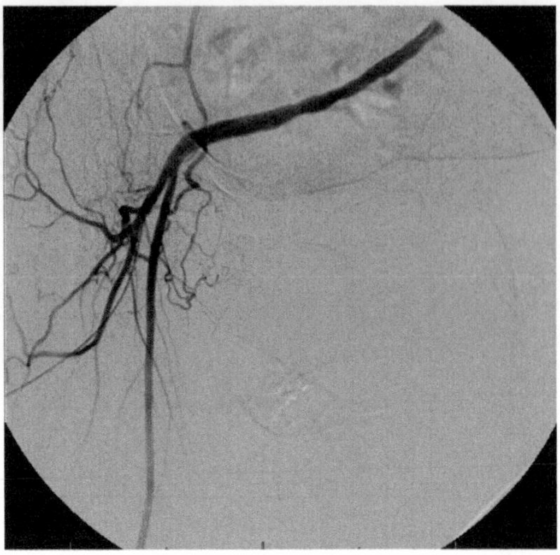

Fig. 14.4 Aortogram showing patent distal anastomosis of right limb thoracofemoral bypass to common femoral artery bifurcation

healed with relief of ischemic rest pain. She died 14 months later from progressive respiratory failure with a patent crossover femoral–femoral graft.

Discussion

In contemporary vascular practice, thoracofemoral bypass for aortoiliac occlusive disease is rarely performed. It is a challenging operation best suited for a subset of patients who have developed repeated occlusions following a prior aortobifemoral bypass graft, or in a patient with a hostile abdomen, with multiple prior laparotomies, or with an infected aortic prostheses following AFB graft. For patients who can tolerate a thoracofemoral bypass, this reconstruction is superior to the extra-anatomic, axillofemoral bypass because of its better cumulative 5-year patency rates of 81% vs. 63% with axillofemoral bypass [1, 2]. Axillofemoral bypass graft is usually reserved for higher-risk patients with a limited life expectancy. The patient should undergo risk stratification and medical optimization, including noninvasive cardiac testing and pulmonary function tests [1, 2]. For evaluation of the descending thoracic aorta, a thin-section CTA of the chest, abdomen, pelvis, and lower extremity is obtained to ensure that the distal thoracic aorta is free of any aneurysmal dilatation or circumferential calcification [1, 2]. Relative contraindications include severe chronic obstructive pulmonary disease and prior left thoracotomy with residual dense intrathoracic adhesions [1, 2].

Operative Description

Positioning A vacuum bean bag from the shoulder to the proximal thigh is placed under the patient on the operating table. A double-lumen endotracheal tube is placed under general anesthesia, and the left hemithorax is elevated 45–65 degrees while the pelvis is maintained in a nearly flat position; this facilitates the thoracotomy and the femoral artery exposure. The left upper extremity is supported on an arm cradle, helping to extend the lower thorax and avoid brachial plexus traction injury. Pillow rests are placed under the knees and between the legs to prevent hyperextension of the legs.

Groin Incision and Retroperitoneal Access A standard incision is made for the exposure of the femoral arteries in both groins. The left groin incision is extended approximately 10 cm cephalad above the inguinal ligament. At the cephalad end of the groin incision, the retroperitoneum is accessed carefully to facilitate the creation of a tunnel connecting the left groin to the left thorax. A 10 cm long incision is made through the aponeurosis of the external oblique and internal oblique muscles on the left, extending parallel to the inguinal ligament approximately 2 cm cephalad to its caudal border. The external oblique muscle fascia is divided along the line of its fibers, the internal oblique muscle fibers are divided, and the transverse abdominus muscle fascia is divided in the direction of its fibers. The retroperitoneal space is entered medial to the anterior superior iliac crest, which is the caudal end of the graft tunnel. This incision is used to route the right limb of the graft from its retroperitoneal location to a preperitoneal space and brought into the right groin for the right femoral artery anastomosis.

Exposure of the Descending Thoracic Aorta A limited left posterolateral thoracotomy through the eighth intercostal space (ICS) is performed. The skin incision is extended laterally just beyond the margin of the latissimus dorsi muscle. The intercostal muscles are incised along the superior border of the inferior rib of the selected ICS. The pleural cavity is entered, and a rib spreader is inserted and opened gradually to prevent rib fractures on entering the thoracic cavity.

Tunneling A 2 cm incision is made in the posteromedial aspect of the left diaphragm over the ribs through the open thoracic incision. The site of aortotomy and the exit site through the diaphragm should be in satisfactory alignment to avoid kinking of the graft. To make a satisfactory tunnel. The left hand is advanced through the left retroperitoneal incision, aiming cephalad and slightly medial over the external iliac vessels and the psoas major, posterior to the left kidney, and proximomedial to the spleen, to approximate with the right hand through the left thoracic cavity.

A long tunneling device is then guided through the tunnel and is used to pass an umbilical tape, facilitating the passage of the graft. The main body of the graft and its two limbs are tunneled through the retroperitoneal channel. A preperitoneal tunnel is created for the passage of the graft to reach the right groin. Two "figure of eight" sutures are placed in the center of the diaphragm using a 0 silk suture, and these are brought through the inferior and anterior chest wall and secured to retract the diaphragm to allow adequate exposure of the distal descending thoracic aorta. The inferior pulmonary ligament is taken down to the level of the inferior pulmonary vein, and the lung is retracted superiorly. The pleura surrounding the distal descending thoracic aorta is incised, and a 6–7 cm segment of aorta immediately proximal to the diaphragm is exposed. A "soft" spot relatively free of atherosclerotic disease is selected. The aorta is dissected circumferentially both proximally and distally. The umbilical tapes are passed around the aorta and used as a "handle" to stabilize the aorta so that a clamp can be placed. Intercostal arteries between the 8th and 12th thoracic vertebrae should be preserved. Tunneling of the graft is done from the left chest to the left groin using a previously placed tunneler. The opening must be sufficiently large through the diaphragm to prevent constriction of the graft, with correct orientation and tension on the limbs to prevent twisting or kinking. The site of aortotomy is carefully selected. The site of aortotomy should be high enough above the crus of the diaphragm to avoid lateral kinking of the proximal portion of the graft passing through the tunnel. Proximal anastomosis is performed to the thoracic aorta using a partially occluding side-biting clamp (Cobra aortic Clamp, Swantia Medical, Sialkot, Pakistan). If the distal descending thoracic aorta is of a smaller caliber, complete clamping of the distal thoracic aorta with a proximal vertical clamp and a distal lower-angled vascular clamp is performed because a partially occluding clamp may not be adequate.

Anastomoses & Choice of Grafts An appropriately sized graft is chosed to match the size of the aorta and femoral arteries. When a bifurcated graft is used, a 16 x 8 mm or 14 x 7 mm graft is appropriate. When a vertical limb from the thoracic aorta to the left groin with a left to right crossover femoral-femoral graft it is preferable to use a 10 mm graft for the vertical limb and an 8 mm for the crossover graft. Both Dacron and PTFE grafts are suitable alternatives. The aortotomy is created and the body of the graft is appropriately spatulated. When a bifurcated graft is used it is better to leave the main body of the graft in its entire length to make certain that the right limb of the graft will reach the right groin without excessive tension. If the graft is not long enough to reach the right groin easily, excess graft from the left limb can be used to construct a composite limb (graft-graft composite). A tension-free aortic anastomosis is created in a continuous fashion using 2′ 0″ or 3′ 0″ CV polypropylene suture. After completion the proximal anastomosis, a vascular clamp is applied to the body of the graft a few centimenters beyond the proximal anastomosis to check for bleeding at the suture line. The thoracic and groin incisions are closed in layers using standard techniques. A large chest tube (36F) is placed through a separate incision inferior to the thoracotomy incision with its tip in the apex of the thoracic cavity. The lung is reinflated under direct vision. The ribs are approximated using an interrupted absorbable suture in a figure-of-eight configuration. The chest wall muscles are closed with running absorbable suture closed suction drain may be left in the subcutaneous space.

The major complications include bleeding, respiratory failure, cardiac complications, renal failure, and paraplegia.

Multiple Choice Questions

1. Thoracofemoral bypass is best indicated for
   A. Juxtarenal aortic occlusion in a 52-year-old man with bilateral hip claudication and erectile dysfunction
   B. Aortic occlusion at the level of the inferior mesenteric artery with associated bilateral common femoral artery occlusive disease
   C. Infrarenal aortic occlusion in a patient with prior sigmoid resection with bilateral hip claudication
   D. Failed aortobifemoral bypass graft in a 52-year-old woman with prior multiple celiotomies for Crohn's disease, presenting with ischemic rest pain in both feet

2. An absolute contraindication for thoracofemoral bypass is
   A. Stable coronary artery disease
   B. Mild aortic valve stenosis
   C. Circumferential distal thoracic aortic calcification
   D. Left ventricle ejection of 50%
3. Thoracofemoral bypass is planned for a 62-year-old man with juxtarenal aortic occlusion and a failed aortobifemoral bypass with an ischemic ulcer of the right big toe with a history of suprapubic prostatectomy. The optimal routing of the right limb of a thoracofemoral bypass graft is
   A. Right limb of the graft should be tunneled in the space of retzius
   B. Thoracic aorta to left femoral bypass graft with right axillo-femoral bypass graft
   C. Right limb of the graft is tunneled through the right obturator foramen and anastomosed to the right superficial femoral artery
   D. A crossover subcutaneous femoral-femoral graft with its origin from one limb of the thoracofemoral bypass (unilateral)

Answers: 1(D), 2(C), 3(D)

References

1. Pippinos I, Hernandez H. Thoracofemoral bypass. In: Long G, Weaver M, Bove P, Hans SS, editors. Endovascular and open vascular reconstruction: a practical approach. Boca Raton: CRC Press; 2017. p. 307–11.
2. McCarthy WJ, Mesh CL, McMillan WD, Flinn WR, Pearce WH, Yao JS. Descending thoracic aorta-to-femoral artery bypass: ten years' experience with a durable procedure. J Vasc Surg. 1993;17(2):336–47; discussion 347-338. PMID:8433429

15 Repeat Aorto-Bifemoral Graft Using a Retroperitoneal Approach for Recurrent Symptoms of Lower Extremity Ischemia

Presentation

A 68-year-old man presented to the vascular clinic with ischemic rest pain in June 2024. He had a limited range of motion of the right ankle with associated paresthesia of the right foot. He had undergone an aortobifemoral bypass graft 6 years earlier, for symptoms of intermittent claudication at an outside hospital. The surgeon at an outside hospital performed a left axillobifemoral graft 4 years later, following occlusion of the aortobifemoral graft; medical records from the outside hospital were not available. Medical comorbidities included hypertension, coronary artery disease, and hyperlipidemia. He was a current smoker (50 pack-year). ABI (Right) 0.42, ABI (Left) 0.38 with severely decreased perfusion of the toes and toe brachial index of 0.2 (right) 0.24 (left). A CTA of the abdomen and pelvis showed a juxtarenal aortic occlusion; patent axillofemoral graft with stenosis at the origin of the crossover femoral-femoral graft (Figs. 15.1 and 15.2).

A repeat aortobifemoral graft using the retroperitoneal approach was planned following cardiopulmonary risk assessment. The patient underwent cystoscopy and bilateral ureteral stent placement by the urology team. The patient was positioned in the right lateral decubitus position using the bean bag, and an incision was made in the left 10th intercostal space (ICS) (Fig. 15.3). A vertical incision was made in the left groin and a transverse incision was made in the right groin. A small incision is made for the retroperitoneal approach to expose the axillofemoral graft in the left flank. Proximal and distal vascular clamps were applied to the axillary limb of the axillofemoral graft, and the graft was divided. A 24 F chest tube was used as a shunt to maintain perfusion through the graft and the patient was administered intravenous heparin by the anesthesia team. An incision was made in the 10th ICS and deepened through the muscle layers. The retroperitoneal dissection was started, and the pleural cavity was entered. The diaphragm was divided approximately 2–3 cms. Away from the costal margin in a circumferential fashion to preserve the branches of the phrenic nerve. The diaphragm ends were tagged with polypropylene suture for orientation. The peritoneal cavity was mobilized medially and dissected down to the psoas major posteriorly. The paravisceral aorta, the left renal artery, the SMA, and the celiac artery were dissected and encircled with silastic vessel loops. The right renal artery was identified. The retroperitoneal tunnels were created by using blunt dissection and passage of an aortic "C" shaped clamp, and dissection was kept posterior to the ureters. The umbilical tapes were passed through the retroperitoneal tunnels. After systemic heparinization by the anesthesia team, a proximal aortic clamp was placed at the supraceliac level. A longitudinal aortotomy in the posterolateral wall of the aorta from just inferior to

S. S. Hans, *Secondary and Tertiary Arterial Reconstructions*,
https://doi.org/10.1007/978-3-032-21214-6_15

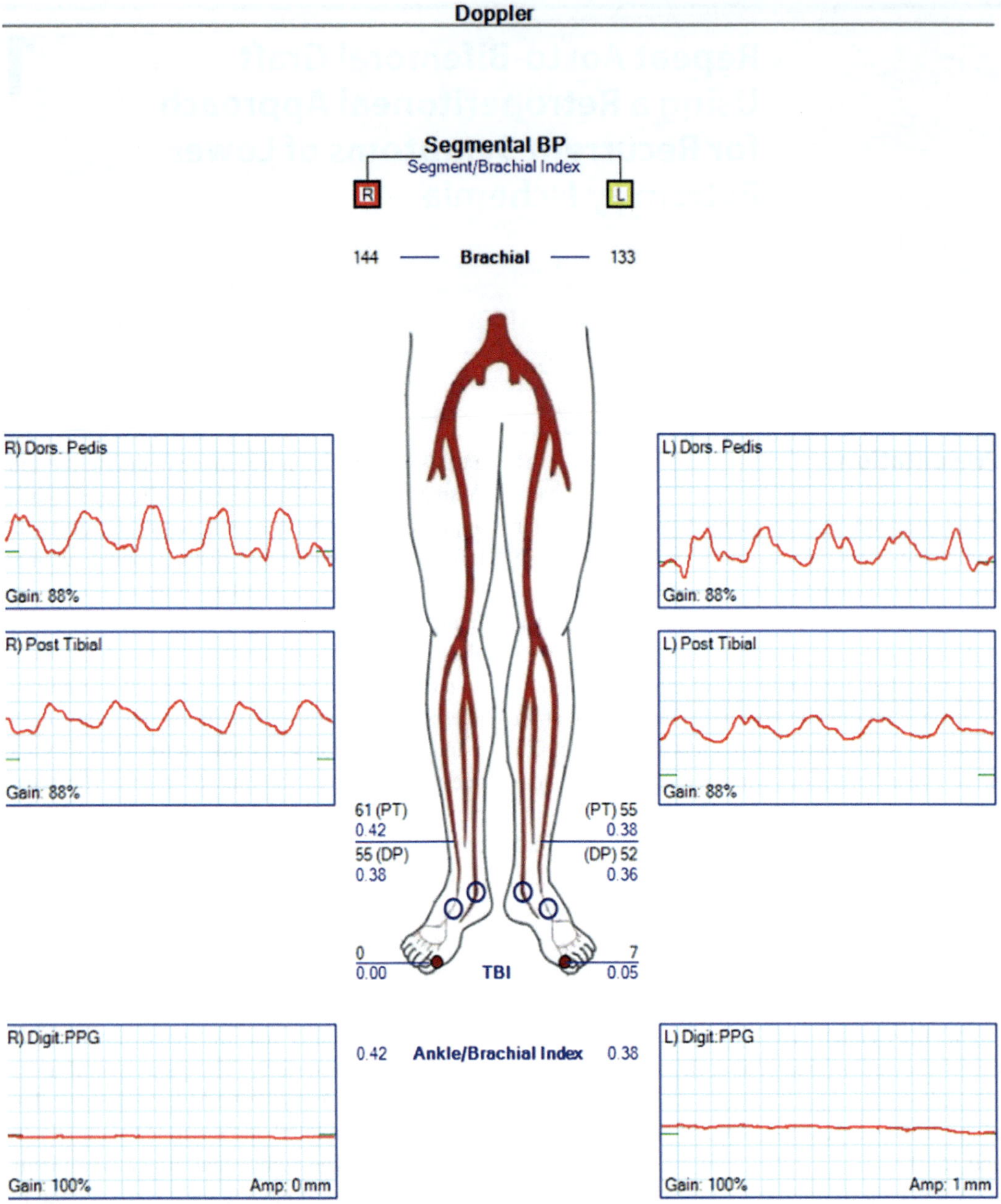

Fig. 15.1 Arterial Doppler study before repeat aortobifemoral graft

the origin of the celiac artery to the infrarenal aorta was made. The infrarenal aorta was transected. The occluded ABF graft was removed. The thrombus and plaque were removed from the paravisceral aorta. The divided distal aorta was closed with a 2′0′ CV polypropylene suture in a running fashion. The visceral arteries and the aorta were vented. The supraceliac clamp was moved to the infrarenal location. A 16 × 8 mm PTFE graft was selected, and the main body of the graft was anastomosed in an end-to-end fashion to the divided aorta using a running 4′ 0″ CV polypropylene suture. The right limb of the graft was tunneled under the ureter with the aid of a previously placed umbilical tape. The previously placed axillofemoral

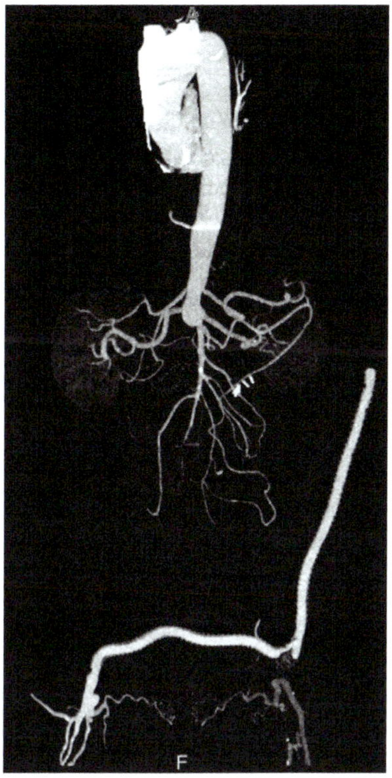

Fig. 15.2 Preoperative CTA chest, abdomen, and pelvis showing juxtarenal aortic occlusion Patent left axillofemoral and crossover femoral–femoral graft with stenosis near its take-off

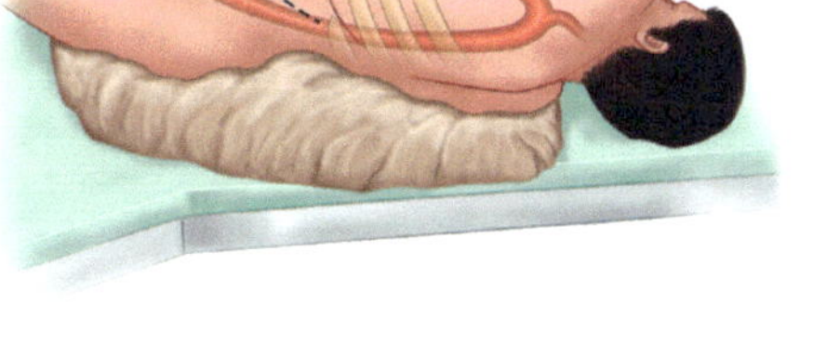

Fig. 15.3 Positioning of the patient and the line of the incision for the retroperitoneal exposure of the aorta

graft was divided in the groin, and the right limb of the ABF graft was anastomosed to the axillofemoral graft limb, which had been anastomosed to the profunda femoris artery at the time of axillofemoral grafting. Similarly, the left limb of the

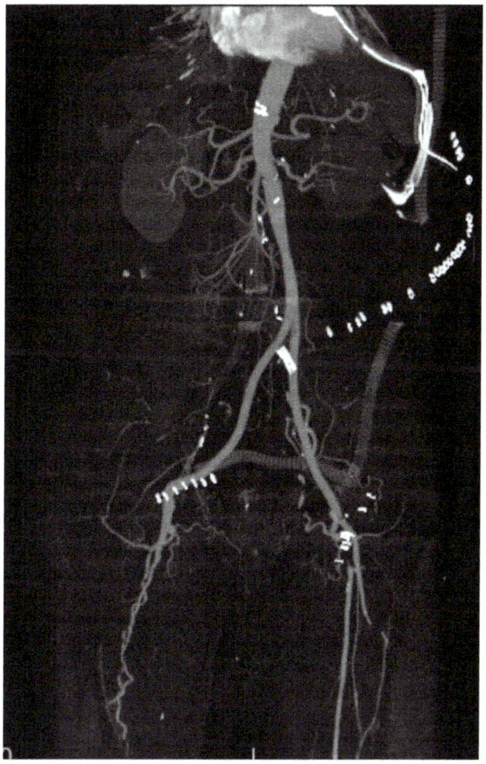

Fig. 15.4 Postoperative CTA showing patent repeat ABF graft with right SFA occlusion

ABF graft was tunneled under the ureter and anastomosed to the left profunda femoris artery with 5′0″ CV polypropylene suture. Heparin was reversed with protamine sulfate. A 20 F chest tube was inserted in the left pleural cavity in the mid-axillary line, just superior to the proximal aspect of the thoracoabdominal incision peritoneal envelope was brought back into its anatomic location. The diaphragm was reconstructed with an interrupted polypropylene suture. The ribs were approximated with PDS sutures in a "figure eight" pattern using a blunt needle. The abdominal muscle and fascial layers were closed with number "1" PDS suture starting from either end, and the groin incision were closed in layers.

Postoperatively, his left foot showed significant improvement, but the right foot pain persisted. Postoperative CTA showed redundancy of the right groin anastomosis from the previous axillofemoral graft to the recently performed aortobifemoral graft, as well as right SFA occlusion (Fig. 15.4). Antegrade access of the previously placed axillofemoral graft was performed with a micro-puncture needle, followed by placement of a 5F sheath.

The right lower extremity arteriogram demonstrated right superficial femoral artery occlusion. The tibioperoneal trunk reconstituted with occlusion of the anterior tibial artery. The distal peroneal artery was occluded in the distal left. The posterior tibial artery was patent with filling of the plantar artery. There was no suitable autologous vein available to be used as a bypass conduit. A 6 mm ringed PTFE graft was selected. The right tibioperoneal trunk was exposed using a medial longitudinal incision below the knee. The redundant position of the right axillofemoral graft anastomosis was resected with end-to-end anastomosis using a 5′0″ CV polypropylene suture. A new PTFE ringed graft was anastomosed end-to-side as a jump graft from the recently placed aortofemoral graft and tunneled into the upper calf.

The distal popliteal tibioperoneal trunk and proximal posterior tibial artery and peroneal artery were exposed, and silastic vessel loops were passed. An arteriotomy incision was made in the tibioperoneal trunk (Fig. 15.5). A vein cuff was tailored from the GSV in the upper thigh was sutured circumferentially to the tibioperoneal trunk. The PTFE graft was sutured to the vein cuff in an end-to-end (beveled) anastomosis. The incision was closed in layers. The patient had a palpable posterior tibial pulse. The patient was last seen in July 2025 at the clinic with a right ABI (0.87) and left (0.56).

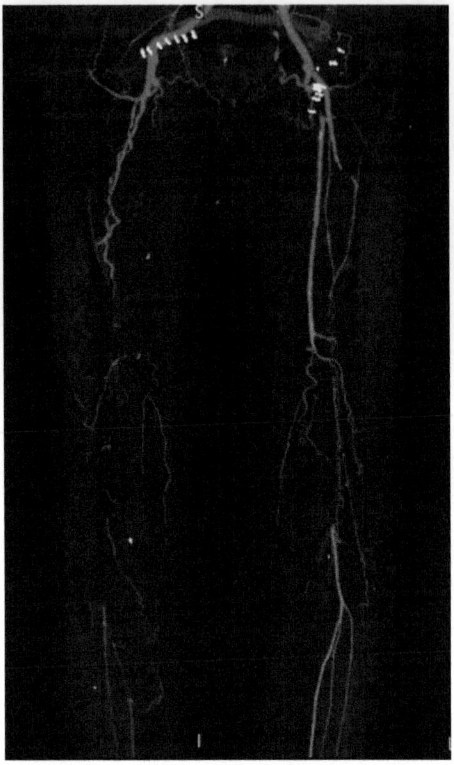

Fig. 15.5 Postoperative CTA showing right SFA and popliteal artery occlusion with poor runoff. Left SFA near occlusion at its origin. Proximal popliteal artery occlusion

Discussion

Aortobifemoral grafting is one of the most effective and durable vascular reconstructions for patients with symptomatic aortoiliac occlusive disease. Aorto-bifemoral grafting is associated with a significant perioperative morbidity (3.8–21.3%) and perioperative mortality (3.5%). The reported 5-year and 10-year graft patency is 87–91%, and 80–87% respectively. Early graft limb occlusion (within 24 months) occurs due to intimal hyperplasia. Late graft limb stenosis/occlusion occurs as a result of progressive atherosclerosis at the distal anastomosis, with stenosis at the origin of the deep femoral artery and/or progressive superficial femoral artery occlusive disease. Occlusion of both limbs with the body of the ABF graft is relatively uncommon. Repeat aortobifemoral graft can be offered to a select group of good-risk patients with an expected longer life expectancy following failure of the primary ABF grafting. Both transabdominal and retroperitoneal approaches can be used. Scali et al., reported that 19 patients who underwent repeat aortobifemoral bypass grafting had greater blood loss, received a larger volume of intraoperative fluids, and a longer procedure time as compared to primary ABF grafting. Patients undergoing repeat ABF grafting had similar perioperative morbidity, mortality, and midterm survival as compared to primary ABF grafting [1]. He was seen in the clinic August 2025, complaining of a bulge in the left flank likely due to injury to intercostal nerves during the retroperitoneal exposure of the aorta (Fig. 15.6). Non-invasive Doppler arterial study showed ABI of 0.91 (right) and 0.96 (left).

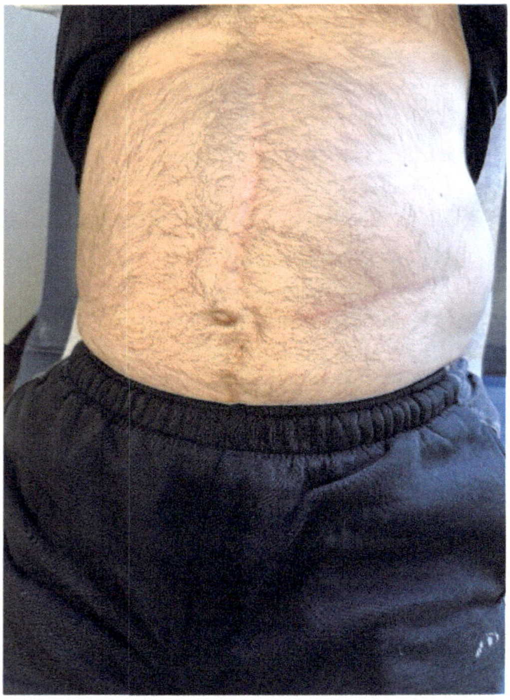

Fig. 15.6 Bulge in the left flank following redo aorto femoral graft using retroperitoneal approach

Multiple Choice Questions

1. Compared to the primary ABF graft, repeat ABF is associated with
   A. Longer operative time
   B. Greater blood loss
   C. Use of a large volume of intravenous fluids in the OR
   D. All of the Above
2. A 65-year-old woman had a failed primary ABF graft 6 years following the index operation. She complains of ischemic rest pain and symptoms of short-distance intermittent claudication. She's a former smoker and had a satisfactory cardiopulmonary evaluation. The best option is
   A. CERAB procedure
   B. Axillofemoral graft
   C. Repeat aortobifemoral bypass graft
   D. Thoracofemoral bypass
3. Repeat ABF graft should be performed using
   A. Transverse abdominal incision and bilateral groin incisions
   B. Left retroperitoneal incision and bilateral groin incisions
   C. Midline abdominal incision and bilateral groin incisions
   D. Using either a midline abdominal incision or a retroperitoneal incision with bilateral groin incisions

Answers: 1(D), 2(C), 3(D)

Reference

1. Scali, S. T., Schmit, B. M., Feezor, R. J., Beck, A. W., Chang, C. K., Waterman, A. L., . . . Huber, T. S. (2014). Outcomes after redo aortobifemoral bypass for aortoiliac occlusive disease. J Vasc Surg, 60(2), 346–355.e341.. PMID:24657290.

16 Repeat Aorto-Bifemoral Graft Using Transabdominal Approach

Presentation

A 65-year-old woman was seen in the clinic for symptoms of lifestyle-limiting bilateral lower extremity claudication on walking (50 yards) and ischemic rest pain in the left foot in May 2002. She had undergone aorto-bifemoral graft reconstruction 15 years earlier at an outside hospital, and review of the old records revealed that her symptoms were pain in the legs on walking 100 yards at that time. An aorto-bifemoral graft reconstruction was performed with a Dacron graft, with an end-to-side proximal anastomosis. An arterial Doppler study of the lower extremities showed an ankle brachial index of 0.5 on the right and 0.38 on the left. She underwent MRA of the abdominal aorta and lower extremities, which showed occlusion of the aorto-bifemoral graft with reconstitution of common femoral and profunda arteries with diffuse mild-to-moderate occlusive disease of both superficial femoral and popliteal arteries. She had diminished pulse in the left upper extremity secondary to left subclavian artery occlusive disease, but was asymptomatic. Medical comorbidities included hypertension and nicotine abuse (60 pack-years). Past surgical history included left carotid endarterectomy in 1999. In June 2002, the patient underwent redo aorto-bifemoral grafting. Proximal aortic anastomosis was carefully dissected using sharp dissection, and incisions were made in each groin to expose the limbs of the Dacron graft for the femoral anastomoses. A silastic vessel loop was passed around the left renal vein and retracted cephalad. Proximal anastomosis of the divided aorta just above the previously end-to-side anastomosis was performed in an end-to-end fashion with a 14 × 7 mm knitted Dacron Gelsoft graft (Terumo Aortic, Inchinnan, Renfrewshire, Scotland) using a 4-0 cardiovascular polypropylene (Ethicon, Raridon, NJ) running suture. The occluded aorto-bifemoral graft was well incorporated, and there was no evidence of perigraft infection. The occluded ABF graft was removed without difficulty. The distal end of the aorta above the aortic bifurcation was sutured with 3-0 cardiovascular polypropylene suture. The left limb of the Dacron graft was brought through the previously created tunnel under the ureter and anastomosed to the common femoral and deep femoral artery as a long-spatulated anastomosis using 5-0 cardiovascular polypropylene running suture. We encountered difficulty in passing the graft limb through the tunnel on the right side. We used an 8 mm arterial dilator to create the tunnel, but there was a tear in the left common iliac vein during this maneuver, which was controlled with a 5-0 cardiovascular running polypropylene suture. This was likely the result of scarring from the index operation. There was a sudden loss of about 500 cc of blood from the tear of the left common iliac vein. Hemostasis was obtained using manual compression proximally and distally from the tear with a folded

S. S. Hans, *Secondary and Tertiary Arterial Reconstructions*,
https://doi.org/10.1007/978-3-032-21214-6_16

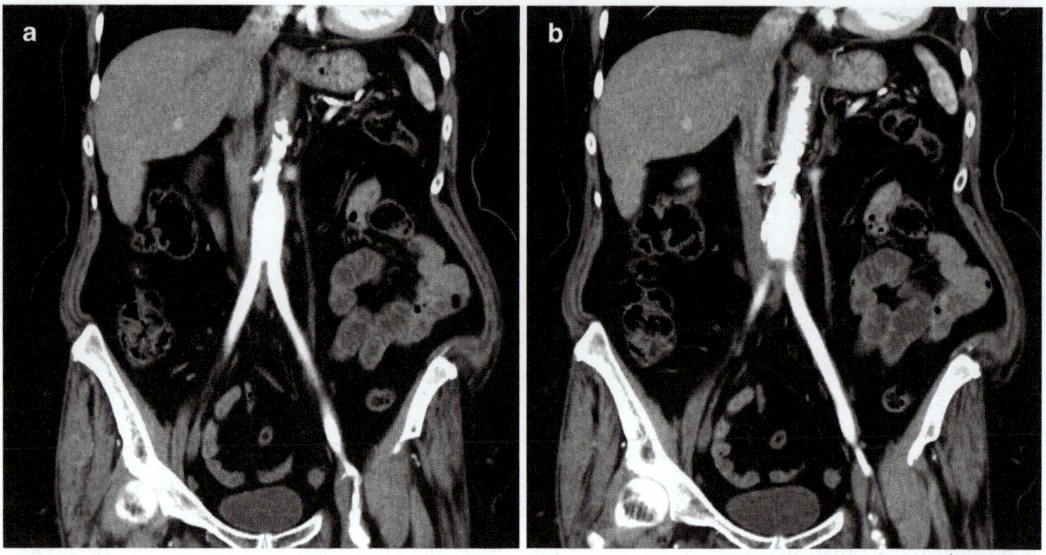

Fig. 16.1 (**a**) Postoperative CTA abdomen and pelvis showing patent repeat aorto-bifemoral bypass graft (**b**) Postoperative CTA abdomen and pelvis showing patent repeat aorto-bifemoral bypass graft

4 × 4 on a sponge stick with lateral venorraphy. The right limb of the Dacron graft was brought under the ureter, in the rectoperitoneal plane and brought into the groin beneath partially divided shelving edge of the inguinal ligament. The graft was anastomosed to the common femoral and deep femoral artery with a running 5-0 cardiovascular polypropylene suture, in an end-to-side fashion. Her postoperative course was uneventful; she was discharged on the sixth postoperative day in satisfactory condition. She was followed for 17 years after the repeat ABF bypass graft, and her last ankle brachial index (October 2018) was 0.89 on the right and 0.77 on the left. A follow-up CTA of the abdomen and pelvis with runoff in November 2018 showed 50% stenosis at the origin of the celiac artery, multifocal stenosis of the superior mesenteric artery, and a patent aorto-bifemoral bypass graft (Figs. 16.1, 16.2 and 16.3). Both femoral anastomoses were widely patent; there was evidence of atherosclerotic plaque at the origin of the right superficial femoral artery, as well as mild to moderate stenosis throughout the remainder of the mid and distal superficial femoral artery. The left superficial

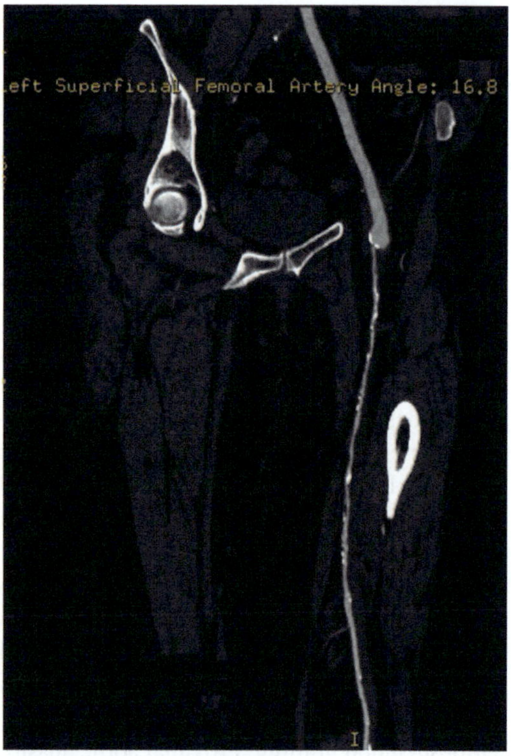

Fig. 16.2 CTA with run-off study showing patent left limb of the graft with diffuse stenosis of left SFA

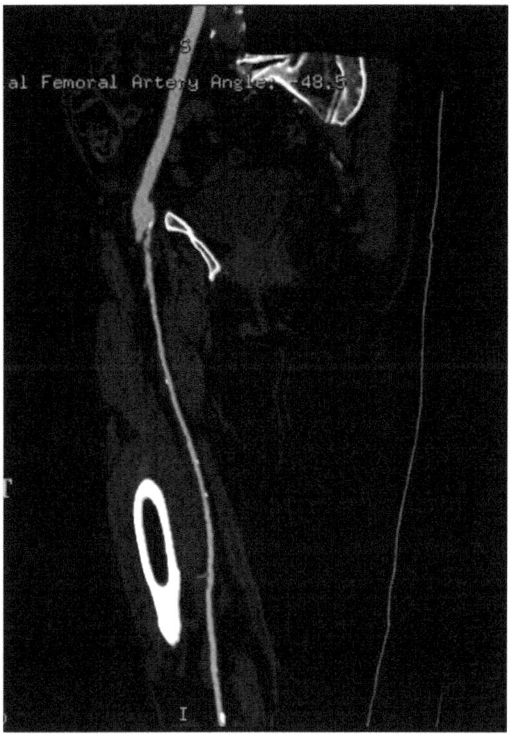

Fig. 16.3 CTA with run-off showing patent right limb of the graft with less than 50 % stenosis of the proximal portion of the SFA

femoral artery also showed diffuse, irregularly mixed atherosclerotic plaque with severe stenosis throughout its course in the distal thigh. No further intervention was offered to the patient because of minimal symptoms of lower extremity ischemia. The patient underwent left lower lobectomy in 2010 for carcinoma of the lung. At a follow-up in December of 2019, the patient was doing well, with a patent ABF graft. Doppler arterial study showed ABI 1.03 (right) and 0.84 (left). She passed away in October 2022 from complications of dementia.

Discussion

Aorto-bifemoral grafting is one of the most effective and durable vascular reconstruction options for patients with symptomatic aorto-iliac occlusive disease. However, this procedure is associated with significant perioperative mortality (3%–5%). Aorto-bifemoral graft is also associated with significant perioperative morbidity (3.8%–21.3%). Surgical site infection in the groin and/or lymphatic leak occurs in 3.5%–22% of patients [1]. The five-year patency of aorto-bifemoral graft ranges from 87%–91%, and the ten-year patency from 80%–87% [1]. We have previously reported a patency of 93% of aorto--bifemoral graft at 48 months [2]. Scali et al. reported 19 patients who underwent redo aorto-bifemoral graft operation for occlusive disease between 2002 and 2012 [3]. Patients undergoing redo aorto-bifemoral bypass experienced greater blood loss, received more intra-operative fluids, and had a longer overall procedure time [3]. They concluded that redo aorto-bifemoral bypass procedures has a higher procedural complexity as compared to primary aorto-bifemoral bypass graft [3]. However, they reported similar perioperative morbidity/mortality and midterm survival. In this patient, there was a left common iliac vein injury during dissection for the tunnel for the passage of the right limb of the graft. This resulted in a sudden loss of blood, and the patient needed two units of packed cells. However, satisfactory hemostasis was obtained with lateral venography. The aorto-bifemoral bypass has remained patent for the past 17 years. The patient had developed bilateral superficial femoral artery occlusive disease with minimal symptoms.

Repeat aorto-bifemoral graft should be considered only in selected patients who are otherwise acceptable candidates for a repeat major arterial reconstruction. Other options, such as axillo-femoral bypass graft for patients with occluded aorto-femoral graft have a poor long-term patency. If the patient has a hostile abdomen, a retroperitoneal aorto-unifemoral, and a crossover femoral–femoral through a retroperitoneal approach, or alternatively, a thoracic aorta-to-femoral bypass may be considered [4]. Repeat aorto-femoral bypass graft should only be considered in good-risk patients, and axillofemoral bypass in poor-risk patients following failure of a primary aorto-femoral bypass grafting in patients with critical limb ischemia. Patient's comorbidities, experience of the surgeon, and life expectancy of the patient should be taken into consideration before undertaking a repeat aorto-bifemoral graft reconstruction.

In patients with repeated occlusions of the ABF graft and without circumferential distal thoracic calcification, thoracofemoral bypass can be a consideration, in good risk patients. However, thoracofemoral bypass reconstruction is technically challenging.

Multiple Choice Questions

1. Repeat aorto-bifemoral graft is associated with a mortality of
   A. <5%
   B. 5–7%
   C. 8–10%
   D. 10% or higher
2. During tunneling of the limb of the ABF graft, venous bleeding is encountered secondary to a tear in the common iliac vein. The best management option is
   A. Manual compression and Heparin reversal
   B. Intraluminal control with balloon insertion via the common femoral vein
   C. Lateral venorraphy
   D. Lateral venorraphy with bovine pericardial patch grafting
3. The most common cause of late occlusion of the ABF graft is
   A. Technical factors during the conduct of the operation
   B. Myointimal hyperplasia at the anastomotic sites
   C. Progression of the disease in the Profunda femoris artery and the SFA
   D. Progression of the disease at the Profunda femoris artery

Answers: 1(A), 2(C), 3(C)

References

1. de Vries SO, Hunink MG. Results of aortic bifurcation grafts for aortoiliac occlusive disease: a meta-analysis. J Vasc Surg. 1997;26(4):558–69. PMID:9357455
2. Hans SS, DeSantis D, Siddiqui R, Khoury M. Results of endovascular therapy and aortobifemoral grafting for transatlantic inter-society type C and D aortoiliac occlusive disease. Surgery. 2008;144(4):583–9; discussion 589-590. PMID:18847642
3. Scali, S. T., Schmit, B. M., Feezor, R. J., Beck, A. W., Chang, C. K., Waterman, A. L., . . . Huber, T. S. (2014). Outcomes after redo aortobifemoral bypass for aortoiliac occlusive disease. J Vasc Surg, 60(2), 346–355.e341. PMID:24657290.
4. Passman MA, Farber MA, Criado E, Marston WA, Burnham SJ, Keagy BA. Descending thoracic aorta to iliofemoral artery bypass grafting: a role for primary revascularization for aortoiliac occlusive disease? J Vasc Surg. 1999;29(2):249–58. PMID:9950983

17 Aorto-Bifemoral Graft Following a Failed Crossover Femoral–Femoral Graft

Presentation

A 57-year-old woman was seen in 2014 in the Vascular Surgery clinic for symptoms of right hip and calf claudication on walking 50 yards for the past 6–9 months. There has been a gradual progression of her symptoms of intermittent claudication. She was a current smoker (35 pack-years). In June 2000, the patient underwent a laparoscopic gynecologic procedure for endometriosis and sustained an iatrogenic perforation of the small intestine and a right common iliac artery laceration at an outside hospital. She underwent a small bowel resection with primary anastomosis and ligation of the right common iliac artery to control bleeding. She also underwent a crossover femoral–femoral graft following ligation of the right common iliac artery. Examination at her clinic visit revealed absent pulses in the right lower extremity, including the femoral pulse. All pulses were palpable in the left lower extremity. A Doppler arterial study revealed ABI right (0.63) and left (1.0). CTA of the abdomen and pelvis run-off showed occlusion of the right common iliac artery at its origin, reconstitution of the right external and internal iliac arteries via mesenteric collaterals. The femoral–femoral graft was occluded. Left common, external iliac, common femoral, superficial femoral, deep femoral, and runoff arteries in the left lower extremity were patent without stenosis (Figs. 17.1, 17.2, and 17.3).

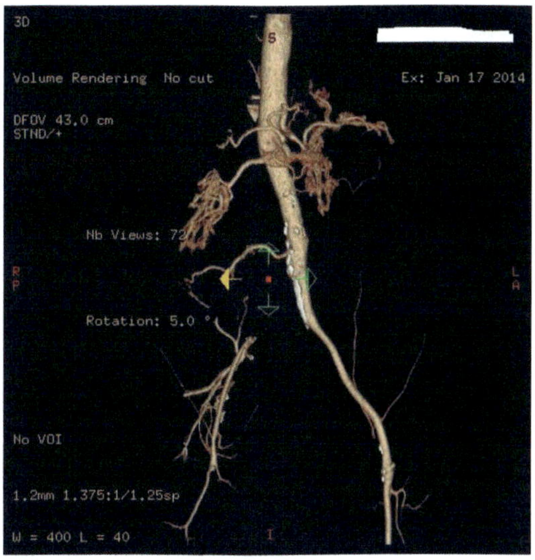

Fig. 17.1 Preoperative CTA showing right common iliac artery occlusion and occlusion of crossover femoral–femoral artery and reconstitution distal right common iliac, external iliac, and hypogastric arteries via collaterals

In September 2014, the patient underwent aorto-bifemoral graft with a 16 × 8 mm knitted Dacron with proximal anastomosis being end-to-end. Dissection was done in each groin by making a vertical skin incision through the previous scar. The dissection was challenging because of the occluded femoral–femoral graft. The graft was partially removed from each groin to about 4 cm toward the lower abdomen, leaving the remaining occluded graft in the suprapubic subcutaneous plane. The distal anastomoses of the

S. S. Hans, *Secondary and Tertiary Arterial Reconstructions*,
https://doi.org/10.1007/978-3-032-21214-6_17

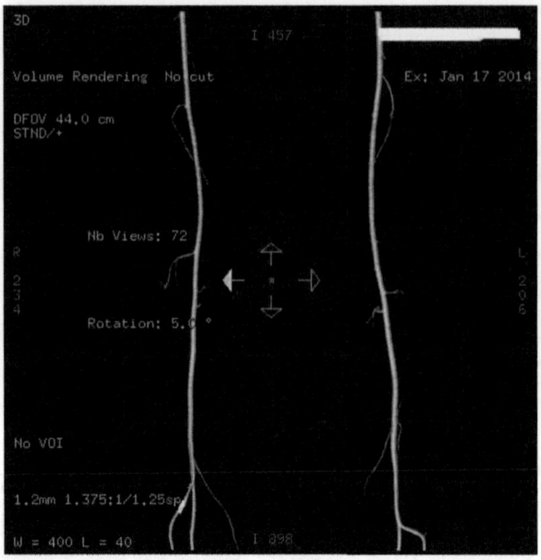

Fig. 17.2 CTA with run-off showing patent bilateral superficial femoral arteries and popliteal arteries

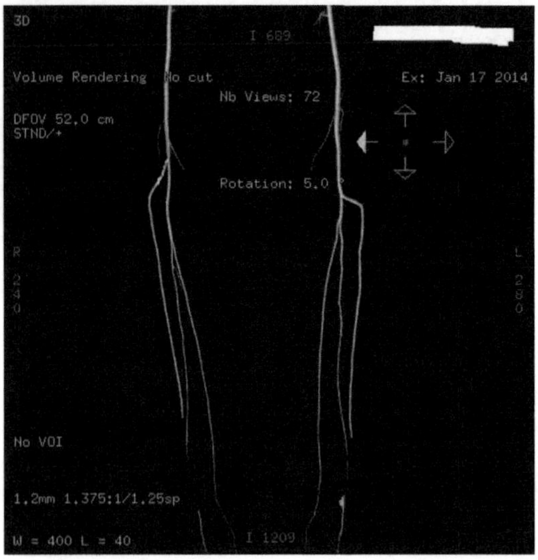

Fig. 17.3 CTA showing patent infrapopliteal arteries with high origin of right interior tibial arteries

limbs of the aorto-bifemoral graft was performed to the common femoral arteries in an end-to-side manner. Patient has an uneventful postoperative course and discharged on the sixth postoperative day. The patient has been followed for 10 years with palpable pulses in each foot, with an ABI of 1.0 on both sides. A follow-up CTA of the abdomen and pelvis showed patent ABF graft (Fig. 17.4a–d).

In 2017, she was diagnosed with carcinoma of the lung, but she has been cancer-free for the past 8 years following lung surgery and chemotherapy.

Discussion

Vascular injuries during laparoscopy are rare (0.2/1000). However, such injuries are associated with 6–13% morbidity and mortality. The injuries commonly occur at the entry of a Veress needle or during insertion of a Trocar. Most patients become hemodynamically unstable and require 1:1:1 resuscitation (packed cells, FP plasma, and platelets) transfusion [1]. Laparotomy is necessary in most patients to control bleeding. In hemodynamically stable patients, an arteriogram and control of bleeding with deployment of a covered stent can control the bleeding; however, this is usually not feasible [1]. In patients with laparoscopic vascular injury, associated perforation of the bowel should also be suspected.

In this patient, a crossover femoral–femoral graft with ligation of the right common iliac artery was required during management of arterial injury with perforation of the small intestine. Occlusion of the crossover femoral–femoral graft with symptomatic lifestyle-limiting claudication necessitated ABF graft reconstruction. The ABF graft had remained patent for 10 years. Schneider et al., reported superior patency of ABF graft as compared to crossover femoral–femoral graft (85% vs. 60% at 3 years $p < 0.01$) [2]. Progression of distal disease is the most common factor resulting in the occlusion of the femoral–femoral crossover graft [3].

In many patients, there is a subclinical trend toward donor iliac artery hemodynamic deterioration following femoral–femoral graft. It can become hemodynamically significant and may not be reflected in the deterioration of the ankle brachial index (ABIs) on the noninvasive study. It may threaten graft patency with a recurrence of ischemic symptoms.

Vascular injuries following urologic, gynecologic, thoracic, general surgery, and robotic procedures often result in a significant increase in

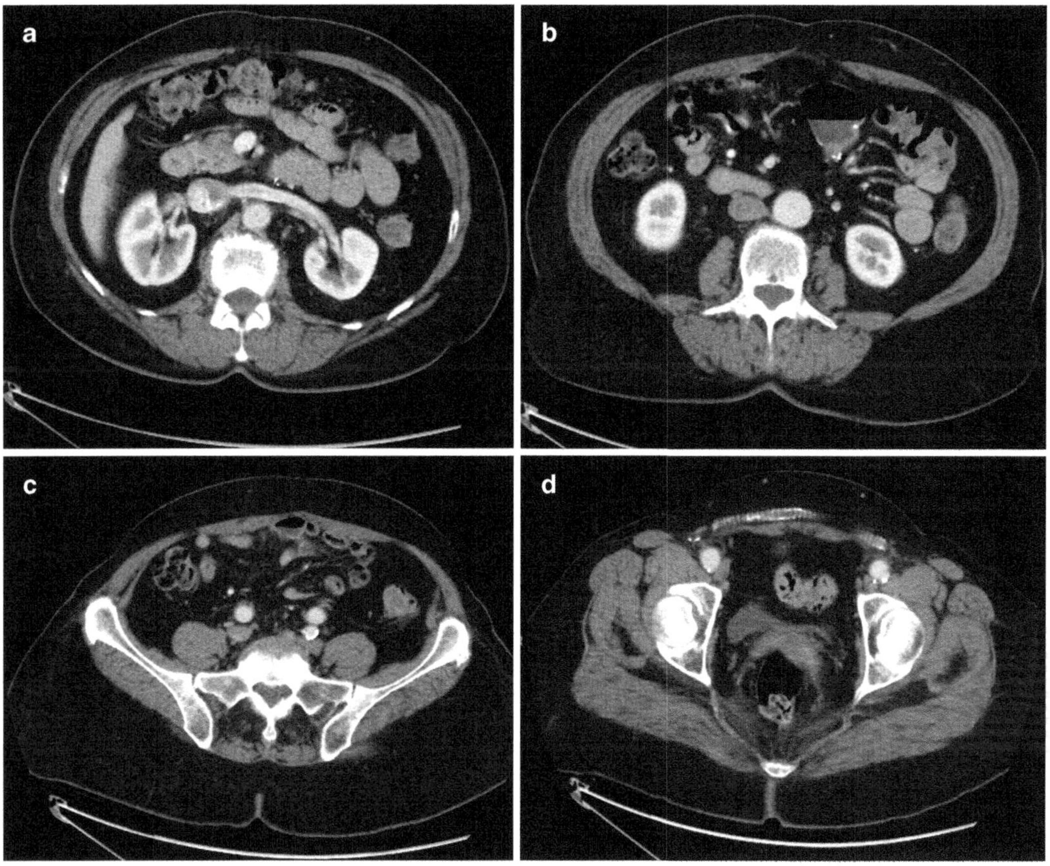

Fig. 17.4 (**a**) Follow-up CTA abdomen and pelvis showing patent ABF graft (**b**) Follow-up CTA abdomen and pelvis showing patent ABF graft (**c**) Follow-up CTA abdomen and pelvis showing patent ABF graft (**d**) Follow-up CTA abdomen and pelvis showing patent ABF graft

morbidity and mortality of the primary operation, and all precautions should be undertaken to prevent such injuries during the insertion of Trocar or Varess needle in laparoscopic and robotic surgery.

Multiple Choice Questions

1. During laparoscopic/robotic gynecologic surgery, there was a Trocar injury to the right common iliac artery with severe bleeding and hypotension. The next best option is
   A. Endovascular repair with stent graft
   B. Fluid resuscitation and exploratory laparotomy
   C. Laparoscopic/robotic repair of common iliac artery injury
   D. Immediate proximal control with passage of an aortic balloon using femoral artery access
2. In the aforementioned patient, with a small bowel injury and a right common iliac artery laceration with loss of 60% circumference of the artery. The best option for repair is
   A. Proximal and distal control and repair with application of a vein patch graft
   B. Endovascular repair with a covered iliac stent using right femoral artery access
   C. Ligation of the right common iliac artery and crossover femoral–femoral graft
   D. Ligation of the right common iliac artery and infrarenal aorta to proximal external iliac bypass graft with Rifampin-soaked PTFE graft

3. The morbidity and mortality of vascular injuries that occurred during laparoscopic surgery are
   A. 1–3%
   B. 3.1–5.9%
   C. 6–13%
   D. 13.5–15%

Answers: 1(B), 2(C), 3(C)

References

1. Asfour V, Smythe E, Attia R. Vascular injury at laparoscopy: a guide to management. J Obstet Gynaecol. 2018;38(5):598–606. PMID:29620475
2. Schneider JR, Besso SR, Walsh DB, Zwolak RM, Cronenwett JL. Femorofemoral versus aortobifemoral bypass: outcome and hemodynamic results. J Vasc Surg. 1994;19(1):43–55; discussion 55-47. PMID:8301737
3. Criado E, Dewhirst N, Burnham SJ, Johnson G Jr, Keagy BA. Progression of occlusive disease following femorofemoral crossover bypass graft. Ann Vasc Surg. 1993;7(1):63–7. PMID:8518121

18 Near Occlusion of the Distal Anastomosis of the Aortofemoral Graft for Occlusive Disease in a Patient with a Prior Renal Transplant

Presentation

A 59-year-old woman had a partial amputation of the left big toe due to osteomyelitis of the phalanx at an outside hospital in September 2023. The healing of the amputation was delayed. She had Type I Diabetes mellitus, coronary artery disease (CAD), hyperlipidemia, morbid obesity (BMI 40.5), and chronic kidney disease (CKD). The patient was a former smoker (35 pack-years). In 2004, she underwent aorto-bifemoral graft at an out-of-state hospital for iliac artery occlusive disease. She underwent a live donor renal transplant in 2009, with the kidney placed in the right iliac fossa, and renal artery anastomosis was performed to the right limb of the aorto-bifemoral graft. She had a coronary bypass graft in 2005 and a left CEA in September 2020. A noninvasive arterial Doppler study showed ABI 0.68 (right) and 0.30 (left). Because of diminished GFR (27), she underwent noncontrast MRA of the abdomen, pelvis, and lower extremities in November 2023, which showed a patent aorto-bifemoral graft with complete occlusion of the right SFA and reconstitution of the popliteal artery with three vessel runoff and moderate stenosis of the posterior tibial artery (Figs. 18.1 and 18.2). There was complete occlusion of the left distal common femoral artery, and the superficial femoral artery. There was reconstitution of the left popliteal artery with three-vessel runoff and severe stenosis of the posterior tibial artery (Fig. 18.3).

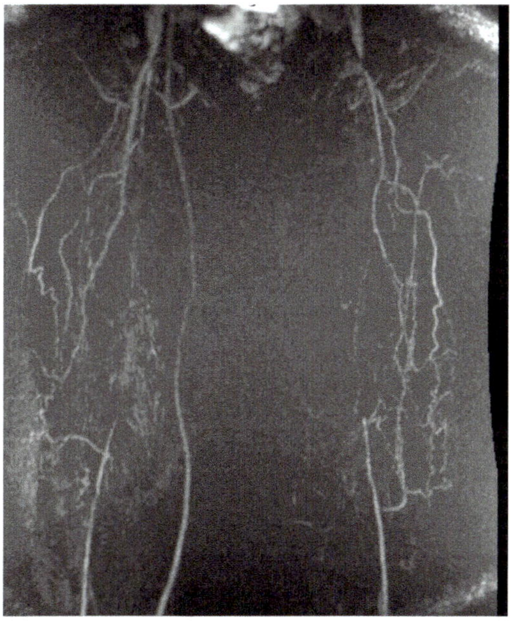

Fig. 18.1 MRA showing near occlusion of the left femoral anastomosis of the ABF graft

In March 2024, the patient underwent a revision of the left limb of the aorto-bifemoral graft with endarterectomy of the near-occlusion of the left distal CFA. A bovine pericardial patch was sutured to the distal portion of the left limb of the ABF graft and the proximal profunda femoris artery. The exposure of the left femoral anasmostosis of the ABF graft was obtained by exposing the medial border of the sartorius and mobilizing the lymphatics, inguinal lymph nodes, arte-

S. S. Hans, *Secondary and Tertiary Arterial Reconstructions*,
https://doi.org/10.1007/978-3-032-21214-6_18

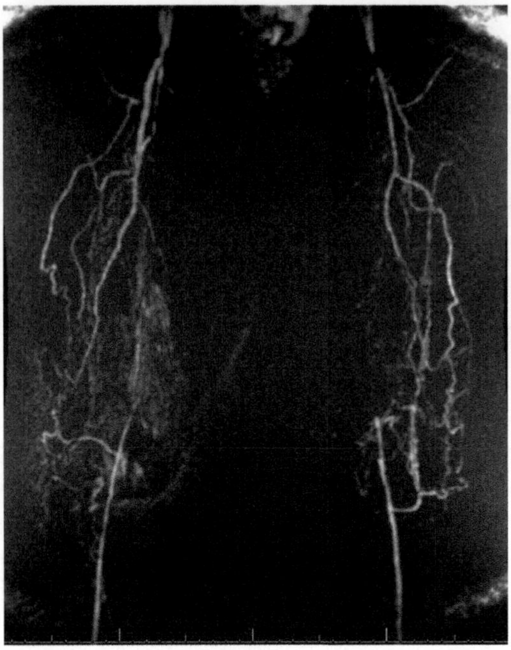

Fig. 18.2 MRA showing near occlusion of the left limb graft anastomotic site to the common femoral artery and bilateral SFA occlusions with reconstitution of popliteal arteries with large collateral in the thigh

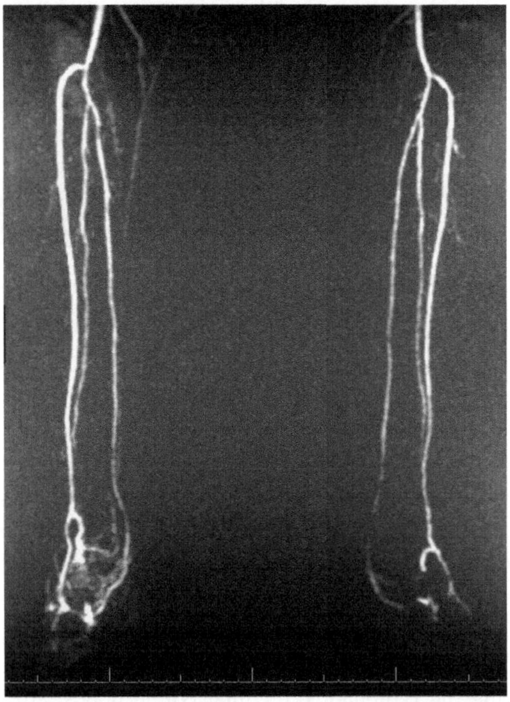

Fig. 18.3 MRA showing 3 vessel runoff with stenotic PTA on both sides

rial and venous branches from lateral to medial side. Her post-operative course was uneventful. A follow-up Doppler arterial study showed an ABI of 0.65 (right) and an increase in ABI from 0.30 to 0.68 on (left) side.

Discussion

The most common etiology of a failure of ABF is due to progressive disease at the femoral anastomosis, with the development of neointimal hyperplasia during healing of the anastomosis during the first 24 months, and a late development of atherosclerotic disease at the femoral artery bifurcation encompassing the orifice of the profunda femoris artery and the progression of infrainguinal arterial occlusive disease. In rare instances, thrombosis of the anastomotic aneurysms at the femoral anastomosis may also result in occlusion of the graft. Unilateral limb complications of the ABF graft are usually managed with thrombectomy, revision of the femoral anastomosis, with patch grafting, interposition grafting, or a crossover femoral–femoral bypass. Axillofemoral bypass is reserved for high-risk patients with limited life expectancy. Proximal aortic anastomotic complications leading to graft failure are infrequent.

In patients with prior ABF and long-standing left SFA occlusion with stenosis at the femoral anastomosis, revision of the femoral anastomosis and extended profundoplasty are usually sufficient to improve arterial flow to aid in healing of ischemic ulceration [1]. Simultaneous femoral popliteal bypass is usually not necessary except in a patient with advanced critical limb ischemia (CLI). In this patient, there was significant improvement in symptoms and hemodynamic parameters (ABI) following revision of femoral anastomosis and profundoplasty without the need of a distal bypass. Occasionally, renal transplantation and open aortoiliac reconstruction can be performed simultaneously. Bonnin et al., performed 22 aorto-bifemoral grafts, 12 in symptomatic patients with claudication or critical limb ischemia with significant aortoiliac occlusive disease with severe calcification, and in 10 patients without ischemic symptoms, but with severe calcification [2]. They reported zero mortality and a morbidity of 22.7% [2].

A similar anatomic consideration may arise in patients with pelvic kidney and associated AAA or aortoiliac occlusive disease because arterial supply to the kidney needs to be preserved at the time of arterial reconstruction.

Multiple Choice Questions

1. In a patient with a nonhealing ulcer of the left big toe, with a history of ABF graft, a renal transplant, ABI 0.68 (right) and 0.30 (left). An MRA shows near occlusion of the distal anastomosis of the ABF graft with bilateral SFA occlusions, with reconstitution of the popliteal artery on both sides with good run-off. The best management option is
   A. Revision of distal anastomosis of left limb of graft with femoral endarterectomy and patch graft
   B. Revision of the left limb with endarterectomy of the common femoral artery and simultaneous left femoral popliteal bypass graft
   C. Balloon angioplasty of the left femoral anastomosis
   D. Interposition graft from the distal portion of the left limb ABF graft to the popliteal artery
2. The most common cause of stenosis at the distal anastomosis of the aorto-bifemoral graft within 24 months of reconstruction is due to
   A. Technical error at the time of initial femoral anastomosis
   B. Myointimal hyperplasia at the distal anastomosis
   C. Progression of atherosclerotic disease in the distal arterial bed
   D. Thrombosis of the femoral anastomotic aneurysm
3. Exposure of the distal anastomosis in the common femoral artery during challenging groin dissection is best achieved by
   A. Suprainguinal incision and retroperitoneal exposure of the femoral limb of the graft
   B. Exposure of the superficial femoral artery
   C. Medial to lateral mobilization in the groin
   D. Lateral to medial mobilization with exposure of the medial border of the sartorius

Answers: 1(A), 2(B), 3(D)

References

1. Salvatore T, Scali Bradley M, Schmit Robert J, Feezor Adam W, Beck Catherine K, Chang Alyson L, Waterman Scott A, Berceli Thomas S, Huber. Outcomes after redo aortobifemoral bypass for aortoiliac occlusive disease. J Vasc Surg. 2014;60(2):346-355.e1. https://doi.org/10.1016/j.jvs.2014.02.002
2. Bonnin P, Kuntz S, Caillard S, Chakfé N, Lejay A. Aortobifemoral bypass in kidney transplant candidates: a ten-year experience. Transpl Int. 2024;37:12085. PMID:38379606

19 Infected Graft Limb of Aortobifemoral Graft

Presentation

A 69-year-old man presented to the ER with acute ischemia of the right lower extremity in June 2024. The patient was a current smoker (60 pack-years) with a history of hypertension and hyperlipidemia. The patient had undergone multiple arterial reconstructions during the previous 22 years. In 2002, the patient underwent bilateral common iliac artery stenting using balloon--expandable bare-metal stents (Palmaz® Genesis™, Cordis, Miami Lakes, FL). By 2003, stenting had failed, and the patient underwent an aortobifemoral graft (ABF) using a 16 × 8 mm knitted Dacron graft for progressively worsening symptoms of intermittent claudication. Proximal aortic anastomosis was performed end-to-end.

In 2009, the patient presented with acute left graft limb thrombosis requiring thrombectomy and revision of the left femoral anastomosis. In 2010, the patient underwent right superficial femoral artery angioplasty and stent deployment for mid-right SFA occlusion with symptoms of intermittent claudication. Due to thrombosis of the right SFA stent 1 year later, the patient presented with acute ischemia of the right lower extremity (Rutherford 2B) and underwent an emergent right femoral–popliteal in situ bypass.

In 2015, the patient presented with recurrent thrombosis of the left limb of the aortobifemoral graft and underwent thrombectomy of the left limb of the ABF graft with removal of the thrombus from the SFA and profunda femoris artery. In 2016, the patient presented with a recurrent cold, painful left lower extremity secondary to left SFA occlusion and occlusion of the main branches of the profunda femoris artery. The patient underwent left superficial femoral artery to above the knee non-reversed great saphenous vein bypass graft.

In August 2016, the patient presented with left groin wound dehiscence with a small amount of serosanguinous drainage. Cultures grew coagulase-negative Staphylococcus aureus and Streptococcus viridans. On the following day, the patient had significant bleeding from the left groin. There was a 2 cm left groin skin dehiscence without an exposed graft limb with surrounding induration. Computerized Tomography Arteriography (CTA) demonstrated a patent ABF bypass graft, with a slight dilatation of the left femoral limb, including surrounding inflammatory change, but without extravasation of the contrast.

During his hospital stay, the patient presented with secondary hemorrhage from the left groin. He underwent an emergent debridement of the left groin. The proximal anastomosis of the left femoral-popliteal bypass was taken down and, a new anastomosis was reconstructed approximately 3cm distal to the previous site. A sartorius muscle flap and application of negative pressure wound therapy was performed. He was discharged on the 10th postoperative day with stable

S. S. Hans, *Secondary and Tertiary Arterial Reconstructions*,
https://doi.org/10.1007/978-3-032-21214-6_19

hemodynamic parameters. The deep wound cultures were negative. He received a systemic course of cefazolin and rifampin along with negative pressure wound therapy for the left groin.

The patient presented to the emergency room 7 days from recent discharge with active arterial bleeding from the left groin and Class III hemorrhagic shock. He was taken to the operating room immediately and was bleeding from the left femoral limb graft anastomosis of the ABF graft. Removal of the infected limb of the aortofemoral graft was performed with ligation of the proximal end of the left limb of the aortobifemoral graft. Intravenous vancomycin was started. Cultures of the perigraft fluid had growth of vancomycin-resistant Enterococcus faecalis (VRE) and Candida Parapsilosis.

Following ligation and partial excision of the left limb, there were no Doppler signals in the foot (Dorsalis pedis (DP) and posterior tibial artery). There was limited motor function of the left lower extremity. The patient was started on intravenous heparin and a left axillo-popliteal bypass with an 8 mm Interring PTFE graft (WL Gore, Newark, DE), routing laterally over the iliac crest.

The patient continued IV antibiotics. A CT angiogram on the 9th post-operative day showed a patent left axillo-popliteal artery bypass. He was discharged with negative pressure wound therapy on IV daptomycin and oral Diflucan for an additional 4 weeks. He was ambulatory with a palpable DP pulse during his 6 week follow-up visit in the clinic.

The patient presented to the emergency room 9 months later (May 2017), with occlusion of the left axillo-popliteal bypass resulting in a cold pulseless extremity. He underwent a crossover right femoral to left proximal popliteal bypass graft with an 8 mm Interring PTFE graft. The graft was routed in a suprapubic subcutaneous route. The right limb of the ABF graft and the hood of the right femoral–popliteal in situ bypass were exposed. The popliteal artery just proximal to the knee joint was exposed following the transection of the medial head of the gastrocnemius muscle. The proximal portion of the crossover femoral-popliteal bypass graft was anastomosed to the hood of the right femoral–popliteal in situ bypass in an end-to-side fashion and distal anastomosis to the above knee popliteal artery in an end-to-side fashion as well. The left dorsalis pedis pulse became palpable. The patient presented to the clinic 3 weeks later with an exposed graft in the left groin, and a gracilis muscle flap with a split-thickness skin graft was performed, with satisfactory healing of the left groin. At follow-up in June 2019, in the clinic, the right ABI was 0.85 and the left 0.69. In March 2020, the patient underwent left above-knee amputation following thrombosis of the cross-over right femoral to left popliteal bypass. He continued to ambulate with a left above-knee prosthesis.

On June 24, 2023, the patient came to the ER with acute ischemia of the right lower extremity secondary to a thrombosed femoral anastomotic aneurysm and thrombosis of the right femoral popliteal bypass with thrombosis of the infrapopliteal arteries (Figs. 19.1, 19.2, 19.3 and 19.4). The right femoral anastomotic aneurysm was resected and repaired with interposition of a new 8 mm knitted Dacron graft (Vascutek, Inchinnan, Renfrewshire, Scotland) from the previously placed right limb of the aorto-bifemoral graft at the origin of right femoral–popliteal in situ bypass with reimplantation of the profunda femoris artery into the posterolateral opening in the interposition graft as a Carrell patch. The right femoral in situ bypass was exposed in the right lower thigh and just below the knee by two separate incisions placed in the healed scars of the previous bypass. There were atherosclerotic

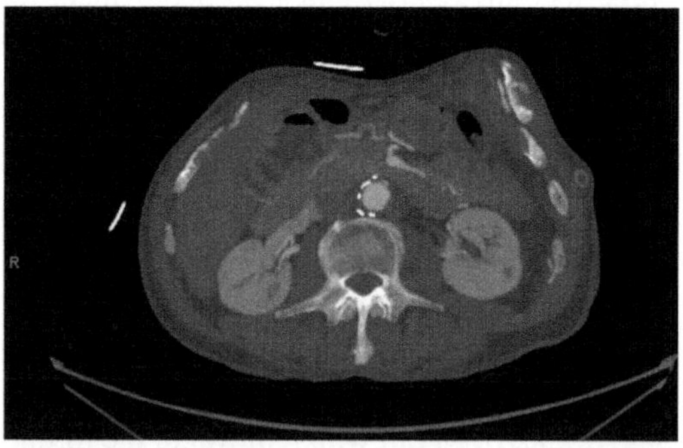

Fig. 19.1 CTA Abdomen showing main body of the ABF graft without perigraft fluid

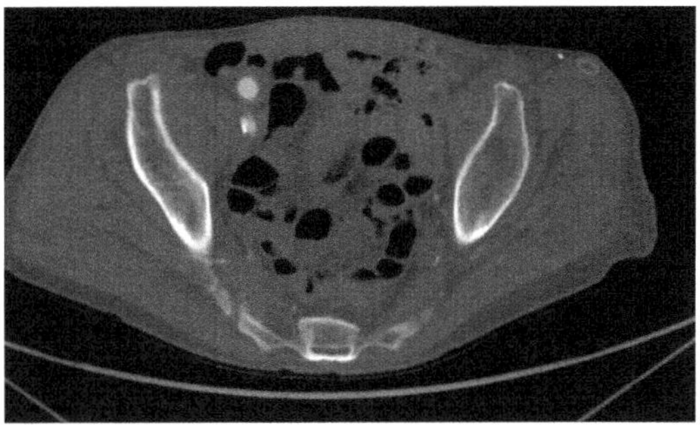

Fig. 19.2 CTA showing patent right limb of the ABF graft and surgical removal of the left limb of the ABF graft

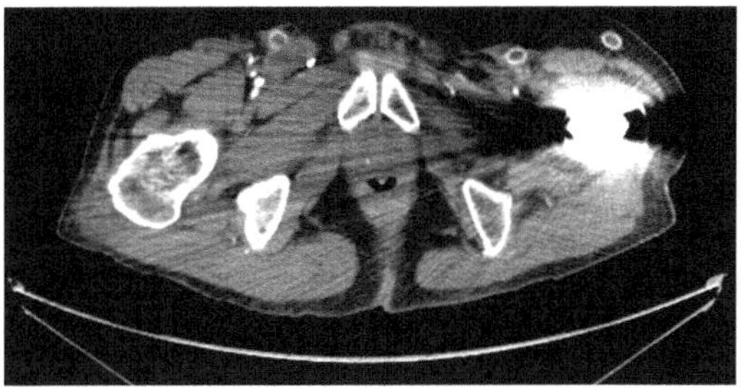

Fig. 19.3 CTA pelvis showing thrombosed right femoral anastomotic aneurysm and thrombosed crossover femoro-popliteal graft and left axillopopliteal bypass graft

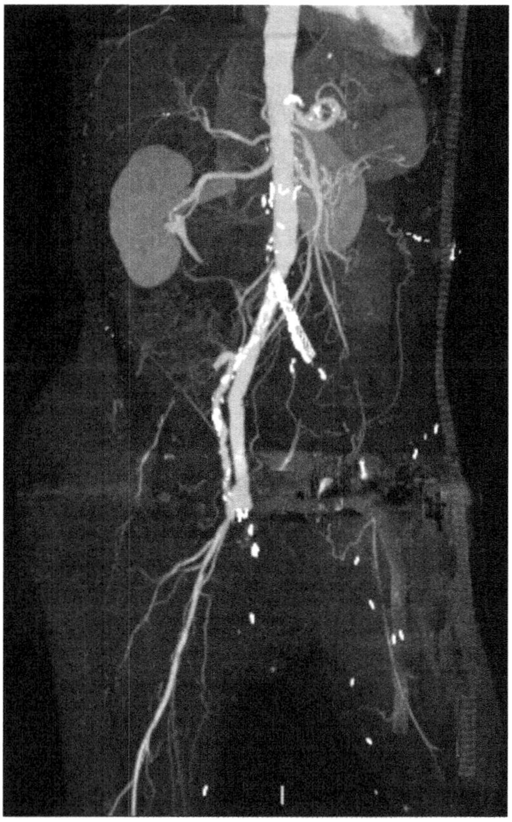

Fig. 19.4 Coronal view of CTA abdomen, pelvis, showing patent right aortofemoral graft occluded right femoral popliteal bypass. Surgical removal of left limb of the ABF graft and left above knee amputation

plaques in the intima of the in situ bypass on opening the in situ bypass. Thrombectomy of the right femoral–popliteal bypass and infrapopliteal arteries with passage of a number 3 Fogarty balloon catheter was performed.

Duplex imaging of the in situ bypass 4 days later showed stenosis in the right mid and lower segments of the right femoral popliteal in situ bypass (Fig. 19.5, 19.6 and 19.7). On June 29, 2023, the patient underwent percutaneous balloon angioplasty of the two areas of stenosis in the in situ bypass using ultrasound-guided left brachial artery access. Completion arteriogram showed a filling defect in the tibial peroneal trunk, most likely due to distal embolization during the procedure.

The patient was emergently taken to the operating room and underwent thrombectomy via distal popliteal arteriotomy at the hood of the distal anastomosis of the femoral–popliteal bypass using a Fogarty balloon catheter. Because of the recurrent thrombosis of the right femoral in situ bypass, the patient underwent exploration of the right groin. He was found to have a thrombosed 8 mm interposition Dacron graft (June 30, 2023).

Following the graftotomy incision and passage of a #5 Fogarty catheter proximally, pulsatile flow was obtained; the graftotomy incision was closed. However, the patient was oozing blood continuously from the interstices of the graft. Despite local application of BioGlue, Floseal, and Gelfoam soaked in thrombin, bleeding persisted. Thrombectomy of the previous femoral–popliteal bypass was performed. Passage of #3 Fogarty catheter into the tibioperoneal trunk did not retrieve any thrombi. Despite administration of fresh frozen plasma, packed red cells, bleeding from the interstices of the Dacron graft persisted. The interpostion Dacron graft was removed and replaced with an 8 mm standard-

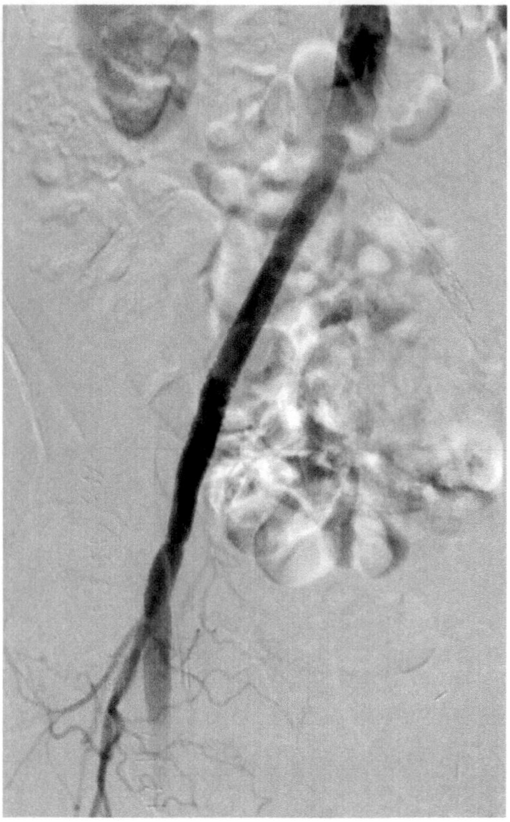

Fig. 19.5 Arteriogram showing patent right aorto limb of the ABF graft patent, interposition femoral graft, and proximal segment of right femoropopliteal bypass

wall PTFE graft (WL Gore, Newark, DE) with control of bleeding.

A basilic vein was harvested from the medial upper arm and was used as a bypass from the distal portion of the femoral–popliteal bypass to the mid-peroneal artery in a non-reversed fashion with lysis of the valves. Excessive bleeding stopped following four units of fresh frozen plasma and protamine sulfate administration. Approximately 3 weeks following composite bypass to the peroneal artery, the patient developed secondary hemorrhage from the groin site, necessitating explantation of the PTFE graft and the proximal portion of the right femoral-popliteal bypass, as this anastomosis was the source of the bleeding. The patient subsequently underwent right above-knee amputation in August 2023, secondary to ischemia of the right lower extremity, and was transferred to a rehabilitation unit. He was subsequently fitted with a right above-knee prosthesis (with prior left AK prosthesis). The patient died 1 year and 7 months later (in March 2025), most likely from a cardiac cause.

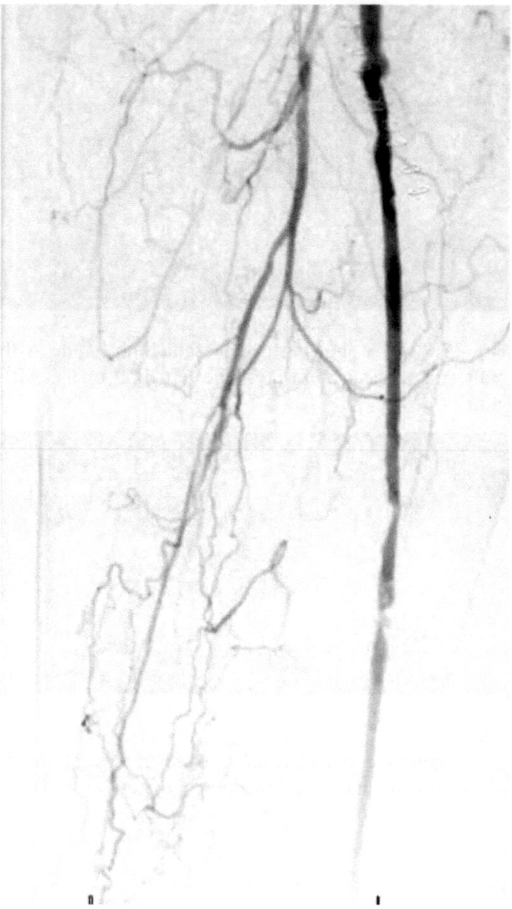

Fig. 19.6 Arteriogram showing stenosis in the mid and distal segment of right femoral popliteal in situ bypass

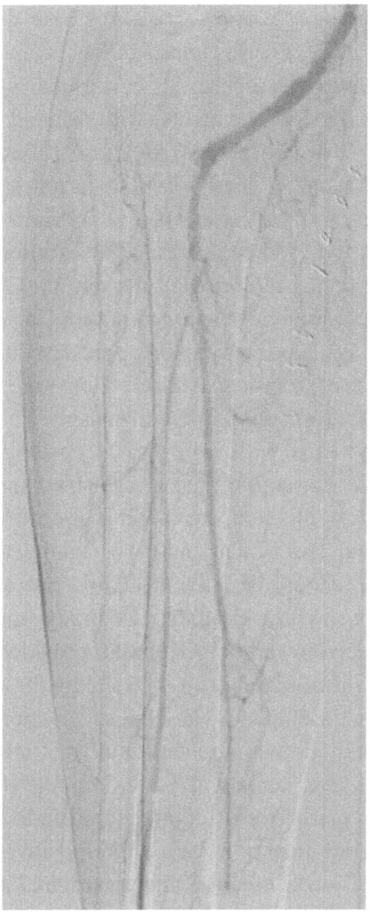

Fig. 19.7 Arteriogram showing patent right femoral infrapopliteal in situ bypass with filling defect in the tibioperoneal trunk

Discussion

From the patient's first presentation in 2002 to his ultimate demise in 2025, the patient underwent more than 10 arterial reconstructions. One of the important risk factors for graft infection is repeated arterial reconstructions. He continued to smoke cigarettes from age 15 to age 70 (55 pack-years). He died at age 71. This was probably an important risk factor for the progression of atherosclerosis and repeated graft failure.

Aortic graft infections can be classified as (1A) early infection, which is defined as manifesting less than 4 months from the time of initial surgery. These infections tend to be of a higher grade with high virulence, or (1B) late infection is defined as occurring more than 4 months from the time of initial surgery and is usually of low grade with lower virulence. Graft infection is the result of either direct infection or hematogenous seeding or direct extention from a superficial wound infection [1–4]. A vast majority of these infections are caused by micro-organismas already colonized on patient's skin. Bacteria also can travel from a surface level incision infection with extension into deeper perigraft tissues. Micro-organisms present in the artheroscleoritic plaque and/or arterio-thrombus may contaminate the graft may contaminate the procedure. Micro-organisms can also be introduced via transected lymphatics particularly in patients with concommitant infection in the distal lower extremity. Groin complications following aorto-femoral grafting poses risks because of moisture and high bacterial count at that site. Although perioperative contamination is a frequent cause of infection, almost 50% of infections occur 25–70 months following arterial reconstruction [5–7]. The most common organisms are gram-positive cocci and Staphylococcus aureus. Other common organisms are coagulase-negative staphylococci, streptococci, enterococci, and other gram-negative organisms (Pseudomonas, E. coli, Bacteroides).

The risk factors for aortic graft infection include but are not limited to: prolonged operative time (greater than 4 h), perioperative infection at a different site, nasal carrier of staphylococci, older age, female gender, reconstruction critical limb ischemia, and patient risk factors such as obesity, chronic obstructive pulmonary disease, hyperglycemia, malnutrition, end stage renal disease, immunodeficiency, an infected thrombus within an aortic aneurysm, inadequate choice/dosing/timing of perioperative antibiotics, break in sterile technique, tissue trauma, bacteremia, and a postoperative surgical site infections.

Multiple classification systems have been presented to delineate the type of aortic graft infection. The two most common classifications used are by Szilagyi and Samson. According to Szilagyi's classification, Grade I infection represents superficial infection with cellulitis involving the wound, Grade II deep infection involving subcutaneous tissue, and Grade III graft infections [8]. Samson classification: Grade I infection limited to dermis, Grade II infection involving subcutaneous tissue, Grade III infection of the graft not involving the anastomosis, Grade IV infection involving the anastomosis but no bleeding or bacteremia present, and Grade V infection involving the anastomosis with bleeding and/or hemorrhage [6].

The main principle in the treatment of aortic graft infection is debridement of surrounding infected tissue, excision of the graft, and secondary revascularization. Antibiotics play a key role in the treatment of these patients and are usually administered for a period of 6 weeks. The gold standard in the past for aortic graft infection was removal of the graft with revascularization using axillary-bifemoral bypass reconstruction. Axillary–bifemoral bypass following explant of ABF graft is associated with a mortality of 25–40%, risk of aortic stump blowout (mortality 30%), graft thrombosis, poor long-term patency rates, and a reinfection rate of 5–15%. In lieu of these outcomes, more recent literature has shown that in situ reconstruction, debridement with or without muscle flap, is superior in terms of perioperative mortality, decrease in limb amputations, and reinfection rates [9]. The in situ revascularization can be performed with a cryopreserved allograft, autologous femoropopliteal veins (deep veins), spiral vein grafts, rifampicin-soaked or silver-coated Dacron or PTFE grafts. Nonetheless, extra-anatomical bypass grafts can be utilized in patients with a hostile abdomen and the presence of severe comorbidities.

In patients with severe comorbidities, a more conservative approach with antibiotics, local debridement, muscle flap, and negative pressure therapy may be undertaken. To attempt to salvage the graft, it should be surrounded by healthy, non-infected, viable tissue. In a retrospective study by Ryu et al., the sartorius muscle flap provided coverage in the setting of soft tissue groin infections following a lower extremity revascularization [5]. In patients with non-availability of sartorius muscle flap (as was the case with this patient), the gracilis muscle flap is a suitable alternative. Morasch et al. performed a gracilis muscle flap in 18 patients, with a failed muscle flap graft in two patients. A mean follow-up of 40 ± 10 months. There was no recurrence of graft infection in their series [10]. Other muscle flaps that can be used for coverage of exposed grafts are the rectus femoris and the tensor fascia lata flap. Anastomotic aneurysm suture line hemorrhage, systemic sepsis, or aggressive bacterial infections (gram-negative infections) are contraindications to conservative management.

In patients with a history of aortobifemoral graft reconstruction presenting with a unilateral graft limb infection, a unilateral graft limb excision with revascularization or complete graft removal should be attempted. In a retrospective study, Crawford et al. demonstrated unilateral limb excision can be performed, provided infection is infra-inguinal. In their study, 50% of the patients developed a subsequent infection in the main body or a contralateral limb at a median of 2 years after unilateral graft limb excision [2]. Factors predictive of contralateral limb or main body graft infection are culture-positive suprainguinal graft infection and an original aortobifemoral graft placed for aortoiliac occlusive disease. Although microbes cultured in suprainguinal infections were unique from microbes causing recurrent graft infections in their study, raising suspicion for a new infection in the contralateral limb.

In patients with an inaccessible groin (either secondary to infection or multiple previous interventions), an in situ bypass or extra-anatomic bypass to the groin cannot be performed. Met et al. performed 30 extra-anatomical bypass on 24 patients over a period of 11 years. In 23 limbs, the indication was persistent groin infection from a previous reconstruction. In seven limbs, it was not possible to perform anastomosis in the groin. The primary patency after one year was 64% (n=9). The secondary patency after one year was 77%. Seven amputations were performed, six for ischemia and one for persistent infection. They reported limb salvage at one year of 84%. They also reported 29% mortality after one year [3]. In a small study by Seeger et al., there was 100% graft thrombosis with 0% primary patency at 7 months [7]. However, there is limited data regarding one-year patency rate of axillopopliteal bypass. In our patient, the axillopopliteal bypass remained patent for 9 months. The patient subsequently underwent crossover right femoral– left popliteal bypass graft, which maintained patent for 27 month without any evidence of infection involving the main body or the right limb of the ABF graft. Most patients with an infected limb of an aortobifemoral graft, will require removal the entire graft. However, the patient in this report had a well-incorporated right limb ABF and there was no evidence of infection until his demise. Therefore, the main body and the limb of the ABF graft may occasionally be feasible salvaged in patient's with a unilateral graft limb infection of ABF graft.

Multiple Choice Questions

1. The optimal muscle for coverage of the exposed Dacron graft in the groin in a patient who had a prior sartorius muscle flap is:
   A. Rectus femoris
   B. Gracilis
   C. Rectus abdominis
   D. Tensor fascia lata
2. Following thrombectomy of the left limb of aortobifemoral bypass graft for pulsatile groin mass, the patient had a small amount of serosanguinous drainage. Mass is non-pulsatile. Cultures grew Staphylococcus aureus (coagulase-negative) and Streptococcus viridians. The optimal imaging test to be obtained is:
   A. Duplex ultrasound left groin
   B. MRA left groin, abdomen, and pelvis
   C. CTA abdomen and pelvis
   D. Arteriography
3. Patient has dilatation of the left limb of the graft at the anastomotic site with perianastomotic fluid collection. The optimal management is:
   A. Aspiration of fluid in IR and appropriate parenteral antibiotics
   B. Exploration of groin, muscle flap, and parenteral antibiotics immediately
   C. Partial removal of the left limb of the graft and extra-anatomic bypass routed laterally over the iliac crest through the obturator foramen
   D. Antibiotics course for 6 weeks and followed by either excision of the left limb with extra-anatomic bypass or total removal of the graft.

Answers: 1(B), 2(C), 3(C)

References

1. Calligaro KD, Veith FJ, Yuan JG, Gargiulo NJ, Dougherty MJ. Intra-abdominal aortic graft infection: complete or partial graft preservation in patients at very high risk. J Vasc Surg. 2003;38(6):1199–205. PMID:14681612
2. Crawford JD, Landry GJ, Moneta GL, Mitchell EL. Outcomes of unilateral graft limb excision for infected aortobifemoral graft limb. J Vasc Surg. 2016;63(2):407–13. PMID:26482992
3. Met R, Hissink RJ, Van Reedt Dortland RW, Steijling JJ, Verhagen H, Moll FL. Extra-anatomical reconstruction in the case of an inaccessible groin: the axillopopliteal bypass. Ann Vasc Surg. 2007;21(2):240–4. PMID:17349372
4. O'Connor S, Andrew P, Batt M, Becquemin JP. A systematic review and meta-analysis of treatments for aortic graft infection. J Vasc Surg. 2006;44(1):38–45. PMID:16828424
5. Ryu DY, Jung HJ, Ramaiah VG, Rodriguez-Lopez JA, Lee SS. Infected groin (graft/patch): managed with Sartorious muscle flap. Vasc Specialist Int. 2016;32(1):11–6. PMID:27051655
6. Samson RH, Veith FJ, Janko GS, Gupta SK, Scher LA. A modified classification and approach to the management of infections involving peripheral arterial prosthetic grafts. J Vasc Surg. 1988;8(2):147–53. PMID:3398172
7. Seeger JM, Pretus HA, Welborn MB, Ozaki CK, Flynn TC, Huber TS. Long-term outcome after treatment of aortic graft infection with staged extra-anatomic bypass grafting and aortic graft removal. J Vasc Surg. 2000;32(3):451-459; discussion 460-451. PMID:10957651
8. Szilagyi DE, Smith RF, Elliott JP, Vrandecic MP. Infection in arterial reconstruction with synthetic grafts. Ann Surg. 1972;176(3):321–33. PMID:4262892

9. Armstrong PA, Back MR, Bandyk DF, Johnson BL, Shames ML. Selective application of sartorius muscle flaps and aggressive staged surgical debridement can influence long-term outcomes of complex prosthetic graft infections. J Vasc Surg. 2007;46(1):71–8. PMID:17606124
10. Morasch MD, Sam AD 2nd, Kibbe MR, Hijjawi J, Dumanian GA. Early results with use of gracilis muscle flap coverage of infected groin wounds after vascular surgery. J Vasc Surg. 2004;39(6):1277–83. PMID:15192569

20 Early Graft Limb Occlusion Following EVAR for a Large Abdominal Aortic Aneurysm

Presentation

A 68-year-old man was sent to the emergency room after his primary care physician palpated an asymptomatic pulsatile mass on the left side of the abdomen and obtained an urgent ultrasound of the abdomen, which showed a 10 × 10 cm abdominal aortic aneurysm (AAA). Comorbidities included stable coronary artery disease (CAD), hypertension, and hyperlipidemia.

He was referred to the emergency room by his primary care physician. An emergent CTA of the abdomen and pelvis in March of 2023 revealed an 11 × 10 cm AAA without periaortic stranding (Figs. 20.1 and 20.2). The anatomy of the AAA was suitable for an endovascular aneurysm repair (EVAR), which was performed emergently with an Endurant stent graft (Medtronic, Dublin, Ireland). The main body, 28 × 14 x 103 mm, was deployed from the right side, and a contralateral--iliac limb 16 × 16 × 156 mm and an ipsilateral extension limb 16 × 16 × 156 mm were deployed. Completion aortogram showed satisfactory exclusion of the aneurysm (Fig. 20.3). There was narrowing of the proximal right limb of the endograft, which, in retrospect, was overlooked. The patient was discharged on postoperative day one (Fig. 20.4).

Three weeks following EVAR, the patient was seen in the vascular clinic with symptoms of intermittent claudication involving the right lower extremity for the past week. He had an absent right femoral pulse; however right lower extremity did not show any evidence of acute ischemia. Ankle-brachial index on the right was 0.39 and 0.93 on the left. CTA abdomen and pelvis showed occlusion of the right limb of the endograft with extension of thrombus into the proximal external iliac artery with reconstitution of flow into the right hypogastric artery and distal external artery and common femoral artery, and profunda femoris artery (Figs. 20.5, and 20.6 b).

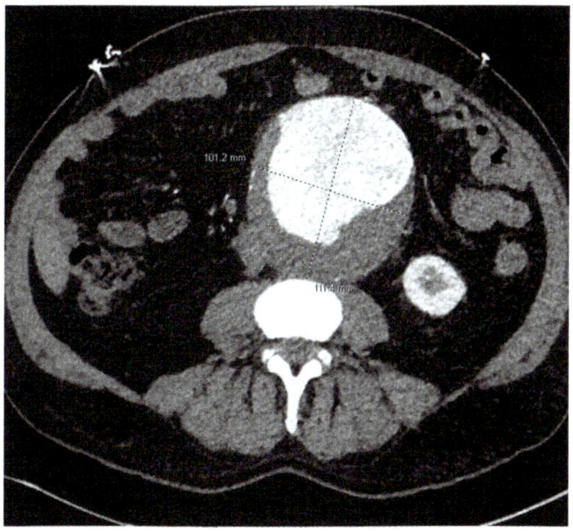

Fig. 20.1 CTA abdomen showing 11 × 10 cm infrarenal AAA

In April 2025, the patient underwent thrombectomy of the right limb using superficial femoral artery access obtained via bilateral groin using

S. S. Hans, *Secondary and Tertiary Arterial Reconstructions*,
https://doi.org/10.1007/978-3-032-21214-6_20

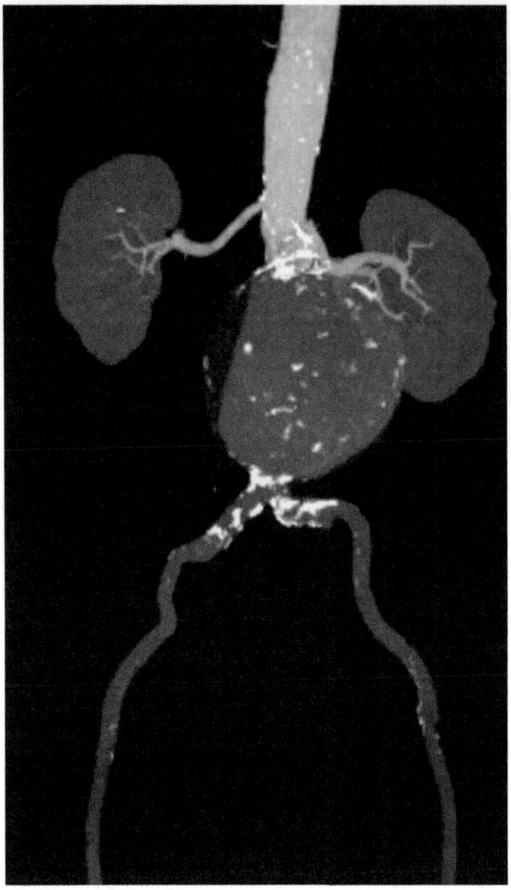

Fig. 20.2 MIP images showing large AAA with narrow distal aorta: left renal artery inferior to right renal artery with narrow distal aorta

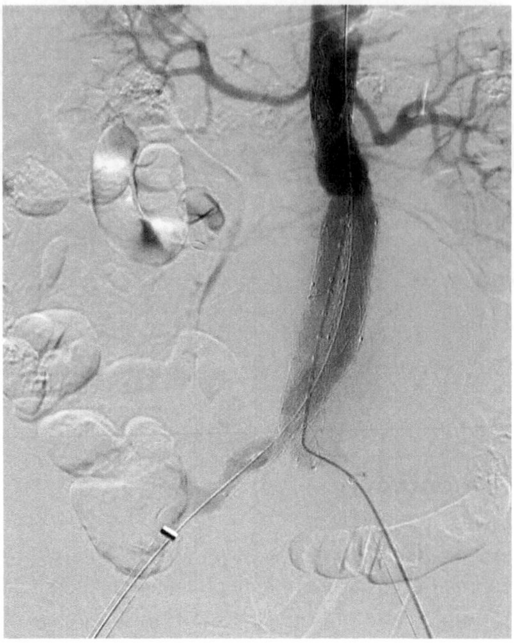

Fig. 20.3 Completion aortogram showing satisfactory exclusion of AAA

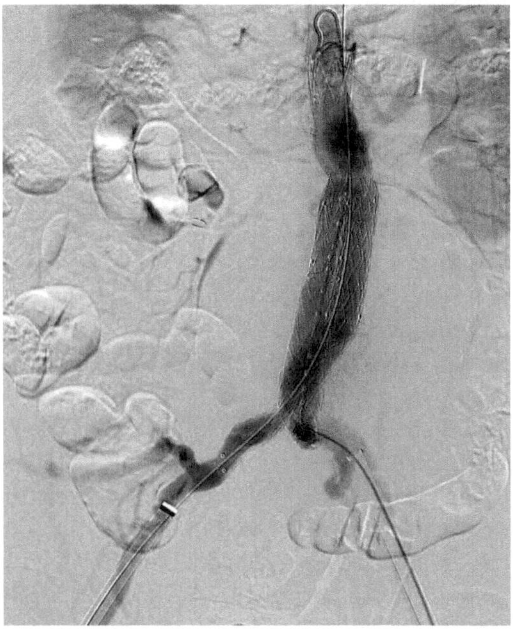

Fig. 20.4 Completion aortogram showing exclusion of AAA. There is moderate stenosis of the right iliac limb of the endograft at the aortic bifurcation

a short hockey stick incision from the groin crease to the upper thigh. A 12 × 20 mm Armada balloon was used to occlude the left limb just inferior to the flow divider during Rotarex™ thrombectomy (BD Franklin Lakes, NJ) to prevent distal embolization in the contralateral lower extremity. A channel was created in the thrombosed iliac limb. A 16 × 16 × 93 mm iliac limb was deployed to exclude the adherent thrombus in the occluded iliac limb. Two VBX 11 mm × 59 mm covered stents (WL Gore, Newark, DE) were deployed as kissing stents in the distal aorta, both iliac limbs, and postdilated using a 10 × 20 mm angioplasty balloon (Fig. 20.7). Contrast injection through the right femoral sheath revealed stenosis at the origin of the external iliac artery. A balloon-expandable Omnilink stent 10 × 39 mm (Abbott, Chicago, IL) was then deployed in the external iliac artery.

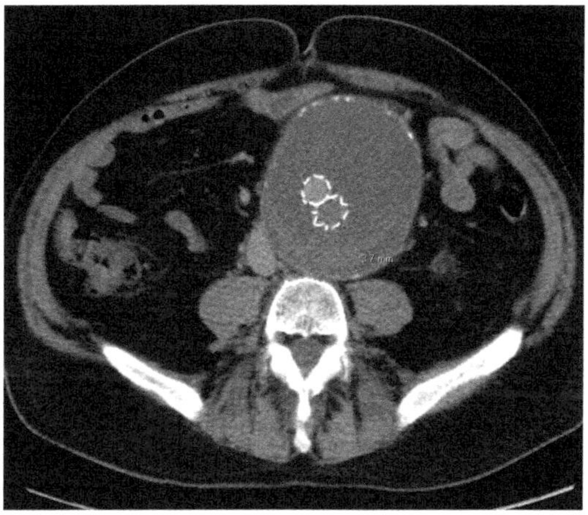

Fig. 20.5 Postoperative CTA abdomen and pelvis shows occlusion of the right limb of the endograft

Completion angiogram showed satisfactory ex clusion of the AAA (Fig. 20.8). There was a diffuse narrowing of the left limb, probably secondary to a trapped thrombus between the two limbs. The patient had palpable post-tibial artery and Dorsalis pedis pulse bilaterally. He was discharged on the second postoperative day. In June 2025, a follow-up CTA of the abdomen and pel-

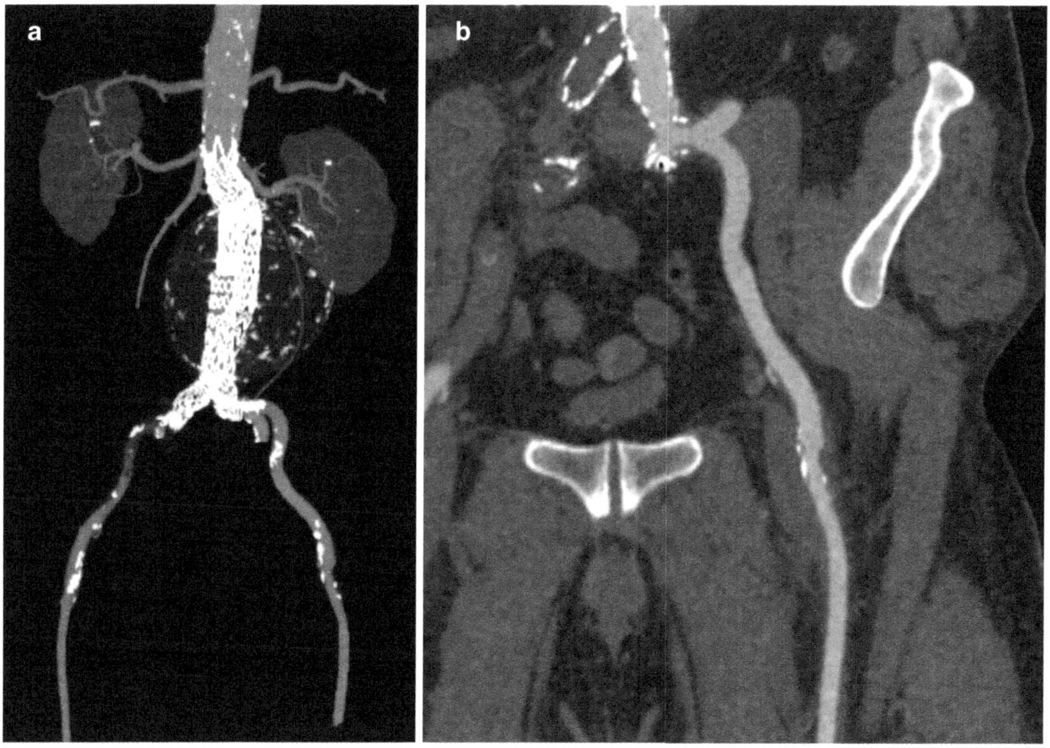

Fig. 20.6 (**a**) MIP images of CTA abdomen and pelvis showing occlusion of right limb of endograft. (**b**) MIP images of CTA abdomen and pelvis showing occlusion of the proximal external iliac artery and right hypogastric artery

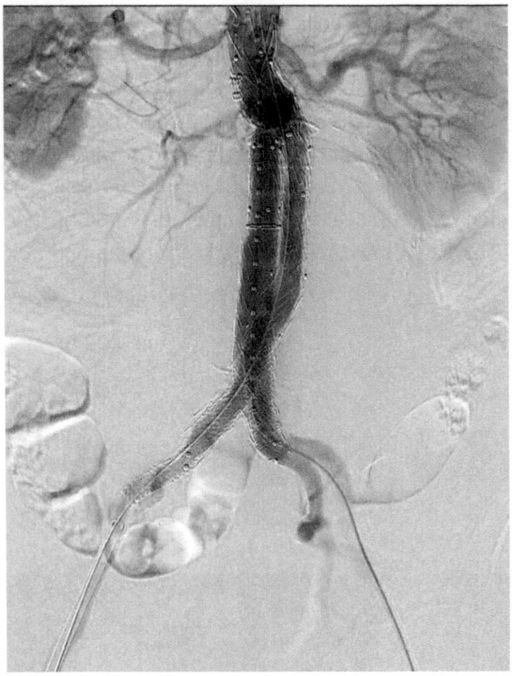

Fig. 20.7 Completion aortogram following graft thrombectomy and placement of kissing bilateral balloon expandable stents in the iliac limbs at the native aortic bifurcation

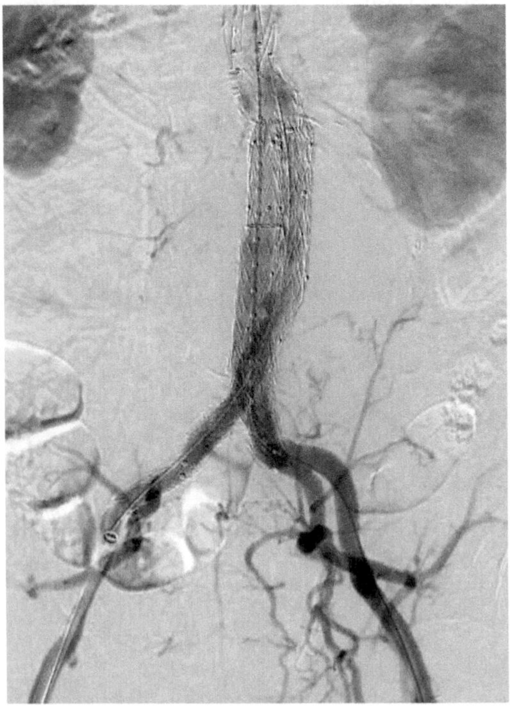

Fig. 20.8 Completion aortogram through right femoral sheath showing normal lumen of both iliac limbs of the endograft

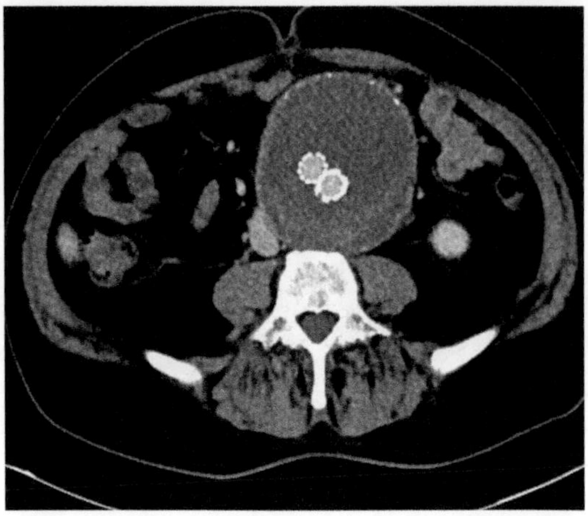

Fig. 20.9 Postoperative CTA following graft thrombectomy and kissing iliac stents showing patency of both iliac limbs

vis showed satisfactory flow in both limbs of the endograft (Fig. 20.9).

Discussion

Graft limb occlusion has been reported in 5.9–7.3% of patients undergoing EVAR [1–5]. Graft limb thrombosis commonly occurs in the first year following EVAR, with most occurring in the first 3 months following EVAR [1–5]. The anatomical risk factors responsible for graft limb thrombosis include angulation, tortuosity, and small-diameter iliac arteries, with associated calcification. Extensive calcification at the aortic bifurcation, narrowing the distal aorta (less than 20 mm), may cause compression of one or both graft limbs [1–5]. There is no correlation between the type of endograft used and the incidence of graft limb occlusion [1–5]. A graft limb deployed in an angulated and tortuous iliac artery anatomy can restrict arterial flow, leading to graft limb thrombosis. The narrowing of the distal end of the endograft can be addressed by a graft limb extension or deployment of an additional self--expanding stent. Inadequate anticoagulation (Heparin) during the procedure, severe angulation, poor outflow, or iliac artery dissection during the insertion of the sheath are other factors causing graft limb occlusion. Graft limb occlusion has been reported to be more common on the side of the main body deployment. Many patients presenting with late graft limb occlusion may be asymptomatic or have symptoms of mild intermittent claudication, and for those, no intervention is necessary. Surveillance with non-invasive Doppler arterial studies is essential.

Both endovascular and surgical options can be used for the management of graft limb occlusion. Endovascular options include mechanical, thrombectomy, pharmacologic, mechanical thrombolysis, and standard thrombolytic therapy. In most endografts, contralateral femoral access and placement of a catheter for thrombolytic therapy (TPA) is impossible because of the acute bifurcation of the commonly used endografts. Patients with severe acute ischemia often require a combination of a pharmacological agent with a mechanical device for thrombectomy. A thrombectomy with a Fogarty balloon catheter is often not successful because the thrombus is usually adherent to the fabric of the endograft.

The surgical options consist of an open surgical endograft limb thrombectomy from the groin or iliac artery with or without iliofemoral bypass. Surgical thrombectomy is often performed over a wire Fogarty balloon catheter or sometimes with an angioplasty catheter. For iliofemoral bypass, proximal control of the limb should be obtained either by a balloon occlusion catheter or a large Garret dilator (No.10 or 12). Direct clamp of the artery with the endograft limb can result in injury to the endograft. An extra-anatomic bypass (crossover femoral–femoral graft or axillo--femoral graft) in high-risk patients is another option in those presenting with severe ischemia. Crossover femoral–femoral graft is preferred in patients with late occlusion of the iliac endograft limb, with normal flow in the contralateral limb, and with significant symptoms of ischemia of the affected extremity. de Guerre et al. identified 21,119 AAA repairs (19,017 EVAR, 2,102 open) of which 15.2% were for large AAAs (diameter greater than 65 mm), and assessed 5-year reintervention, rupture, mortality, and follow-up rates [6]. The 5-year adjusted reintervention, rupture, mortality, and loss to follow-up rates for patients who had undergone large AAA EVAR were higher than those for patients who had undergone small AAA EVAR and large AAA open repair [6]. They concluded that for medically fit patients with large AAA should preferably be treated with open repair [6]. Montelione et al. reported that EVAR in patients with AAA larger than 59 mm with larger volume had higher rates of reintervention and death. Patients also had worse long-term EVAR outcomes [7].

Multiple Choice Questions

1. The most common time period for graft limb occlusion after EVAR is within:
   A. 4 years
   B. 2–3 years
   C. 1–2 years
   D. 1–11 months
2. A 64-year-old man, a former smoker with stable CAD and hypertension, stable COPD, has a 6.3 cm AAA with satisfactory 15 mm neck and 30-degree angulation. Common iliac arteries are satisfactory in size with minimal angulation. The best optimal management is:
   A. Endovascular repair
   B. Open repair
   C. Follow-up in 6 months with aortic ultrasound
   D. Follow-up in 3 months with a CT scan of the abdomen and pelvis
3. A 64-year-old man undergoes EVAR for a 7.0 cm AAA and presents to the clinic 3 weeks postoperative with symptoms of right lower extremity claudication and absent right femoral pulse, ABI right (0.3) left (1.0). A CTA and pelvis show a right graft limb occlusion. The best management option is:
   A. Anticoagulation
   B. Cross over femoral–femoral graft
   C. Pharmacomechanical thrombectomy of the graft limb and relining the graft limb with balloon-expandable covered stents and completion arteriogram
   D. Open thrombectomy of the graft limb with a Fogarty catheter.

Answers: 1 (D), 2 (A), 3 (C)

References

1. Clair DG. Maintaining Stent Graft Limb Patency. Endovasc Today (September); 2015. p. 3–5.
2. Cochennec F, Becquemin JP, Desgranges P, Allaire E, Kobeiter H, Roudot-Thoraval F. Limb graft occlusion following EVAR: clinical pattern, outcomes and predictive factors of occurrence. Eur J Vasc Endovasc Surg. 2007;*34*(1):59–65.
3. Bogdanovic M, Stackelberg O, Lindström D, Ersryd S, Andersson M, Roos H, et al. Limb graft occlusion following endovascular aneurysm repair for infrarenal abdominal aortic aneurysm with the zenith alpha, excluder, and endurant devices: a multicentre cohort study. Eur J Vasc Endovasc Surg. 2021;*62*(4):532–9.
4. Draper K, Choi SHJ, Fung A, Baxter K, Taylor D, Chen JC, Misskey J. Evaluation of factors associated with limb thrombus formation after endovascular aortic aneurysm repair. J Vasc Surg. 2023;*77*(2):440–5.
5. Chacko P, Hans SS, Nahirniak P, Morton K. Clinical patterns, predictors, and results of graft limb occlusion following endovascular aneurysm repair. Ann Vasc Surg. 2023;94:341–6.
6. Guerre L, Dansey K, Li C, Lu J, Patel PB, van Herwaarden JA, et al. Late outcomes after endovascular and open repair of large abdominal aortic aneurysms. J Vasc Surg. 2021;*74*(4):1152–60.
7. Montelione N, Sirignano P, d'Adamo A, Stilo F, Mansour W, Capoccia L, et al. Comparison of outcomes following EVAR based on aneurysm diameter and volume and their postoperative variations. Ann Vasc Surg. 2021;74:183–93.

21 Contained Rupture of Femoral Anastomotic Aneurysm Following Aortobifemoral Grafting for Arterial Occlusive Disease

Presentation

A 56-year-old man was seen in the ER on February 15, 2015, with purplish discoloration of the left 4th and 5th digits, with pain in the left foot, which was cooler than the right foot. All the pulses in the left lower extremity, including the femoral pulse, were absent. The right femoral pulse was palpable, but distal pulses were absent in the right lower extremity. Doppler evaluation of the lower extremities revealed ABI right (0.75) and left (0.50), with an unattainable toe brachial index on the left. The patient underwent CTA of the abdomen and pelvis and run off and catheter based arteriography which showed left external iliac artery occlusion, left common femoral artery (CFA) occlusion, reconstitution of the profunda femoris artery via collaterals, right superficial femoral artery (SFA) occlusion, left SFA occlusion and occlusion of the left proximal popliteal artery with patent distal popliteal artery and faint visualization of the left anterior tibial & peroneal artery. On the right side, there were three vessel runoffs. Medical comorbidities included coronary artery disease (CAD), morbid obesity (BMI 49), hypertension, and hyperlipidemia. The patient was a current smoker with a history of smoking 40-pack-years.

On March 9, 2015, the patient underwent aortobifemoral bypass graft using a 16 × 8 mm knitted Dacron graft with proximal anastomosis end-to-side; distal anastomosis was performed to the common femoral artery and extending into the proximal profunda femoris artery on the left side. The endarterectomy of the common femoral artery and orifice of the profunda femoris artery was performed prior to the performance of the distal anastomosis on the left side. He had an uneventful recovery, and a noninvasive Doppler arterial study on April 21, 2015, showed ABI 0.78 (right) and 0.57 (left). The patient was lost to follow-up for the subsequent 3 years. He came to the emergency room on November 27, 2017, with severe right groin and testicular pain along with significant ecchymosis of the skin of the right groin and suprapubic area (Fig. 21.1). He underwent CTA of the abdomen, pelvis, and run-off study, which showed contained rupture of the right femoral artery anastomotic aneurysm (FAAA) (Fig. 21.2) with bilateral superficial femoral artery occlusion. He underwent repair of the contained rupture of the right femoral anastomotic aneurysm with interposition of an 8 mm knitted Dacron graft with proximal anastomosis to the previously placed right limb of the aortobifemoral (ABF) graft in an end-to-end fashion and distal anastomosis to the main trunk of the profunda femoris artery. At the last follow-up (July 2024), there was no evidence of anastomotic aneurysm in the left groin, and without any recurrence of an anastomotic aneurysm on the right. Noninvasive Doppler arterial study showed an ankle-brachial index of (0.54) on the right and (0.55) on the left.

S. S. Hans, *Secondary and Tertiary Arterial Reconstructions*,
https://doi.org/10.1007/978-3-032-21214-6_21

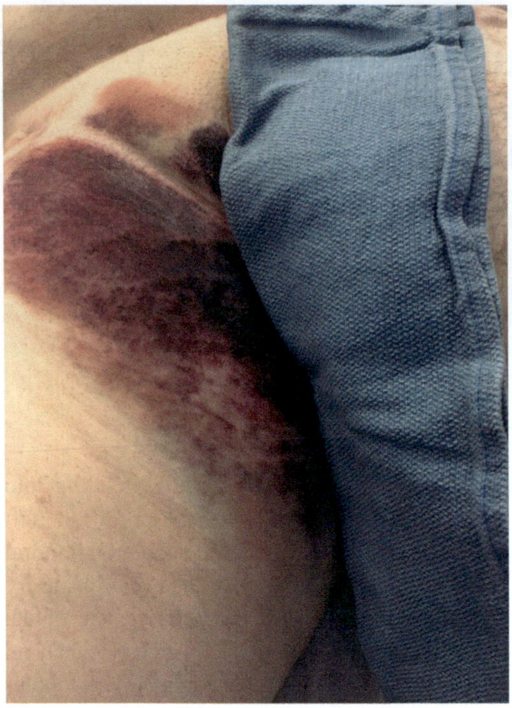

Fig. 21.1 Ecchymosis of the right groin due to hematoma in a patient who developed a right femoral anastomotic aneurysm 5 years after aortobifemoral bypass graft

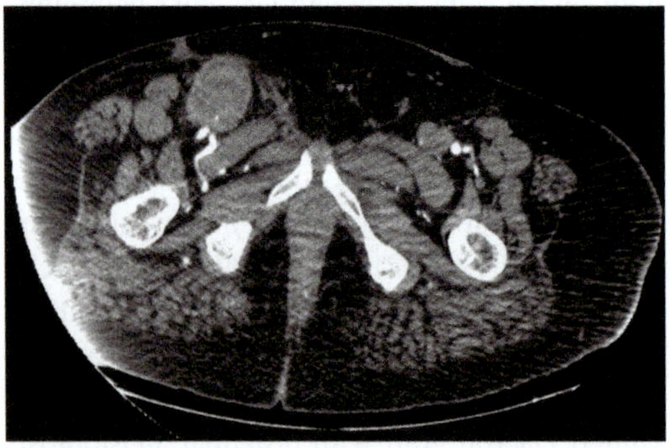

Fig. 21.2 CT angiography demonstrating a contained rupture aneurysm at the right femoral anastomosis of aortobifemoral bypass graft

Discussion

Femoral AA is an uncommon complication of aortofemoral graft reconstruction, and its incidence ranges from 1% to 3% in patients undergoing ABF grafting. Both systemic and local factors have been implicated in the development of FAAA [1]. In the 1960s, the suture material used for anastomosis of the prosthetic graft to the femoral artery was silk, and with the fraying of silk suture material, FAAA was quite common. Since the use of polypropylene suture for prosthetic graft to artery anastomosis, the deterioration of suture material is not a significant factor in the development of FAAA [2]. Local low-grade infection and progressive degeneration of the femoral artery with atherosclerotic plaque and repeated hip movements are considered to be other important factors in the development of a FAAA [3]. After initial aortofemoral reconstruction, a surveillance program with duplex imaging of the groin should be performed at 5 years after reconstruction, and if an aneurysm is detected, a yearly follow-up study should be performed until FAAA reaches 3 cm in its greatest anteroposterior/transverse diameter or becomes symptomatic. The repair of a FAAA should be considered in those circumstances. Untreated FAAA may rupture or develop thrombosis, with possible loss of life or limb [4].

Groin wound infection, reoperation in the groin, and excessive tension at the distal anastomosis are other factors in the development of FAAA. Seabrook et al. reported coagulase-negative staph in 60% of femoral FAAA [6]. Nicotine abuse and COPD are risk factors that increase the activity of matrix metalloproteinase inhibitors and inhibit connective tissue turnover, resulting in the formation of aneurysms [6]. The use of Dacron graft for aortofemoral reconstruction results in a higher incidence of femoral anastomotic aneurysm than with the use of PTFE graft [7]. The overall operative mortality for repair of FAAA should be similar to the primary operation, but for complex aneurysms such as those presenting with rupture, large size, or thrombosis, mortality of 7.6% has been reported [8].

For repair of leaking or recurrent femoral anastomotic aneurysm and those with a large size, proximal control can be facilitated with retroperitoneal exposure of the prosthetic graft limb using a suprainguinal incision.

Multiple Choice Questions

1. The repair of a femoral anastomotic aneurysm should be recommended for an aneurysm the size of:
   A. 1.5 cm
   B. 2.5–3.0 cm
   C. 3.5–4.0 cm
   D. Larger than 4 cm
2. For repair of a contained rupture of a large femoral anastomotic aneurysm, proximal control is preferably obtained by:
   A. Contralateral access of the graft limb and balloon occlusion of the ipsilateral limb
   B. Balloon occlusion of the ipsilateral limb using brachial artery access
   C. Lower quadrant of abdominal incision (suprainguinal) and retroperitoneal exposure of the graft limb
   D. Direct control of the anastomotic aneurysm using prior groin incision
3. The important predisposing factors to the development of femoral anastomotic aneurysm in contemporary practice are:
   A. Use of silk sutures in arterial anastomosis
   B. Low-grade infection
   C. Progressive degeneration of the femoral artery from atherosclerotic plaque and repeated hip movement
   D. Low-grade infection and progressive degeneration of the femoral artery from hip movement and atherosclerotic disease

Answers: 1(B), 2(C), 3(D)

References

1. Demarche M, Waltregny D, van Damme H, Limet R. Femoral anastomotic aneurysms: pathogenic factors, clinical presentations and treatment. A study of 142 cases. Cardiovasc Surg. 1999;7(3):315–22. https://doi.org/10.1016/S0967-2109(98)00161-6.
2. Mulder EJ, van Bockel JH, Haas J, van den Akker PJ, Hermans J. Morbidity and mortality of reconstructive surgery of noninfected false aneurysms detected long after aortic prosthetic reconstruction. Arch Surg. 1998;133(1):45–9. https://doi.org/10.1001/archsurg.133.1.45.
3. Ylonen K, Biancari F, Leo E, et al. Predictors of development of anastomotic femoral pseudoaneurysms after aortobifemoral reconstruction for abdominal aortic aneurysm. Am J Surg. 2004;187(1):83–7. https://doi.org/10.1016/j.amjsurg.2002.09.001.
4. Levi N, Schroeder TV. True and anastomotic femoral artery aneurysms: is the risk of rupture and thrombosis related to the size of the aneurysms? Eur J Vasc Endovasc Surg. 1999;18(2):111–3. https://doi.org/10.1053/ejvs.1999.0842.
5. Seabrook GR, Schmitt DD, Bandyk DF, Edmiston CE, Krepel CJ, Towne JB. Anastomotic femoral pseudoaneurysm: an investigation of occult infection as an etiologic factor. J Vasc Surg. 1990;11(5):629–34. https://doi.org/10.1067/mva.1990.19708.
6. Knuutinen A, Kokkonen N, Risteli J, Vähäkangas K, Kallioinen M, Salo T, et al. Smoking affects collagen synthesis and extracellular matrix turnover in human skin. Br J Dermatol. 2002;146(4):588–94. PMID:11966688
7. Stollwerck PL, Kozlowski B, Sandmann W, Grabitz K, Pfeiffer T. Long-term dilatation of polyester and expanded polytetrafluoroethylene tube grafts after open repair of infrarenal abdominal aortic aneurysms. J Vasc Surg. 2011;53(6):1506–13. PMID:21536404
8. Pansuriya S, Hans SS. Results of open and endovascular repair of complex aortic, iliac, and femoral anastomotic aneurysms. Am Surg. 2025:31348251363809. PMID:40719340

22 Repair of a Giant Femoral Anastomotic Aneurysm

Presentation

A 64-year-old man presented to the emergency room in December 2024 with a large pulsatile mass in the left groin with erythema of the overlying skin (Fig. 22.1). He was a former smoker (40 pack years) and had exclusion and bypass of bilateral popliteal aneurysms in the remote past. He had a left femoral–popliteal bypass more than 20 years ago at an outside hospital. The details of this operation were not available. In May 2016, the patient presented with acute ischemia of the left lower extremity. The operative note indicated exploration of his left below-knee popliteal artery. Thrombectomy of the left anterior tibial artery (ATA), posterior tibial artery (PTA), and peroneal artery, open balloon angioplasty of the left posterior tibial artery, and left femoral below--knee popliteal artery bypass graft (6 mm ringed Propaten PTFE graft) was performed. The patient underwent exclusion of a right popliteal aneurysm and a right femoral below-the-knee popliteal artery bypass (6 mm PTFE) approximately 2 years ago. CTA of abdomen and pelvis run off at this admission showed a 9.4 cms left femoral anastomotic aneurysm (Fig. 22.2) with occlusion of the left SFA and popliteal artery and faint visualization of mid and distal posterior tibial artery. There was visualization of the left profunda femoris artery and occlusion of the left femoral popliteal bypass graft. The right femoral popliteal bypass was patent.

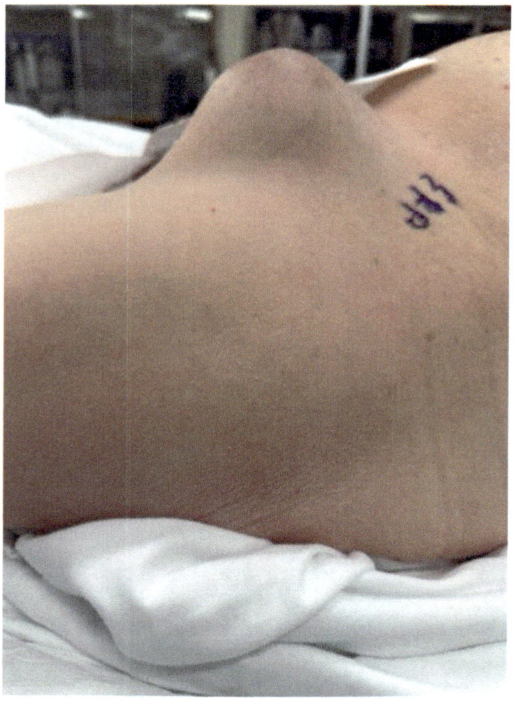

Fig. 22.1 Large pulsatile mass in the left groin with erythema of the overlying skin

Patient underwent urgent repair of a large left femoral anastomotic aneurysm with proximal control of the distal left external iliac artery. Using a left lower quadrant incision, exposure of the distal external iliac artery was obtained using a retroperitoneal approach. A large left femoral anastomotic aneurysm was resected through the

S. S. Hans, *Secondary and Tertiary Arterial Reconstructions*,
https://doi.org/10.1007/978-3-032-21214-6_22

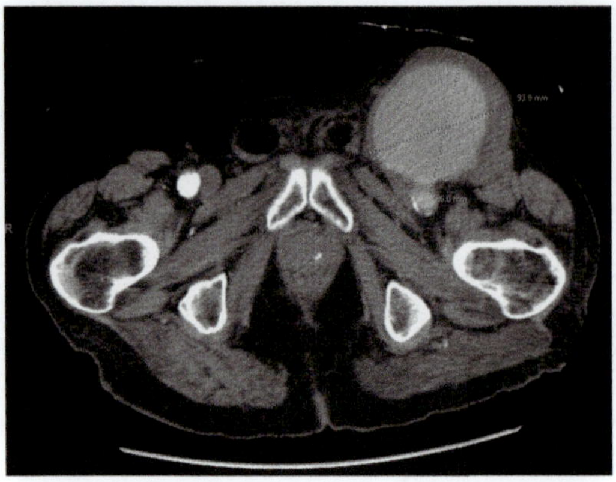

Fig. 22.2 CTA pelvis showing a large left femoral anastomotic aneurysm

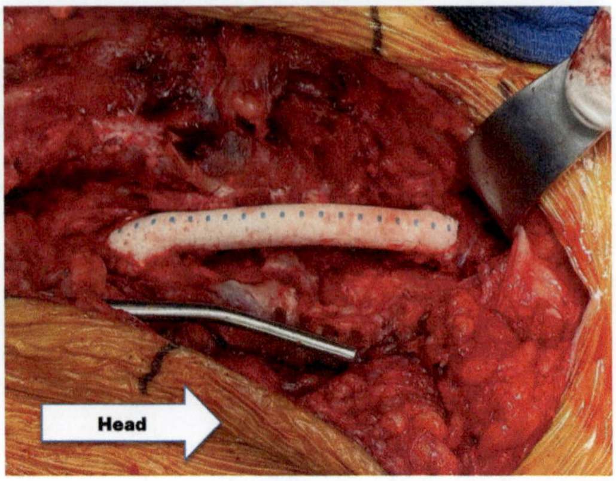

Fig. 22.4 Interposition 8 mm PTFE graft from proximal common femoral artery to distal profunda femoris artery

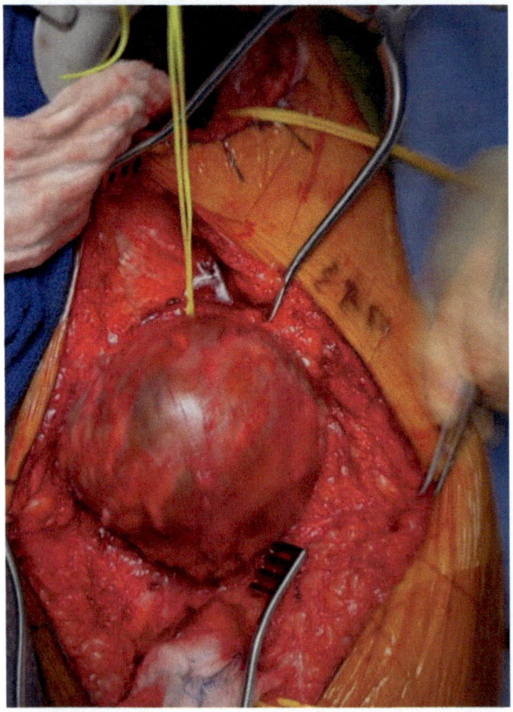

Fig. 22.3 Exposed left femoral anastomotic aneurysm with silastic vessel loops around the left external iliac artery (proximal) and distal around the proximal common femoral artery

previous groin incision scar (Fig. 22.3). A giant left femoral anastomotic aneurysm was mobilized and resected. The previously occluded left femoral–popliteal bypass graft (PTFE) was partially removed, and the distal left profunda femoris artery was exposed and mobilized. The dissection was challenging due to a third arterial reconstruction. Aneurysm was resected with proximal control obtained by an angled vascular clamp and distal control by a number 6 Garrett arterial dilator (Teleflex, Wayne, PA) after the aneurysm was opened, inserted into the orifice of the profunda femoris artery. An 8 mm PTFE graft was anastomosed to the proximal common femoral artery end-to-end and distal anastomosis to the profunda femoris artery in an end-to-end fashion using 5′0″ polypropylene suture for both anastomoses (Fig. 22.4). The patient was discharged on the 5th postoperative day in satisfactory condition. A follow-up noninvasive Doppler arterial study showed an ankle-brachial index of 0.54. The right femoral–popliteal bypass was patent. At a follow-up clinic visit 2 months later, the patient complained of mild discomfort in the left foot, and the ankle-brachial index had decreased to 0.39.

Catheter-based arteriography using right femoral artery access showed a patent left interposition graft to the deep femoral artery, but with filling of only one main branch of the profunda femoris artery (Fig. 22.5). The left SFA, popliteal, and trifurcation were occluded. There was filling of the mid and distal segment of the left posterior tibial artery (PTA) via collaterals. At the last follow-up in June 2025, chronic ischemic symptoms in the form of mild rest pain in the LLE have remained stable. As no satisfactory autologous vein was available for distal posterior tibial artery bypass, further arterial reconstruction was not recommended.

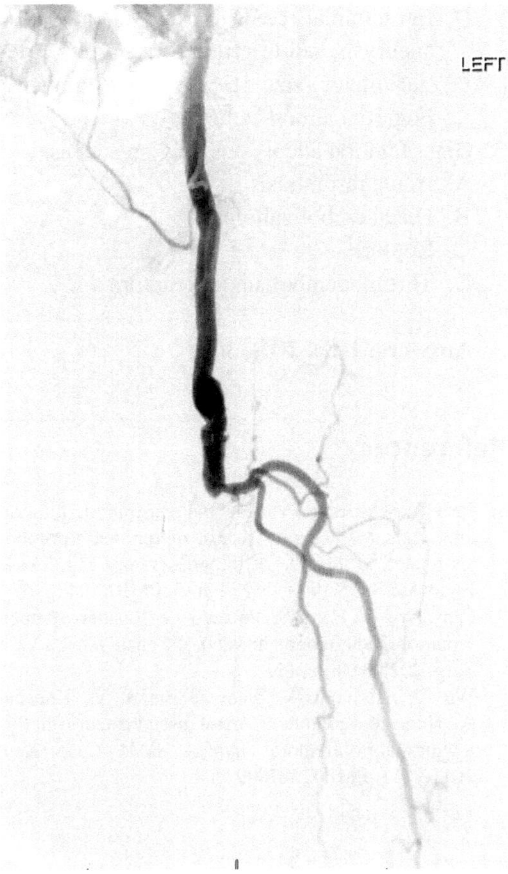

Fig. 22.5 Follow-up arteriography (3 months) patent interposition graft for common femoral artery to main branch of profunda femoris artery

Discussion

Giant femoral anastomotic aneurysm (FAA) may present with acute thrombosis and/or distal embolization, resulting in acute ischemia of the lower extremity. These large aneurysms may occasionally rupture, but rupture is often contained. Patients may complain of discomfort in the groin and testicular area due to compression of surrounding nerves. Additionally, extrinsic compression of the femoral vein may result in swelling of the lower extremity. Femoral anastomotic aneurysms smaller than 4 cm in diameter typically present as asymptomatic masses in the groin [1].

In most patients presenting with a femoral anastomotic aneurysm, the open repair is technically straightforward. Femoral anastomotic aneurysm repair is technically straightforward. However, in patients with large aneurysms and in those presenting with rupture, repair does pose technical challenges. For the repair of complex femoral aneurysms, technical aids should be considered. Proximal control in most femoral anastomotic aneurysms can be obtained using the previous groin incision with exposure of the proximal common femoral artery (CFA) and external iliac artery (EIA) junction under the inguinal ligament. However, in patients with complex aneurysms, proximal control of the distal left external iliac artery using a retroperitoneal approach is helpful. The dissection around the profunda femoris artery with the lateral circumflex femoral vein should be done carefully, as excessive bleeding can occur. Circumferential dissection of the artery with scar tissue and venous branches should be avoided while distal intra-luminal control is obtained using a Garrett's arterial dilator or a balloon occlusion catheter. In this patient, a decrease in left ABI at follow-up study (0.54–0.39) may have resulted from an occlusion of a branch of the left profunda femoris artery.

Due to increasing use of endovascular therapy instead of aortobifemoral graft reconstruction for iliac artery occlusive disease the number of patients requiring repair of femoral anastomotic aneurysm has decreased substantiall during the last three decades. Levi et al. reported that the risk of rupture and thrombosis of true femoral artery aneurysms and FAA was greater in aneurysms measuring 5 cm or more in diameter [1].

Pansuriya et al. reported 16 giant FAAs (greater than 65 mm in diameter) and compared the results of their repair to open repair of 69 conventional femoral anastomotic aneurysms (FAAs) (35 to 64 mm in diameter) from 2000 to 2024 [2]. Clinical outcomes were similar in both groups, but there was increased blood loss and operative time during repair of complex FAAs. Wu et al. also reported a successful open repair of a large (10 × 7 cm) femoral pseudoaneurysm following a remote ABG bypass graft [3].

Multiple Choice Questions

1. As compared to standard-size femoral anastomotic aneurysms (< 6.5 cm), the repair of giant femoral anastomotic aneurysms (>6.5 cm) is associated with:
   A. Increased blood loss
   B. Increased operative time
   C. Increased mortality
   D. Increased blood loss and increased operative time
2. During repair of a giant femoral aneurysm in a patient with significant arterial disease, the control of the profunda femoris artery is best obtained by:
   A. By exposure and mobilization of the profunda femoris artery proximal to the aneurysm
   B. Catheter-based femoral access and balloon occlusion of profunda femoris artery
   C. Distal control is not necessary, and bleeding can be controlled after the aneurysm sac is opened
   D. Intraluminal control after opening the aneurysm and insertion of a Garret's arterial dilator (size 5F or 6F)—a number 5 Fogarty balloon catheter
3. Giant femoral aneurysms may present as:
   A. Acute thrombosis
   B. Distal embolization
   C. Rupture
   D. Thromboembolism and rupture

Answers: 1(D), 2(D), 3(D)

References

1. Levi N, Schroeder TV. True and anastomotic femoral artery aneurysms: is the risk of rupture and thrombosis related to the size of the aneurysms? Eur J Vasc Endovasc Surg. 1999;18(2):111–3. PMID:10426967
2. Pansuriya S, Hans S, Polanco G. Results of open repair of Giant femoral anastomotic aneurysms. J Vasc Surg. 2025;81(6):e212.
3. Wu AY, Al-Jundi W, Ziadi Z, Barkat M, Khushal A. Huge anastomotic femoral pseudoaneurysm following aortobifemoral bypass. BMJ Case Rep. 2011;2011. PMID: 22700937

23 Impending Rupture of Recurrent Right Femoral Artery Pseudoaneurysm

Presentation

An 85-year-old woman presented with impending rupture of a right femoral artery pseudoaneurysm in January 2025 (Fig. 23.1). Past history was significant for lower GI bleeding in November 2016, for which she underwent visceral angiography for possible embolization of the bleeding vessel using right femoral artery access. Following removal of the right femoral sheath, she was found to have Rutherford 2B, ischemia of the right lower extremity. CT angiography showed a moderate amount of thrombus in the common femoral artery extending into the profunda femoris and an occlusion of the distal right SFA. Occlusion of the stent in the superficial femoral artery, popliteal artery, and absent flow in the infrapopliteal arteries. She underwent emergent thromboembolectomy of the right CFA, profunda, SFA, and the distal arterial bed. Due to irreversible ischemia of the right lower extremity patient underwent right above-knee amputation 3 days. She also underwent a Hartmann procedure for lower GI bleeding with sigmoid colostomy during the same admission. Closure of the sigmoid colostomy was performed 8 months later.

In 2020, the patient presented again to the hospital for bleeding in the right groin. A review of medical records showed a right femoral pseudoaneurysm confirmed by CTA of the abdomen and pelvis, for which she underwent an emergent repair. The neck of the pseudoaneurysm was wide, and the defect was in the proximal segment of the SFA. Therefore, proximal and distal ligation of the SFA was performed, and she was discharged to an extended care facility. She developed flexion contracture of the right hip. Medical comorbidities included dementia, ane-

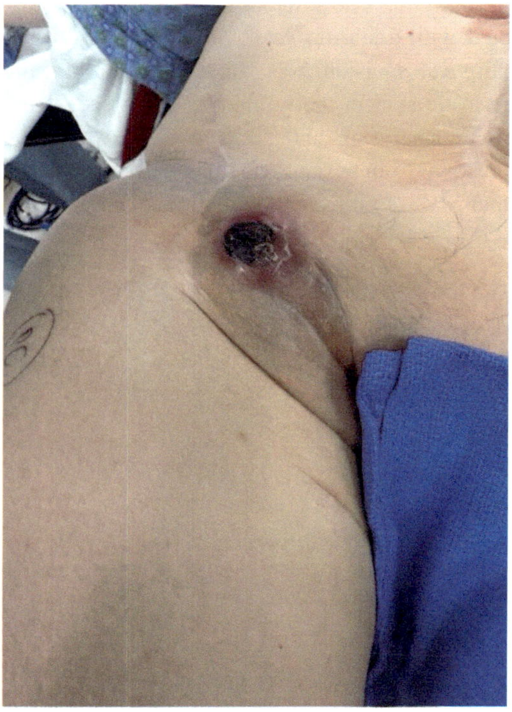

Fig. 23.1 Impending rupture of the right femoral pseudoaneurysmwith overlying skin necrosis

S. S. Hans, *Secondary and Tertiary Arterial Reconstructions*,
https://doi.org/10.1007/978-3-032-21214-6_23

mia, and essential thrombocytosis. CTA of the abdomen and pelvis at this admission showed a large right femoral artery pseudoaneurysm (Fig. 23.2). She was taken emergently to the operating room. A right transverse incision was made, and the right distal external iliac artery was exposed using a retroperitoneal approach. The exposure of the external iliac artery was facilitated by the division of the tendon of the psoas major muscle. The hip contracture had resulted in shortening of the muscle and its tendon with a lateral displacement of the external iliac artery coursing posterior to the tendon of the psoas major. The external iliac artery was encircled with a silastic vessel loop (Fig. 23.3). An elliptical incision was made surrounding the necrotic skin in the groin. The large sac of the pseudoaneurysm entered, and there was brisk bleeding from the anteromedial wall of the proximal SFA in close approximation the previously placed stent. The opening was 5 mm in diameter and was sutured with a continuous 3′0″ CV polypropylene suture. The contents and the sac of the pseudoaneurysm were removed, and the cultures from the wall of the pseudoaneurysm were obtained. After copious irrigation with normal saline, a white and gray sponge was applied, and vacuum-assisted closure was performed (Figs. 23.4, 23.5, 23.6 and 23.7). She was continued on intravenous antibiotics as recommended by the infectious disease consultant.

On February 11, 2015, a plastic surgeon performed debridement of the skin, subcutaneous tissue, muscle, and fascia (30 cm) for adjacent tissue transfer (Figs. 23.8, 23.9 and 23.10). She was transferred to an extended care facility, one week later, on a 10-day course of oral antibiotics for a Pseudomonas infection cultured from the groin wound. The healing of the incision was satisfactory. The patient's durable

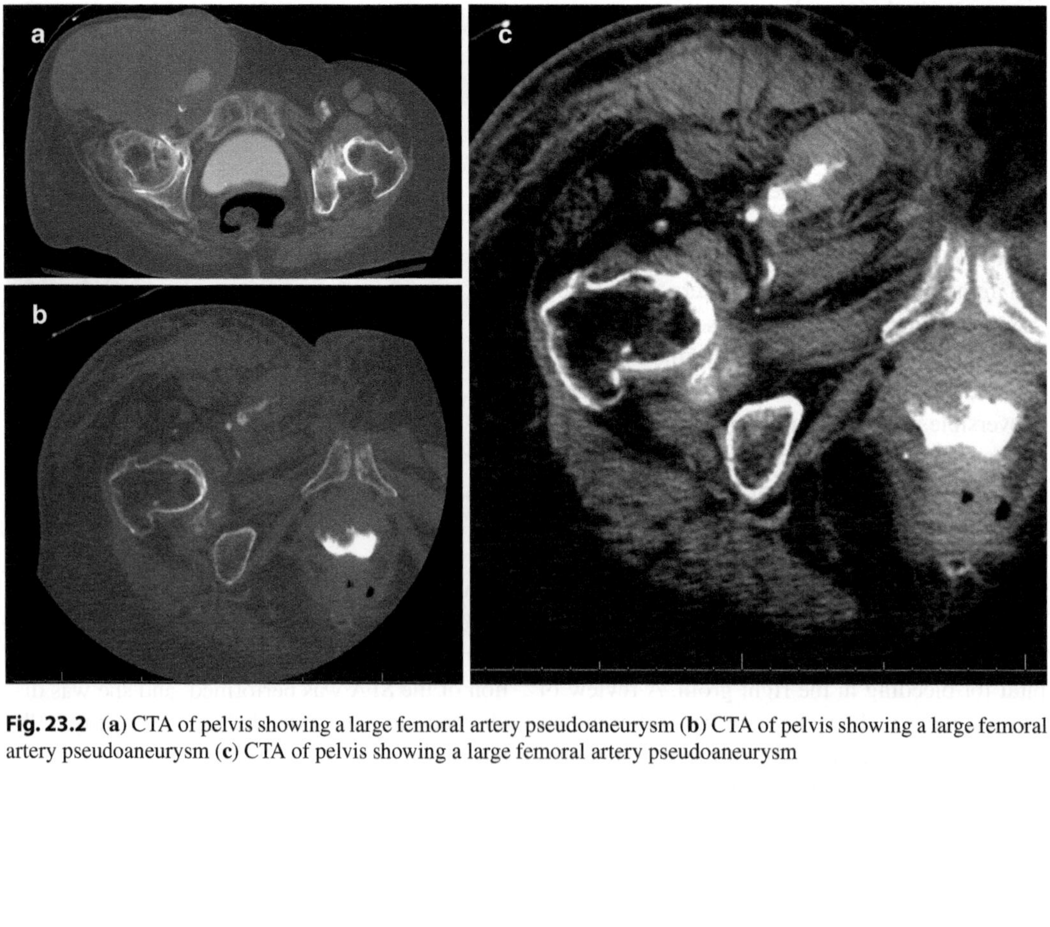

Fig. 23.2 (**a**) CTA of pelvis showing a large femoral artery pseudoaneurysm (**b**) CTA of pelvis showing a large femoral artery pseudoaneurysm (**c**) CTA of pelvis showing a large femoral artery pseudoaneurysm

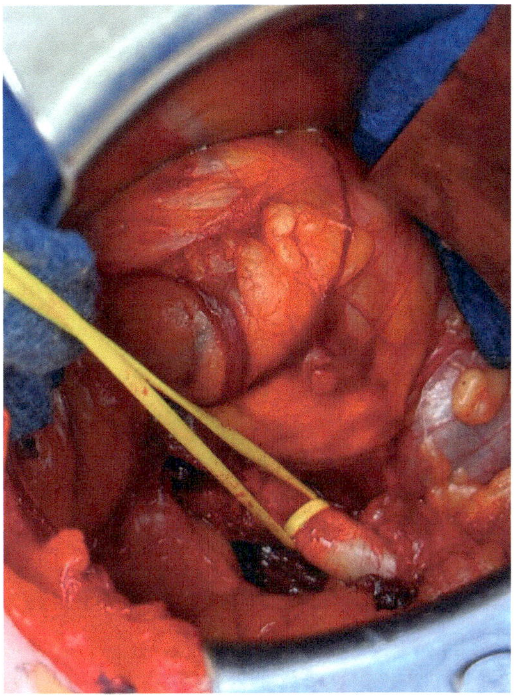

Fig. 23.3 Exposure of the right external iliac artery encircled silastic vessel loop via the right lower quadrant abdominal incision

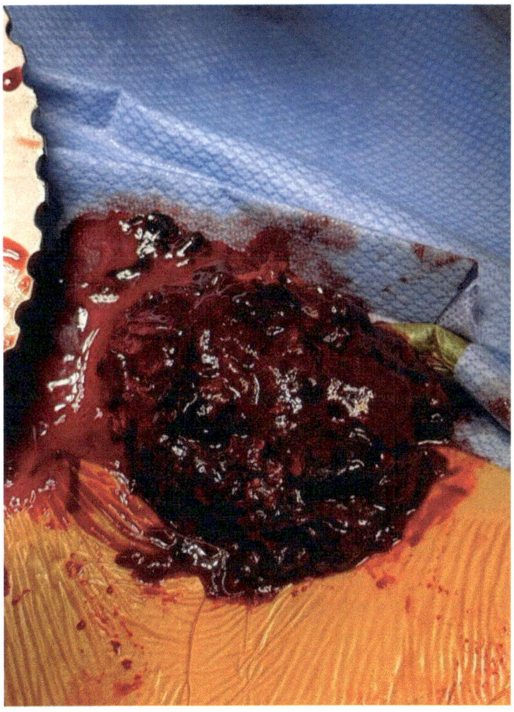

Fig. 23.4 Large amount of blood clots removed from the right femoral pseudoaneurysm

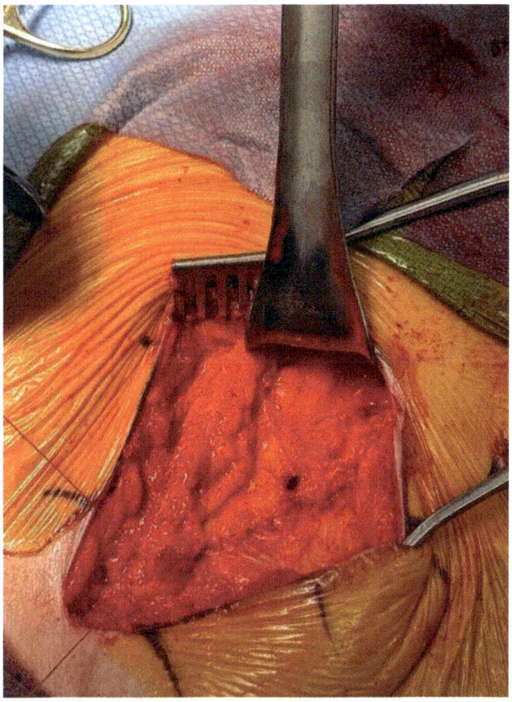

Fig. 23.5 Closure of the right lower quadrant incision in layers following repair of femoral mycotic pseudoaneurysm

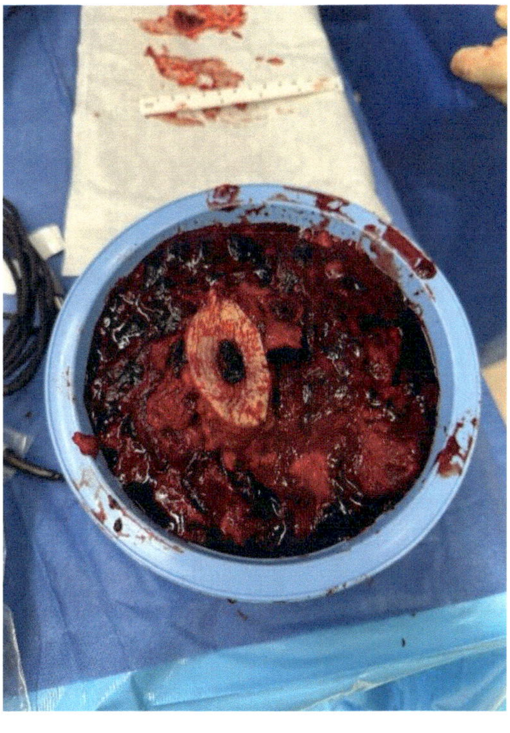

Fig. 23.6 Operative specimen with removal of necrotic skin overlying femoral pseudoaneurysm

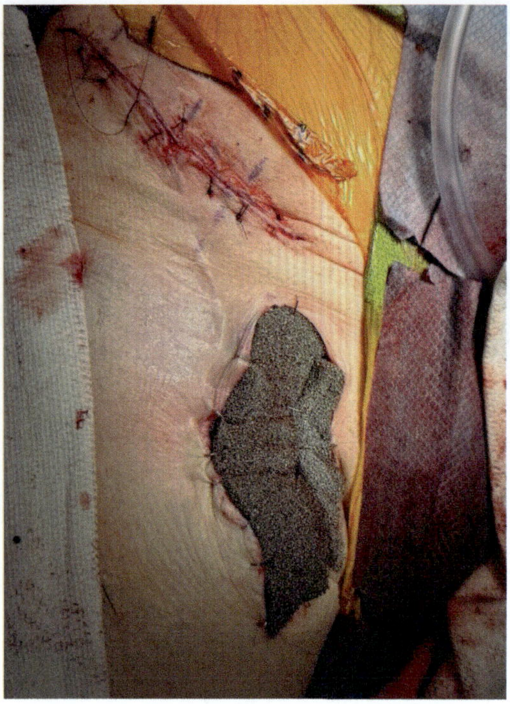

Fig. 23.7 Closure of right lower extremity incision and negative pressure wound therapy over the debrided area in the right groin and upper thigh

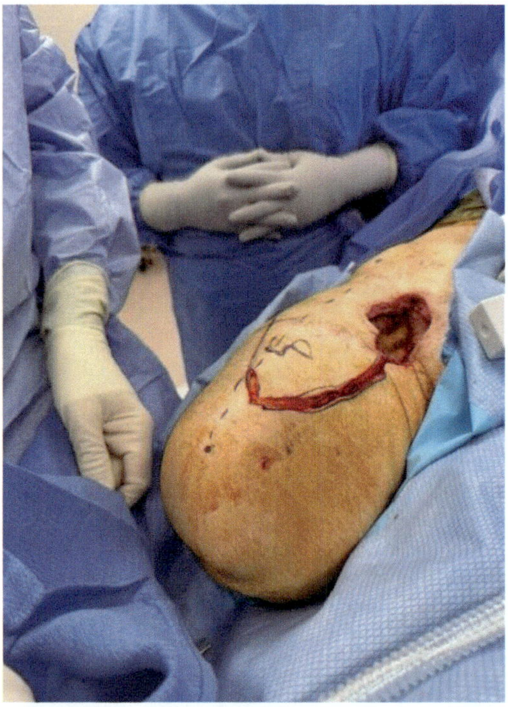

Fig. 23.8 Rotation skin flap planned inferior to the large defect in the right groin for wound closure

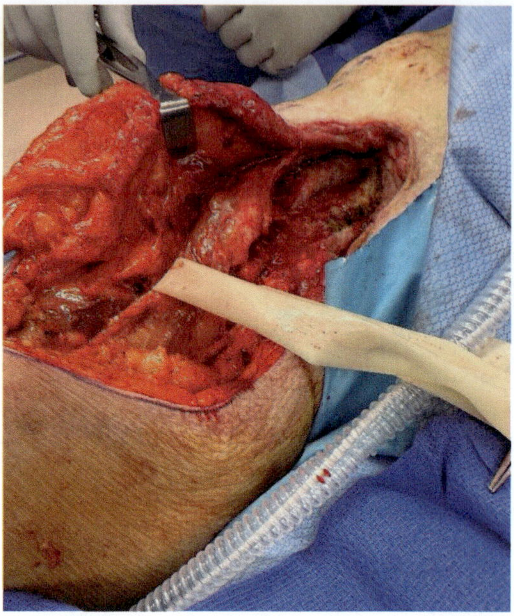

Fig. 23.9 Lateral flap of skin dissected and sartorius muscle mobilized, and a Penrose drain passed around the sartorius

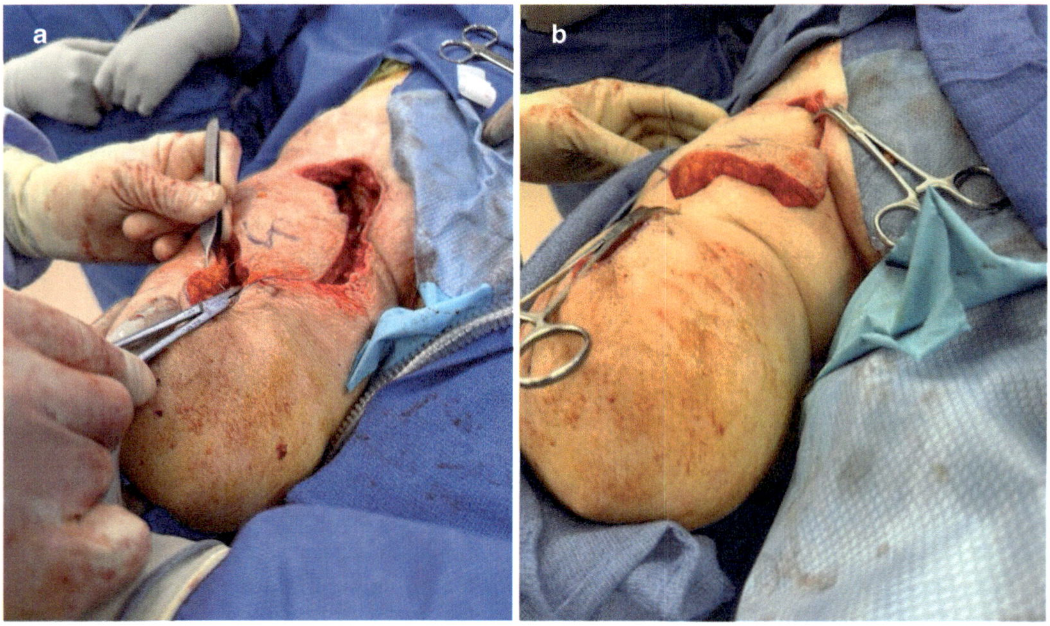

Fig. 23.10 (**a**) Skin flap advanced superiorly, and deeper tissues sutured (**b**) Skin flap advanced superiorly, and skin to be approximated with sutures and staples

power of attorney (DPOA) decided to place her under Hospice Care 2 months following discharge.

Discussion

Recurrent femoral pseudoaneurysms are extremely uncommon in the absence of infection. For iatrogenic femoral pseudoaneurysms, ultrasound-guided compression, ultrasound-guided percutaneous thrombin injection, and operative repair are standard treatment options. Ultrasound-guided compression of a femoral pseudoaneurysm is painful and takes a longer time (average time 33 minutes) and requires concurrent sedation. A success rate of 75–98% has been reported [1].

Ultrasound-guided thrombin injection is the modality of choice for post-catheterization femoral pseudoaneurysm with a success rate of 91–100% [1]. Patients with a large femoral pseudoaneurysm with associated skin necrosis should undergo surgical repair.

The common microorganisms cultured from femoral mycotic pseudoaneurysms are gram-positive, such as Staphylococcus aureus, Staphylococcus epidermidis, and Enterococcus faecalis. Gram-negative, such as E. coli, Salmonella species, Pseudomonas, Bacteroides fragilis, Clostridium, Propionibacterium species, and anaerobic. Gram-negative bacilli are mostly from the Bacteroides fragilis group.

This patient was on intravenous antibiotics for a prolonged period. It is possible that an ongoing low-grade infection in the arterial wall resulted in the recurrence of the pseudoaneurysm. In patients with a large groin wound following repair of a femoral pseudoaneurysm, wound washout, debridement, and consultation with a plastic surgeon should be obtained to achieve satisfactory tissue coverage.

The most used muscle flaps for infected femoral pseudoaneurysms are Rectus femoris, Gracilis, and Rectus abdominis. Some patients may require a rotation flap (fascia) of the skin for wound closure, which was performed in this patient.

Proximal control of the external iliac artery is a valuable aid in the repair of large recurrent, potentially infected femoral pseudoaneurysms. Since this patient had a prior above-knee amputation, revascularization following ligation of the proximal SFA was not necessary.

In patients with non-availability of autologous vein, the great saphenous vein (GSV, a femoral vein), Rifampicin impregnated Dacron graft with proximal anastomosis to the iliac artery and graft tunneled through the obturator foramen with distal anastomosis to the mid superficial femoral artery can be a suitable alternative choice. Ligation of the femoral artery without revascularization results in an amputation rate of 25–35% [2]. The internal iliac artery has also been used as an arterial conduit for interposition in the femoral artery in patients with a mycotic aneurysm. The great saphenous vein (GSV) from the contralateral leg or the superficial femoral vein can also be used as a conduit for bypass [2, 3]. The success rate of revascularization in the presence of infection is poor. Common femoral artery ligation and local debridement are safe modalities for iatrogenic femoral artery pseudoaneurysms in patients with intravenous drug abuse [2, 3]. A multidisciplinary team approach is required in managing complex femoral artery pseudoaneurysms to achieve satisfactory results.

Multiple Choice Questions

1. Ligation of the common femoral artery in patients with mycotic aneurysm of the femoral artery without revascularization results in an amputation rate of:
   A. 40–45%
   B. 35–39%
   C. 25–35%
   D. 15–24%
2. Following repair of an infected femoral pseudoaneurysm with skin breakdown, negative pressure wound therapy, wash outs, and intravenous antibiotics, the tissue coverage is best obtained by
   A. Sartorius muscle flap
   B. Rectus femoris flap
   C. Gracilis muscle flap
   D. Tensor Fascia lata flap
3. The most common microorganisms cultured from mycotic femoral pseudoaneurysms are:
   A. Gram-positive cocci
   B. Gram-negative bacilli
   C. Anaerobic Gram-negative bacilli
   D. Gram-positive cocci, Gram-negative bacilli, and anaerobic Gram-negative bacilli

Answers: 1 (C), 2 (B), 3 (D)

References

1. Webber GW, Jang J, Gustavson S, Olin JW. Contemporary management of postcatheterization pseudoaneurysms. Circulation. 2007;115(20):2666–74. PMID:17515479
2. Arora S, Weber MA, Fox CJ, Neville R, Lidor A, Sidawy AN. Common femoral artery ligation and local debridement: a safe treatment for infected femoral artery pseudoaneurysms. J Vasc Surg. 2001;33(5):990–3. PMID:11331839
3. Hans SS. Mycotic femoral artery aneurysms. In: Springer, editor. Contemporary Management of Lower Extremity Aneurysmal Disease. 1st ed. Berlin: Springer; 2025.

24 Complex Femoral Anastomotic Aneurysm Following Redo Aortofemoral Graft

Presentation

A 62-year-old woman, a former smoker (40 pack years) with a history of hypertension and hyperlipidemia, was seen in the vascular clinic in December 2020 with a large pulsatile mass in the left groin and a smaller pulsatile mass in the right groin. She had undergone an Aortobifemoral graft in 2000 and a repeat aortobifemoral bypass graft in 2005 at an out-of-state hospital. Duplex ultrasound showed a 6.5 cm left femoral and 3.5 cm right femoral artery anastomotic aneurysm (FAAA). CTA of the abdomen and pelvis revealed the aneurysms (Figs. 24.1 and 24.2).

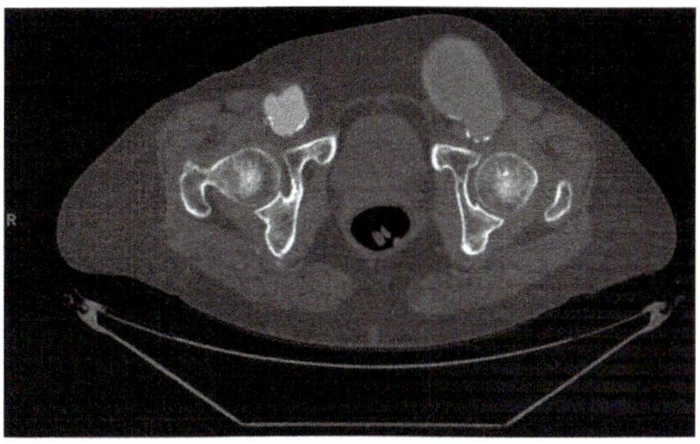

Fig. 24.1 CTA of the abdomen and pelvis demonstrates a 6.5 cm left femoral aneurysm and a 3.5 cm right femoral aneurysm

The patient underwent urgent repair of FAAA using a left lower quadrant transverse incision, about 4 cm above the left groin crease. Retroperitoneal exposure of the left external iliac artery was obtained after the peritoneal envelope with the ureter was retracted medially and cephalad. Two Dacron limbs of the graft (one occluded and one patent) were seen. A Silastic vessel loop was passed around the functioning limb of the Dacron graft. The aneurysm was then exposed using a hockey stick groin incision through the scar tissue resulting from two prior groin incisions. The aneurysm was mobilized using primarily a sharp dissection.

With careful dissection, the proximal superficial femoral artery (SFA) and profunda femoris artery were exposed and mobilized in their proximal segments. No attempt was made to dissect the aneurysm medially. After systemic heparinization, the anastomotic aneurysm was opened following application of proximal and distal vascular clamps. The aneurysm was resected including the distal most portion limb of the aortofemoral graft was transected. The graft was well incorportaed. A new 8 mm Dacron graft was selected and a proximal anastomisis was performed in an end-to-end fashion with a 4′0″ CV polypropelene suture to the transected limb of the remotely placed ABF graft. Because the aneurysm extended into the orifice of the profunda femoris artery, it was divided completely with a 2–3 mm cuff to be used as a Carrel patch for reimplantation into an 8 mm knitted Dacron graft (Vascutek, Inchinnan, Scotland) with 5′0″ CV polypropelene CV suture (Fig. 24.3). The distal anastomosis of the new Dacron graft

S. S. Hans, *Secondary and Tertiary Arterial Reconstructions*,
https://doi.org/10.1007/978-3-032-21214-6_24

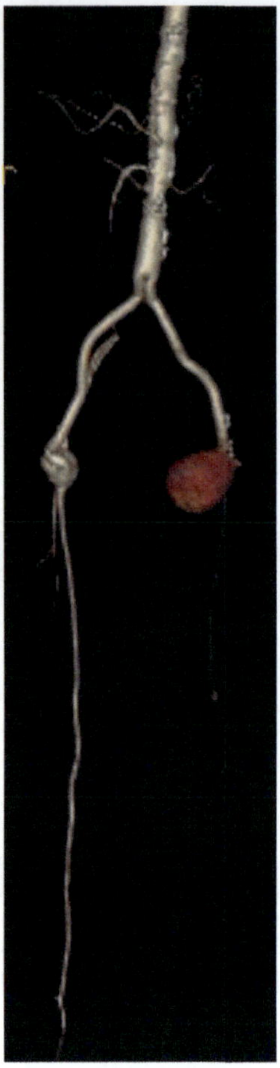

Fig. 24.2 CTA abdomen and pelvis and runoff show patent aortobifemoral graft and a large left femoral artery anastomotic aneurysm and a moderate-sized right femoral anastomotic aneurysm

was performed to the proximal SFA in an end-to-end fashion with 5′0″ CV polypropelene suture just below the site of the reimplantation of the profunda femoris artery.

The patient underwent uneventful repair of the right femoral anastomotic aneurysm in 2021. Follow-up duplex imaging approximately 2 years later showed elevation of the peak systolic velocity in the proximal SFA. A left SFA angioplasty was performed using left brachial artery access. At the last follow-up in January 2025, there was no recurrence of the anastomotic aneurysm by clinical examination and by duplex imaging.

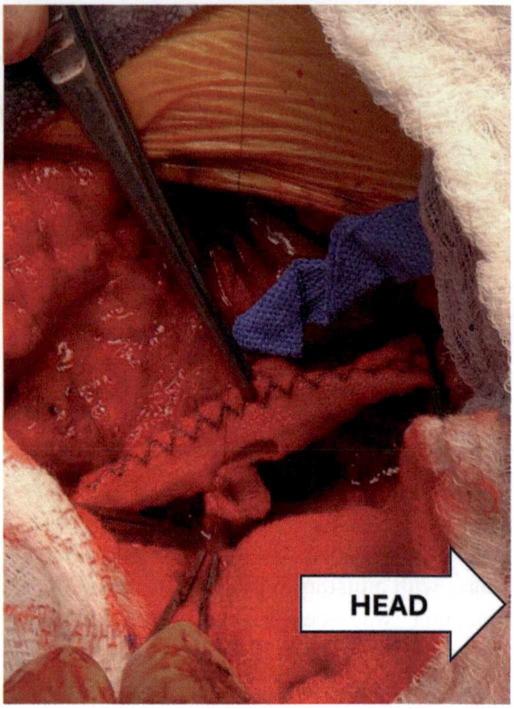

Fig. 24.3 Repair of femoral anastomotic aneurysm with interposition of an 8 mm Dacron graft and reimplantation of profunda femoris artery as a Carrell patch

Discussion

The incidence of FAAAs after AFB grafting ranges from 1% to 5% with higher rates reported in some series with longer follow-up and routine surveillance by imaging studies. Some series have reported an incidence of 23% 15 years after AFS grafting [1]. Progressive degeneration of the femoral artery, local low-grade infection, repeated hip movement, reoperation in the groin, and excessive tension at the femoral anastomosis are important factors in the development of femoral anastomotic aneurysms. [1, 2]

Patients being evaluated for anastomotic femoral aneurysm should undergo duplex imaging of the groin followed by CT angiography of the entire graft to rule out low-grade infection (gas or perigraft fluid) involving the graft. Following repair of femoral anastomotic aneurysm, patients should undergo yearly femoral duplex imaging as recurrence of such aneurysms is not uncommon. The common postoperative complications include hemorrhage, lymphatic leak, and surgical site infection. Surgical site infection is more common following repair of the FAAAs than repair of the common femoral artery aneurysm. Graft occlusion following repair is uncommon.

Patients presenting with large femoral AAAs (greater than 5.0 cm in diameter) often present with pain and compressive symptoms manifesting as femoral cutaneous neuropathy due to compression of the branches of the femoral nerve. This can result in paresthesia and pain in the region of the thigh. Swelling of the limb may occur due to femoral vein compression. Large-sized femoral AAAs may rupture, leading to pain and ecchymosis; hypotension is uncommon due to the contained nature of the rupture.

Repairing large and recurrent femoral aneurysms carries similar morbidity and mortality as compared to uncomplicated femoral AAAs, but has greater blood loss and requires longer operative time. After initial ABF bypass grafting, Duplex imaging should be performed at 5 years and if an aneurysm is detected, surveillance should be performed yearly according to the guidelines of the Society for Vascular Surgeons [3].

Multiple Choice Questions

1. A 68-year-old woman presents with a left groin pulsatile mass 10 years following an aortobifemoral aneurysm. Duplex ultrasound confirms a 6.0 cm left femoral anastomotic aneurysm. She should undergo further evaluation by:
   A. CTA pelvis.
   B. CTA abdomen and pelvis and runoff.
   C. Catheter-based abdominal and pelvic arteriogram.
   D. MRA abdomen and pelvis
2. The incidence of femoral anastomotic aneurysms after 15 years of aortofemoral bypass grafting can be as high as:
   A. 3%
   B. 13%
   C. 23%
   D. 28%
3. The most common complication following repair of the femoral anastomotic aneurysm is:
   A. Lymphatic leak
   B. Hemorrhage
   C. Graft thrombosis
   D. Surgical site infection

Answers: 1(B), 2(C), 3(D)

References

1. Mulder EJ, van Bockel JH, Maas J, van den Akker PJ, Hermans J. Morbidity and mortality of reconstructive surgery of noninfected false aneurysms detected long after aortic prosthetic reconstruction. Arch Surg. 1998;133(1):45–9. PMID:9438758
2. Seabrook GR, Schmitt DD, Bandyk DF, et al. Anastomotic femoral pseudoaneurysm: an investigation of occult infection as an etiologic factor. J Vasc Surg. 1990;11(5):629–34. PMID:2139897
3. Chaikof EL, Dalman RL, Eskandari MK, Jackson BM, Lee WA, et al. The Society for Vascular Surgery practice guidelines on the care of patients with an abdominal aortic aneurysm. J Vasc Surg. 2018;67(1):2–77.e72. PMID:29268916

25 Antegrade Aortic-Superior Mesenteric Artery Bypass Graft for Chronic Intestinal Ischemia Complicated by Retrograde Thoracic Aortic Dissection

Presentation

A 75-year-old woman was evaluated in the emergency room in July 2020 with complaints of abdominal and back pain for the past 3 weeks. The pain was post-prandial and was associated with severe nausea and vomiting. She had loose bowel movements for the last 2 weeks. The patient had lost 20 pounds during the past 3 months. She was a former smoker (quit 10 years prior) with a history of smoking approximately 55 pack-years. Medical comorbidities included hypertension, hyperlipidemia, and chronic kidney disease (stage 3B).

Visceral Duplex imaging showed greater than 70% stenosis of the superior mesenteric artery (SMA) (Fig. 25.1a, b). The patient had a non--contrast CT scan of the abdomen obtained by her primary care physician due to chronic kidney disease (stage 3B). The scan revealed severe calcification at the origin of the superior mesenteric artery (SMA). She had a negative UGI endoscopy. She underwent abdominal aortography using femoral artery access with CO_2 and with 20 cc of contrast (Isovue 250) with selective catheterization of the celiac artery. There was occlusion of the proximal 3 cm of the SMA (Fig. 25.2). The celiac artery was patent with a calcified plaque narrowing the lumen to approximately 50%, and the inferior mesenteric artery (IMA) was patent. There were mesenteric collaterals in the form of an enlarged gastroduodenal artery

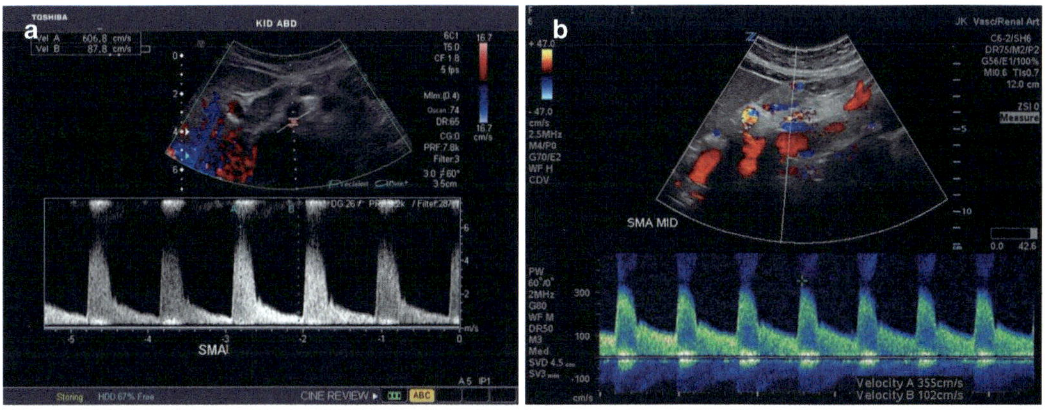

Fig. 25.1 (**a**) Duplex imaging showing greater than 70% stenosis SMA with marked elevation of PSV of the SMA (**b**) Duplex imaging showing greater than 70% stenosis SMA

S. S. Hans, *Secondary and Tertiary Arterial Reconstructions*,
https://doi.org/10.1007/978-3-032-21214-6_25

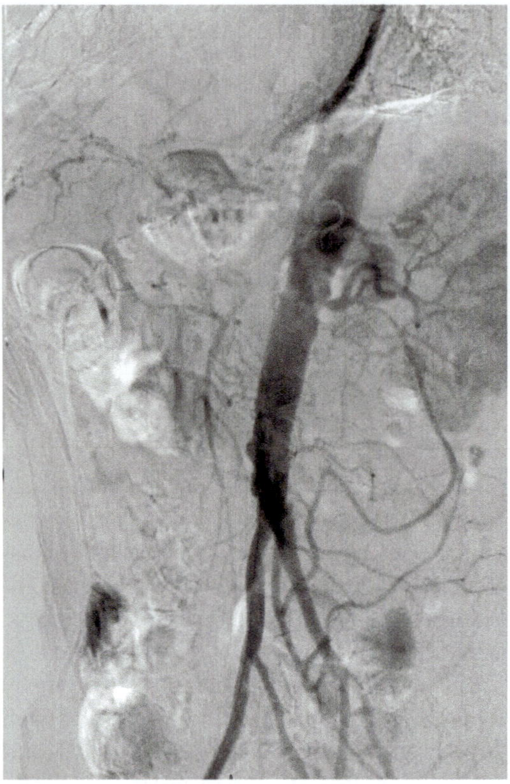

Fig. 25.2 Abdominal and visceral aortography showing proximal 3.0 cm occlusion of the SMA, enlarged gastroduodenal artery and Arc of Riolan as collateral flow

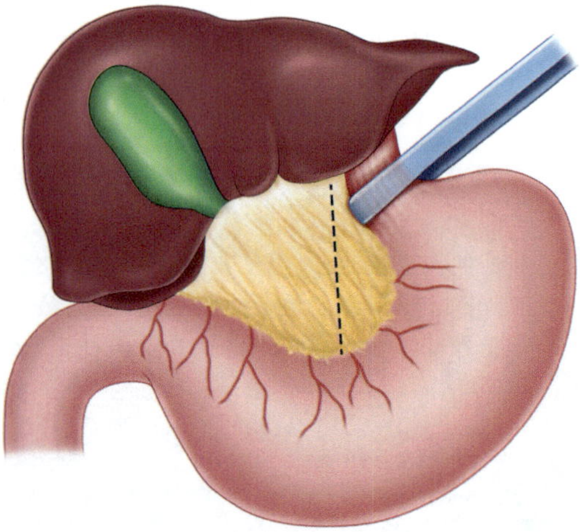

Fig. 25.3 Incision in gastrohepatic omentum for exposure of the supraceliac aorta

and arc of Riolan (Fig. 25.2). She underwent antegrade supraceliac aorta to superior mesenteric artery bypass using a midline laparotomy incision on August 20, 2020. The supraceliac and

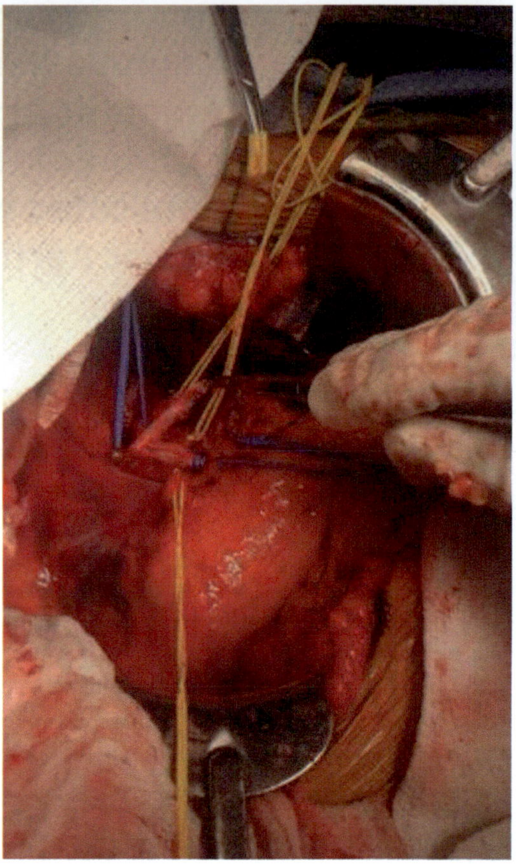

Fig. 25.4 Arteriotomy in the SMA with a blue silastic vessel loop proximally and distally and yellow silastic loops around the jejunal branches

aorta were exposed through an incision in the gastro-hepatic omentum (Fig. 25.3). Aortotomy in the supraceliac aorta revealed a calcified plaque in its inferior portion.

The SMA was exposed in the root of the mesentery artery, and silastic vessel loops were passed around the SMA and its jejunal branches (Fig. 25.4). The superior mesenteric artery was small in caliber. An 8 mm PTFE interring graft was anastomosed to the supraceliac aorta in an end-to-side fashion with a continuous 4′0″ cardiovascular polypropylene suture. The calcified plaque was partially removed from the aorta. A large Satinsky was applied to the supraceliac aorta as a side-biting clamp. The graft was brought posterior to the stomach but anterior to the pancreas (Fig. 25.5) and anastomosed to the SMA distally after it was opened longitudinally and a saphenous vein patch was sutured to the

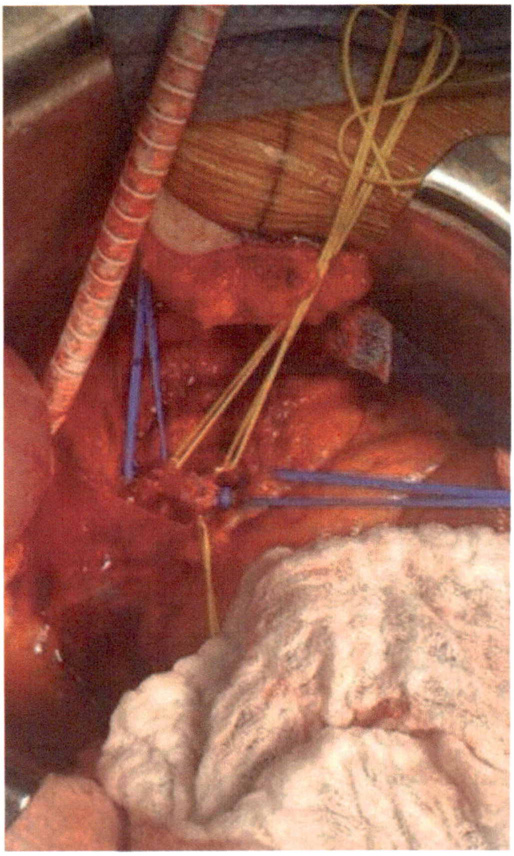

Fig. 25.5 Vein patch graft over the arteriotomy in the SMA and ringed PTFE graft brought anterior to the pancreas in preparation for distal anastomosis to the SMA using an incision in the vein patch graft in an end-to-side fashion

SMA as a patch graft (Fig. 25.5). An incision was made in the vein patch graft, and a distal anastomosis was performed to the vein patch in the SMA in an end-to-side fashion.

She was discharged on the 7th postoperative day and was seen in the clinic 2 weeks later for removal of the sutures. She was readmitted to the hospital on November 16, 2020, with paroxysmal atrial fibrillation and was treated with beta--blockers and Apixaban (Eliquis).

She underwent CTA Abdomen, which showed retrograde Type B Aortic Dissection distal to the origin of the left subclavian artery to the distal thoracic aorta with a false lumen larger than the true lumen with retrograde aortic dissection starting just proximal to the diaphragm (Fig. 25.6a, b). There was rim-enhancing fluid (5.1 × 3.7 cm) around the periaortic region at the proximal anastomosis. The fluid diminished around the origin of the celiac artery in comparison to the prior CT scan. Retrograde dissection probably resulted from calcified plaque separating from the aortic wall at the site of proximal anastomosis (supraceliac aorta).

She was treated conservatively with anti--impulse therapy. A repeat CTA of the chest and abdomen revealed that the false lumen was smaller distal to the origin of the subclavian artery. The connection between the true lumen and false lumen had decreased from 3.4 cm to

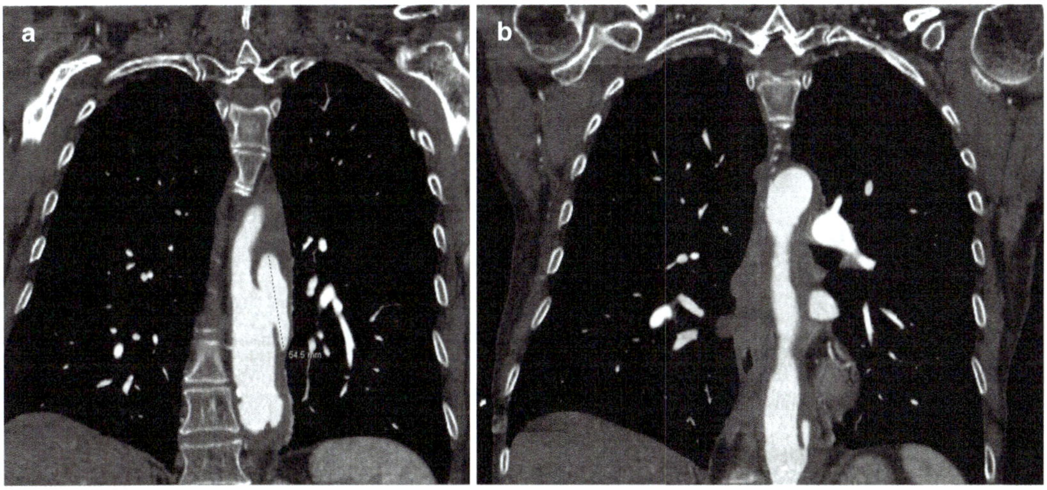

Fig. 25.6 (a) Follow-up CTA chest and abdomen showing retrograde thoracic aortic dissection (b) Follow-up CTA chest and abdomen showing retrograde thoracic aortic dissection originating just above the diaphragm

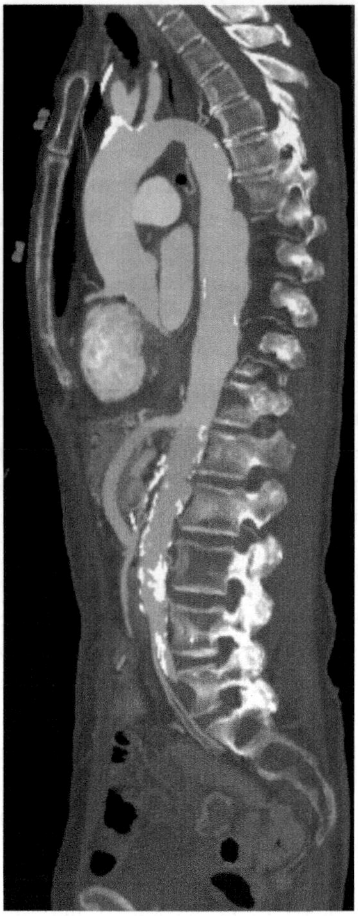

Fig. 25.7 CTA chest and abdomen patent aorto-superior mesenteric artery bypass and aneurysmal changes in the thoracic aorta

3.0 cm. There was a slight aneurysmal dilatation of the thoracic aorta and patency of the supraceliac aorta to SMA bypass graft (Fig. 25.7).

She was seen for follow-up on April 25, 2025. Symptoms of intestinal angina had resolved, and aortic dissection has remained stable, 56 months after aorto-mesenteric bypass.

The patient was seen in the clinic on December 17, 2025, with symptoms of weight loss and dysphagia. She lost 20 pounds of body weight during the last 6 months. She underwent an upper G.I. endoscopy, which was negative for any mass lesions in the esophagus or stomach. On January 6, 2026, she underwent CTA of the chest and abdomen, which showed a stable descending thoracic aortic dissection with the largest transverse diameter of the thoracic aorta measuring 4.2 centimeters. The false lumen of the descending thoracic aortic dissection had completely thrombosed. The perigraft fluid around the origin of the superior mesenteric artery (SMA) bypass had completely resolved. The aortic—SMA bypass was widely patent. Her symptoms were most likely due to a Hiatal hernia per opinion of the gastroenterologist.

Discussion

The diagnosis of chronic mesenteric ischemia is being considered more often because of better awareness of the symptoms of the disease and the readily available visceral duplex imaging for evaluation of patients with suspected mesenteric artery occlusive disease. The optimal method of treatment and type of revascularization (open versus endovascular) and type of surgical repair (transaortic endarterectomy versus aortomesenteric bypass grafting; antegrade versus retrograde bypass) remain controversial [1]. In most series, long-term patency after revascularization with objective means is lacking. Endovascular therapy is significantly less invasive but is mostly successful in patients with stenotic lesions of visceral arteries. Antegrade synthetic aortomesenteric bypass is associated with good long-term graft patency and a satisfactory functional outcome, as reported by Jimenez et al. in 47 patients. They reported in-hospital mortality of 11% and primary assisted and secondary 5-year graft patency of 69% [2]. Most surgeons tunnel the aortic-SMA bypass graft posterior to the pancreas. This author preferentially tunnels the graft anterior to the pancreas in all antegrade SMA bypass grafts.

Type B aortic dissection in this patient was probably a retrograde dissection from the separation of the calcified plaque in the aorta near the origin of the celiac artery. The degree of calcification could not be determined preoperatively because of a non-contrast study of the chest and abdomen was obtained due to low eGFR. A case report of retrograde type B aortic dissection after fenestrated branched endovascular aortic aneurysm repair has been reported [3]. The dissection extends superiorly from the distal descending thoracic or proximal abdominal aorta, potentially causing malperfusion with reduced arterial flow to major branches of the aorta, leading to visceral ischemia. The patient in this report was managed medically because retrograde Type B aortic dissection was asymptomatic without any evidence of associated visceral ischemia. The diameter of the thoracic aorta has remained stable, and the patient has been followed for 4 years without any complications.

Several techniques for mesenteric revascularization are available, including visceral aortic endarterectomy, antegrade arterial bypass, retrograde arterial bypass, and hybrid revascularization. In acute settings, retrograde SMA stenting is being increasingly used for revascularization. In patients with unsatisfactory cardiopulmonary status and significant calcific disease in the supraceliac aorta, a retrograde aortic (iliac) to SMA bypass using an 8 mm ringed PTFE graft in a "lazy C" configuration to the proximal SMA, thus avoiding aortic clamping, is a satisfactory option. Proximal aortic clamping often results in increased afterload, with a decrease in stroke volume and ejection fraction. This has the potential to cause myocardial ischemia and infarction.

Due to the high rate of recurrence, following visceral artery reconstruction, both short-term and long-term follow-up with imaging studies are important to assess the patency of revascularization and plan future intervention if necessary, in patients with symptomatic mesenteric arterial disease.

Multiple Choice Questions

1. The morbidity of Antegrade supraceliac aortic-superior mesenteric bypass for chronic mesenteric ischemia is
   A. 5%
   B. 5–10%
   C. 11–12%
   D. greater than 12%
2. Reported primary and secondary 5-year graft patency of antegrade aortic-superior mesenteric bypass is.
   A. 50%
   B. 51–60%
   C. 61–70%
   D. 71–80%
3. Besides close monitoring for potential complications, Type B aortic dissection should be initially managed by:
   A. Surgery
   B. TEVAR
   C. HYBRID repair
   D. Anti-impulse therapy
4. A 70-year-old woman has classic symptoms of chronic mesenteric ischemia.

   CTA of the abdomen and pelvis shows 50% stenosis of the celiac artery, occlusion of the proximal 3 centimeters of the SMA, and a patent IMA with enlarged collaterals. The supraceliac aorta shows mild atherosclerotic changes. Which procedure will provide the best long-term outcome?
   A. Retrograde aortic-iliac artery to SMA bypass graft
   B. Antegrade aortic-superior mesenteric artery bypass graft
   C. Aortic (visceral) endarterectomy
   D. Stenting of the celiac artery and retrograde aortic-iliac/SMA bypass graft

Answers: 1(C), 2(C), 3(D), 4(B)

References

1. Scali ST, Ayo D, Giles KA, Gray S, Kubilis P, Back M, et al. Outcomes of antegrade and retrograde open mesenteric bypass for acute mesenteric ischemia. J Vasc Surg. 2019;69(1):129–40. PMID:30580778
2. Jimenez JG, Huber TS, Ozaki CK, Flynn TC, Berceli SA, Lee WA, Seeger JM. Durability of antegrade synthetic aortomesenteric bypass for chronic mesenteric ischemia. J Vasc Surg. 2002;35(6):1078–84. PMID:12042717
3. Chen JF, Tan KT, Lindsay TF. Retrograde type B aortic dissection after fenestrated-branched endovascular aortic aneurysm repair. J Vasc Surg Cases Innov Tech. 2024;10(6):101586. PMID:40027268

26 Renal Artery in-Stent Stenosis for Renovascular Hypertension in a Patient with a Solitary Kidney

Presentation

A 52-year-old man was referred by his nephrologist in October 2014 for possible renal artery stenting for uncontrolled hypertension. The patient had a history of hypertension for the prior 10 years and had undergone laparoscopic nephrectomy in 2012 for an atrophic kidney secondary to renal artery occlusive disease with labile hypertension. He's been followed for a small abdominal aortic aneurysm. He was on four blood pressure medications (amlodipine, metoprolol, hydrochlorothiazide, and clonidine). The patient underwent MRA in 2002, which showed occlusion of the right renal artery and moderate stenosis of the left renal artery (Fig. 26.1). In September 2014, the patient underwent a renal duplex study, which showed a normal-sized left kidney with greater than 70% stenosis of the left renal artery. The patient underwent abdominal and renal arteriogram on October 25, 2014, via right femoral artery approach using micropuncture technique followed by insertion of a 5F sheath. Using an Omniflush catheter (AngioDynamics, Latham, NY) over an angle stiff GLIDEWIRE® (Terumo, Tokyo, Japan), (180-cm-long 035 mm) abdominal aortogram showed slight aneurysmal dilatation of the abdominal aorta and 80% stenosis at the origin of the left renal artery (Fig. 26.2). A 5F sheath was replaced with a 6F, 45 cm angled Pinnacle sheath (Terumo, Tokyo, Japan). Using an SOS Omni catheter (AngioDynamics, Latham, NY) and a standard glidewire 0.035″ 180 cm long, the catheter was advanced into the upper pole branch of the left renal artery. The glidewire was exchanged for a 180-cm-long 0.035″ Magic Torque wire (Boston Scientific, Marlborough, MA), and long sheath was advanced near the origin of the left renal artery. A 6 × 19 mm Omnilink

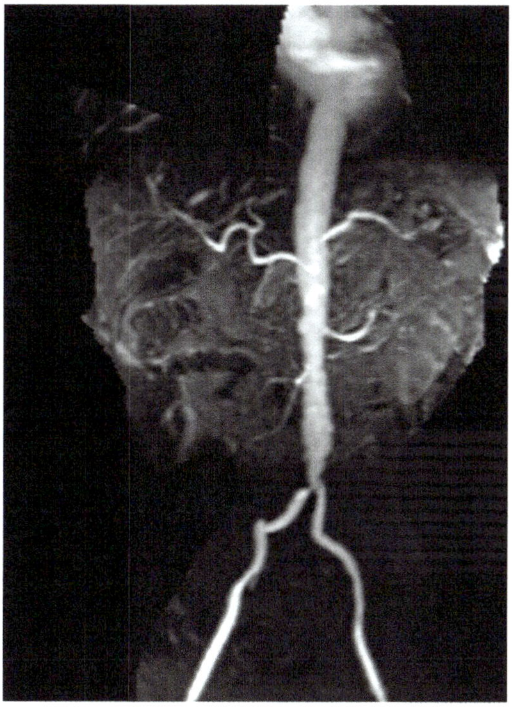

Fig. 26.1 MRA showing right renal artery occlusion and moderate stenosis of the left renal artery in 2002

S. S. Hans, *Secondary and Tertiary Arterial Reconstructions*,
https://doi.org/10.1007/978-3-032-21214-6_26

(Abbott, Abbott Park, IL) balloon-expandable stent was advanced through the sheath. The sheath was retracted, and the stent was deployed with 2 mm of the stent projecting into the lumen of the aorta. 14 atmospheric pressure was used for inflation of the balloon so that the final diameter of the stent was 6.4 cm (Fig. 26.3). The patient was followed for 1.5 years with no evidence of recurrent stenosis with better control of blood pressure.

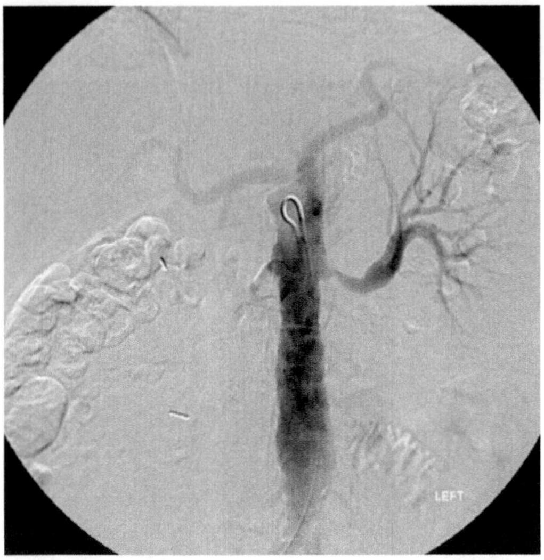

Fig. 26.2 Abdominal aortogram showing greater than 80% left renal artery stenosis in 2014

Follow-up duplex imaging of the left renal artery showed normal peak velocity in November 2014 and in June 2015. In June 2016, a further follow-up renal artery duplex imaging showed greater than 70% left renal artery stenosis with elevation of serum creatinine from 0.9 to 1.2 mg/dL. In July 2016, the patient underwent left renal artery angioplasty for in-stent restenosis (greater than 70%) via percutaneous left brachial artery approach using an exchange-length 260-cm-long 0.035″ glidewire via a 6F 90-cm-long sheath. A 6 mm × 2 cm long balloon was used for angioplasty (Figs. 26.4 and 26.5). During the latter part of the procedure, the patient complained of left flank pain associated with nausea and diaphoresis. He underwent an emergency CT scan of the abdomen, which showed a large subcapsular hematoma of the left kidney with a small retroperitoneal hemorrhage (Fig. 26.6). Since the patient was hemodynamically stable, he was treated conservatively, and his symptoms resolved in 6 h, and he was discharged after a 24-h stay with a stable hematocrit. He was last seen in June 2025, with blood pressure well controlled on Hydralazine and Amlodipine, and serum creatinine 1.7 mg/dL and eGFR 45. Aortic renal duplex study showed normal PSV left renal artery and normal resistive index. Abdominal aortic aneurysm measured 4.8 × 4.8 cm at last follow-up.

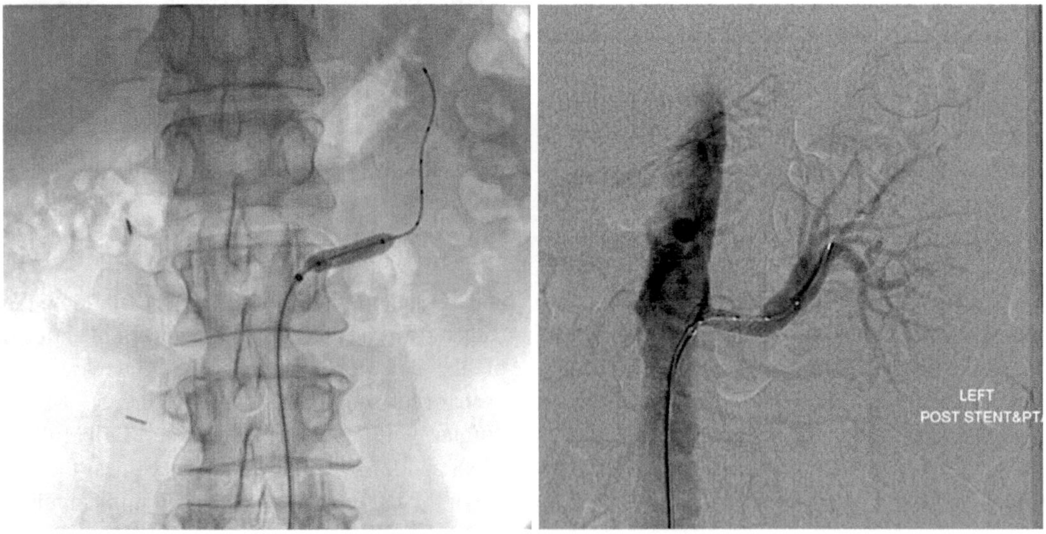

Fig. 26.3 Abdominal aortogram following renal artery stenting

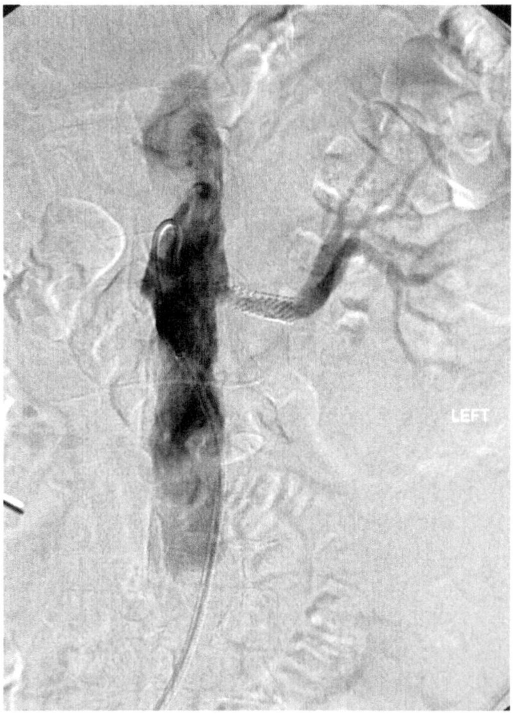

Fig. 26.4 Renal arteriogram showing in-stent stenosis of the left renal artery stent

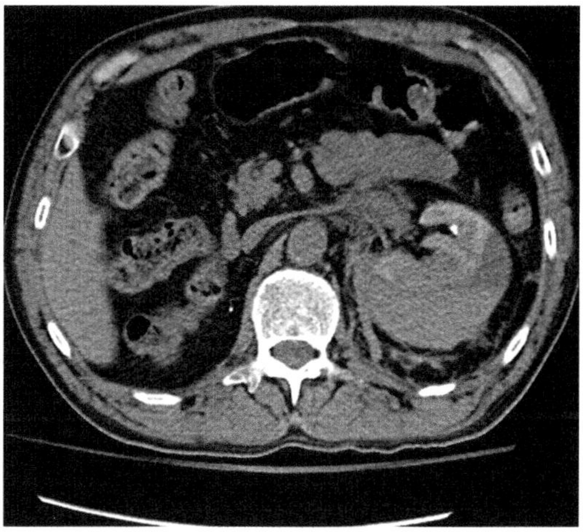

Fig. 26.6 CTA showing left renal subcapsular hematoma

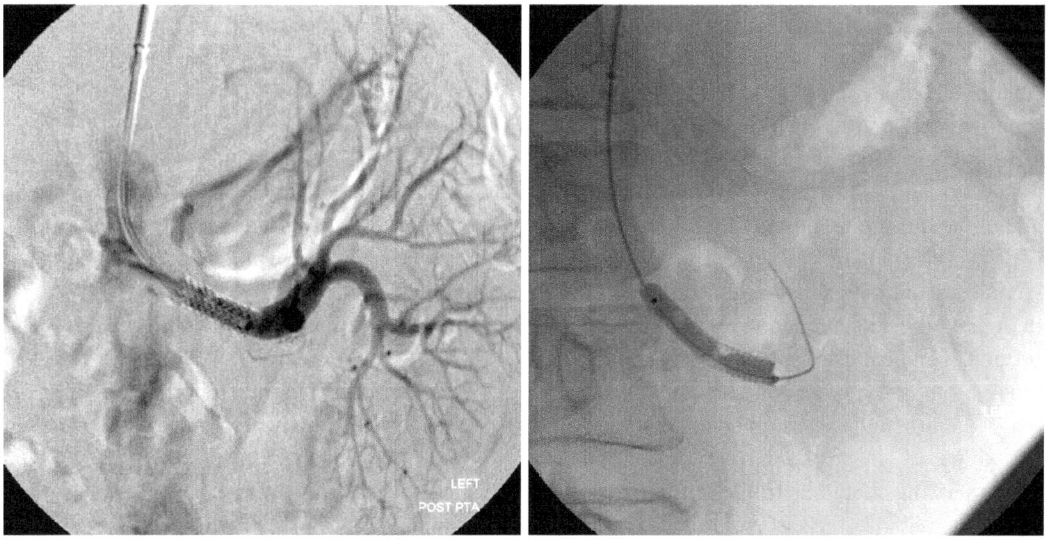

Fig. 26.5 Renal angioplasty via a brachial approach for in-stent restenosis

Discussion

Atherosclerotic renal artery stenosis accounts for greater than 90% cases of renal artery stenosis and most often presents in patients greater than 65 years of age [1]. It may be an independent predictor of death in patients with coronary artery disease [1]. Patients with cardiac destabilization syndromes, renal vascular hypertension, and ischemic nephropathy who are unresponsive to medical therapy are most likely to benefit from renal artery revascularization [1].

The result of the CORAL (Cardiovascular Outcomes in Renal Atherosclerotic Lesions) trial has significantly decreased the indications for renal angioplasty (stenting) for atherosclerotic renal artery stenosis. The CORAL trial did not show a statistically significant reduction in blood pressure following renal angioplasty/stenting when compared with best medical management. Studies evaluating the use of renal angioplasty/stenting for preservation of renal function have been even less promising, with no advantage for renal intervention but with the added possibility of access-related complications [1]. Subgroup analysis of the CORAL trial failed to identify the severity of blood pressure as a good predictor of response to renal artery stenting. The one baseline variable that appears promising for predicting a favorable response to stent intervention is the urine albumin to creatinine ratio, with a low UACR (urine albumin-to-creatinine ratio) portending a favorable response [2]. In this patient, because of uncontrolled blood pressure with a severe renal artery stenosis in a solitary kidney, renal stenting was performed. The benefits of renal artery stenting for renal vascular hypertension and preservation of renal function must be weighed against the complications of intervention. At present, renal artery stenting should be infrequently performed [3]. However, renal artery stenting may need to be performed during or following endovascular aneurysm repair in a select group of patients [3]. In contemporary practice, there are fewer indications of renal artery stenting, and patients should be very carefully selected in close consultation with a nephrologist. Primary patency of renal artery stenting exceeds 80% at 5 years, and surveillance for in-stent restenosis should be done with renal duplex imaging on a yearly basis, with the first follow-up study at 1 month to detect any residual stenosis or any other technical problem.

Multiple Choice Questions

1. Results of the CORAL TRIAL showed that renal angioplasty/stenting for atherosclerotic renal artery stenosis is
   A. Superior to medical management of renovascular hypertension
   B. Inferior to medical management of renovascular hypertension
   C. Equivalent to medical management of renovascular hypertension
   D. Markedly superior in preserving renal function
2. Primary patency of the renal artery, starting at 5 years, exceeds
   A. 70%
   B. 75%
   C. 80%
   D. 85%
3. Management of subcapsular hematoma due to guidewire perforation during renal artery stenting in a hemodynamically stable patient should be managed by
   A. Close observation, serial hematocrit, and CT imaging
   B. Arteriography and embolization
   C. Surgical drainage of hematoma and control of bleeding vessel
   D. Percutaneous drainage

Answers: 1(C), 2(C), 3(A)

References

1. Tafur JD, White CJ. Renal artery stenosis: when to revascularize in 2017. Curr Probl Cardiol. 2017;42(4):110–35. PMID:28325353
2. Gupta R, Assiri S, Cooper CJ. Renal artery stenosis: new findings from the CORAL trial. Curr Cardiol Rep. 2017;19(9):75. PMID:28752274
3. Alexander J, Green D, Sullivan TM. Endovascular intervention for renal artery occlusive disease. In: Hans SS, Shepard AD, Bove P, Weaver MR, Long GW, editors. Endovascular and open vascular reconstruction: a practical approach. Boca Raton: CRC Press; 2017. p. 19–25.

27 Iliac Artery Stenting Complicated by Iliac Artery Rupture

Presentation

A 63-year-old woman was evaluated by a staff vascular surgeon in September 2016 with a history of disabling claudication affecting the left lower extremity on walking 50 yards. Medical comorbidities included coronary artery disease, hypertension, hyperlipidemia, and hypothyroidism. She was a former smoker with a history of smoking 50 pack years. The vascular surgeon performed a retrograde abdominal aortogram using right femoral artery access, which revealed left external iliac artery occlusion (Fig. 27.1). An attempt was made to cross the occluded segment with a glidewire using bilateral femoral access, but intervention was unsuccessful. She was referred to our clinic in September 2022 by her interventional cardiologist for long-segment occlusion of the left iliac artery (both common iliac and left external iliac artery occlusion—TASC II—D), moderate to severe stenosis of the left common femoral artery, and for possible aortobifemoral graft reconstruction. Her symptoms had progressed to ischemic rest pain in the left foot. A Doppler arterial study in September 2022 showed an ABI of 0.77 (right) and 0.38 (left). The Toe Brachial index on the right was 0.54 and 0.33 on the left. Another attempt at percutaneous revascularization was recommended prior to consideration of an open arterial reconstruction.

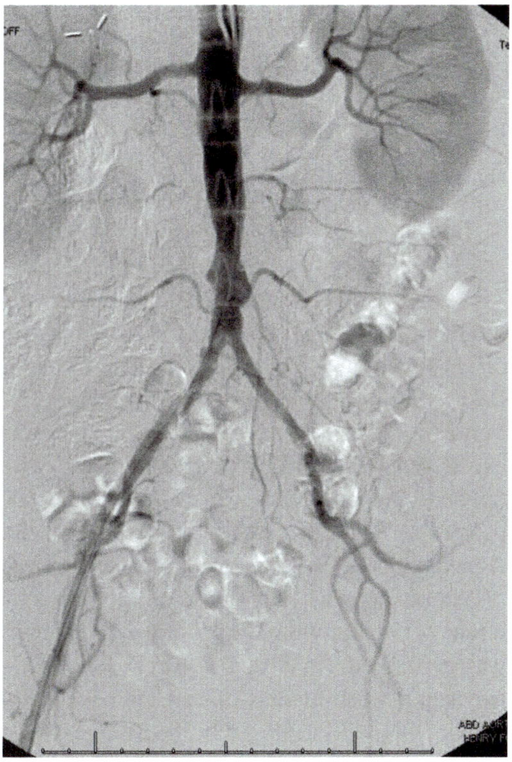

Fig. 27.1 Abdominal and pelvic aortogram in 2016 showed left external iliac artery occlusion and slight aneurysmal dilation of the distal abdominal aorta

In October 2022, under ultrasound guidance left brachial artery was punctured using a micropuncture technique, an abdominal and pelvic aortogram was obtained which showed complete occlusion of left common iliac artery 1 cm from its origin, left external iliac artery occlusion (Fig. 27.2). The lesion was crossed with a long

S. S. Hans, *Secondary and Tertiary Arterial Reconstructions*,
https://doi.org/10.1007/978-3-032-21214-6_27

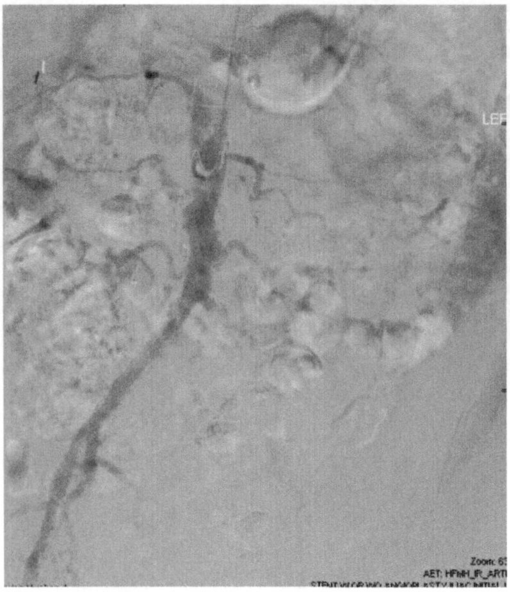

Fig. 27.2 Abdominal and pelvic arteriogram in October 2022 showed progression of arterial occlusion with involvement of the common iliac artery

(260 cm, 0.035″ glidewire) advanced through a 5F Halo sheath (Becton Dickinson, Franklin Lakes, NJ) with the aid of a 125 cm long 5F Vertebral catheter (Fig. 27.3). The glidewire was exchanged for a 300 cm long Spartacore wire (Abbott, Abbott Park, IL). The sheath was upsized to 7F for the passage of a covered stent. A preangioplasty with gradually increasing sizes of Armada balloons (5 mm × 15 cm, followed by 6 mm × 15 cm, followed by 7 mm × 8 cm long) was performed. An 8 mm × 10 cm long self--expanding Smart Stent (Cordis, Cardinal Health, Dublin, OH) was deployed in the distal external iliac artery (just above the acetabulum) and extending proximally. A 7 × 29 mm VBX (WL GORE) was deployed proximal to the Smart Stent with a 1-cm overlap balloon pressure increased to 10 atmospheric pressure so that the final diameter of the stent was 7.5 mm. Our plan was to deploy an 8 × 29 mm VBX stent, but it would not advance through the 7F sheath. After deployment of the VBX stent, the patient became diaphoretic, and systolic BP dropped to 90 mmHg. Contrast injection revealed extravasation of the contrast (Fig. 27.4). The 7F sheath was exchanged for an 8F long sheath. At the site of contrast extravasation, a low-pressure (4 atmospheric pressure) balloon inflation using a 7 × 6 cm Armada balloon, followed by deployment of an 8 × 59 VBX stent extending proximally to the origin of the left common iliac artery (Fig. 27.5a, b), with resolution of contrast extravasation. Patient became hemodynamically stable with satisfactory patency of the left common and external iliac artery. The 8F sheath was removed in the operating room.

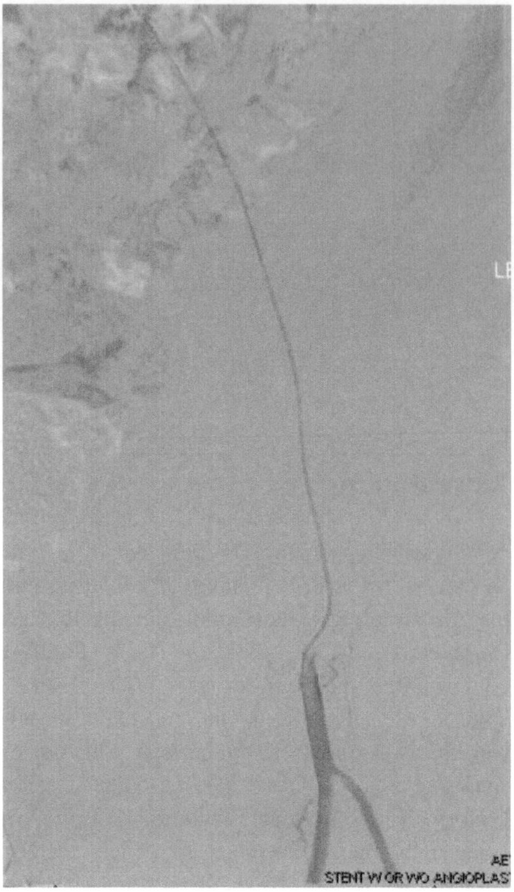

Fig. 27.3 Crossing of the left common and external iliac artery occlusion via left brachial artery access

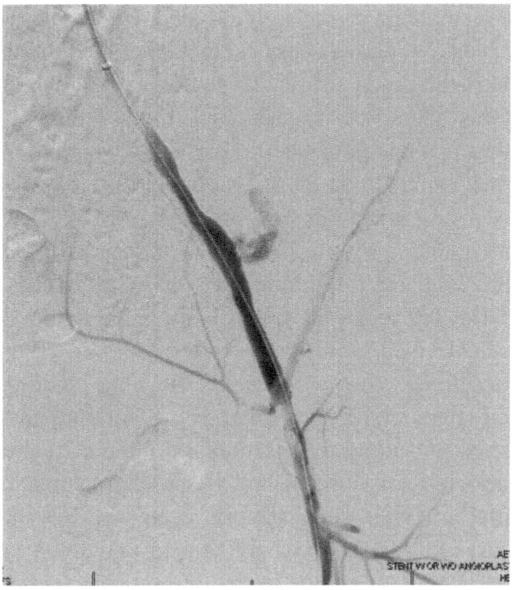

Fig. 27.4 Contrast extravasation at the mid left external iliac artery following angioplasty and stenting

The brachial artery was repaired following open thrombectomy. A vein patch using the basilic vein from the same incision was used over the brachial arteriotomy. Our initial plan was to perform a left femoral endarterectomy at the same time. Since the procedure took significantly longer than anticipated and there was a satisfactory Doppler flow in the foot following left iliac artery intervention, left femoral endarterectomy with bovine pericardial patch was performed 6 weeks later. At her last follow-up in the clinic in October 2024, lower extremity arterial Doppler showed an ABI of 0.85 (right) and 0.98 (left) with complete relief of lower extremity ischemic symptoms.

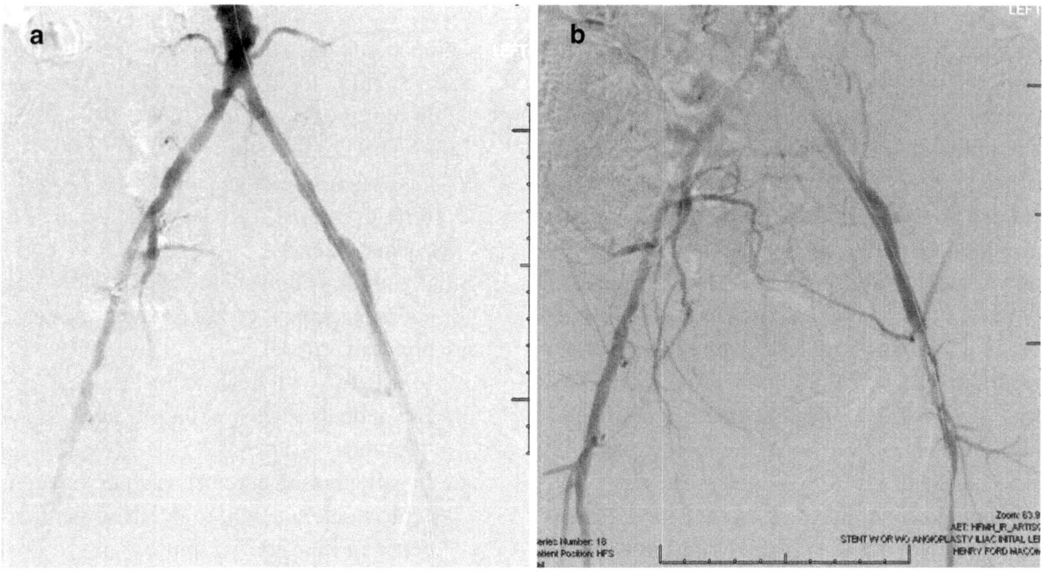

Fig. 27.5 (**a**) Resolution of contrast extravasation following deployment of a covered stent with satisfactory patency of the left common and external iliac artery (**b**) Resolution of contrast extravasation of a covered stent with patency of the left common and external iliac artery and severe calcific stenosis of the left common femoral artery

Discussion

Iliac artery stenting for TASC II A and B lesions is preferred over open arterial reconstruction and is highly successful with good outcomes. For TASC II C and D lesions, iliac artery stenting can be challenging and has an increased risk of serious complications such as iliac artery rupture, dissection, and maldeployment of the stent. Sachwani et al., reported results of iliac stenting in 103 limbs (100 patients) and compared to the results of aortobifemoral grafting in 101 patients with symptomatic iliac artery occlusions [1]. Patients in the iliac stenting group had a lower morbidity, shorter length of stay, and equivalent secondary patency compared to ABS bypass graft. However, primary patency was inferior in the stenting group [1]. At 72 months, the primary patency for ABF grafts was 91% as compared to 73% for the stenting group (p = 0.01) [1]. The length of stay was significantly greater in the ABF graft group (p = 0.001) [1]. There were no peri-procedural deaths in the stenting group and four deaths in the ABF graft group (0.058) [1]. There is a greater risk of iliac artery rupture during angioplasty and stenting in patients with circumferential calcification and long-segment occlusions. Shock wave therapy should be considered prior to stenting in patients with eccentric and circumferential calcification. To prevent rupture of the iliac artery in such lesions, the use of a covered stent as compared to a bare metal stent is preferable. Long-term follow-up of the randomized Covered versus Balloon Expandable Stent trial (COBEST) demonstrated significantly higher patency of covered stents at 5 years [2]. Covered stents may also decrease the risk of distal embolization in complex calcified lesions. During deployment of covered stents, inadvertent coverage of the hypogastric artery should be avoided.

In patients requiring brachial artery access, brachial artery cut-down should be performed if a 6F or larger sheath is required in order to prevent access complications such as brachial artery thrombosis and dissection. In patients with a concomitant common femoral artery and profunda femoris disease, simultaneous common femoral and profunda femoris endarterectomy should be performed to improve the outflow and maintain patency of the intervention. In this patient, common femoral endarterectomy was postponed for 6 weeks because the iliac intervention resulted in rupture of the artery, and brachial artery thrombectomy added extra time following angioplasty and stenting. Therefore, it was decided to postpone the left femoral endarterectomy to a later date. Following stenting inflammatory response manifests in the host artery, resulting in myointimal proliferation and ingrowth of hyperplastic tissue. Symptomatic iliac artery in-stent stenosis occurs in 10% of cases at 1 year and may be more common in patients with complex iliac lesions and with a longer follow-up [3].

Multiple Choice Questions

1. Compared to open aortofemoral grafting, iliac artery stenting for TASC C and D lesions: has:
   A. Better primary patency
   B. Longer hospital stay
   C. Equivalent primary patency
   D. Inferior primary patency but equal secondary patency
2. Stent grafts, as compared to bare metal stents, for the management of iliac occlusive disease are preferable:
   A. In patients with flush occlusions
   B. In patients with a large amount of thrombus
   C. In patients with eccentric plaque with concentric calcification, to decrease the incidence of iliac artery rupture
   D. Stent grafts do not need kissing balloon stents for contralateral common iliac disease
3. Symptomatic iliac artery in-stent restenosis at 1 year occurs at a frequency of:
   A. 5%
   B. 10%
   C. 15%

D. 20%

4. During iliac stenting for a calcified TASC D lesion, there is contrast extravasation with hypotension. The optimal method of treatment is:
   A. Open repair
   B. Prolonged balloon inflation
   C. Covered stent placement
   D. Reverse the heparin, as most perforations will resolve spontaneously

Answers: 1(D), 2(C), 3(B), 4(C)

References

1. Sachwani GR, Hans SS, Khoury MD, King TF, Mitsuya M, Rizk YS, et al. Results of iliac stenting and aortofemoral grafting for iliac artery occlusions. J Vasc Surg. 2013;57(4):1030–7. PMID:23177535
2. Mwipatayi BP, Sharma S, Daneshmand A, Thomas SD, Vijayan V, Altaf N, et al. Durability of the balloon-expandable covered versus bare-metal stents in the covered versus balloon expandable stent trial (COBEST) for the treatment of aortoiliac occlusive disease. J Vasc Surg. 2016;64(1):83–94.e81. PMID:27131926
3. Kudo T, Chandra FA, Ahn SS. Long-term outcomes and predictors of iliac angioplasty with selective stenting. J Vasc Surg. 2005;42(3):466–75. PMID:16171589

Management of Aortoiliac Disease Following Left Common Iliac Artery Stenting

28

Presentation

A 61-year-old woman was seen in the clinic with symptoms of lifestyle-limiting intermittent claudication (IC) affecting the left lower extremity in January 2021. She was a current smoker with history of smoking 45 pack-years. Clinical examination revealed an absent left femoral pulse. The right femoral pulse was easily palpable. Ankle-brachial index (ABI) was 0.76 (right) and 0.62 (left).

CTA of the abdominal aorta and run-off study showed left common iliac artery occlusion (TASC II B). The patient had an unsuccessful percutaneous intervention for iliac artery occlusion using left femoral artery access because the guidewire could not cross the occlusion. Right femoral access was subsequently attempted, but the wire was in the subintimal plane and could not be directed into the true lumen. In May 2021, the patient underwent left common iliac artery (CIA) angioplasty and stenting using a left brachial artery access. An 8 mm × 39 mm Omnilink (Abbott Medical, Abbott Park, IL) balloon-expandable stent was deployed. The final diameter was 8.4 mm as the inflation was increased to 14 atmospheric pressure (Figs. 28.1, 28.2, 28.3 and 28.4). She had a satisfactory result with the resolution of the symptoms of intermittent claudication, and ABI normalized to one on the left side.

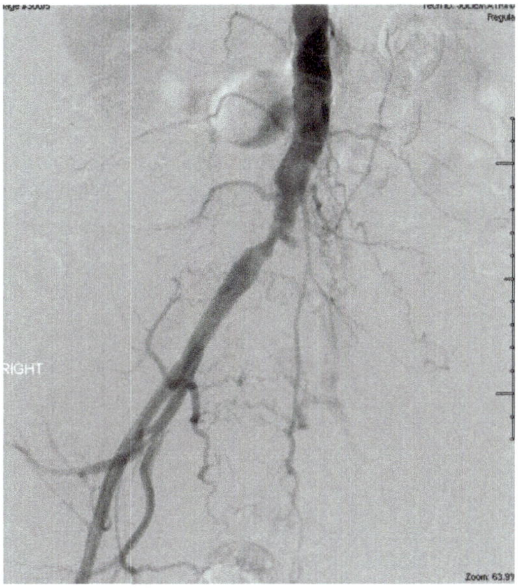

Fig. 28.1 Abdominal and pelvic aortogram showing left common iliac artery with occlusion (TASC B) and moderate right common iliac artery stenosis

S. S. Hans, *Secondary and Tertiary Arterial Reconstructions*,
https://doi.org/10.1007/978-3-032-21214-6_28

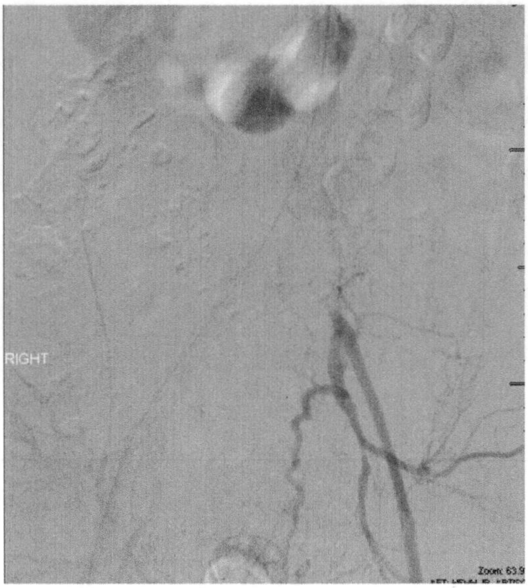

Fig. 28.2 Reconstitution of the distalmost common iliac artery beyond occlusion and a patent left external iliac and hypogastric artery

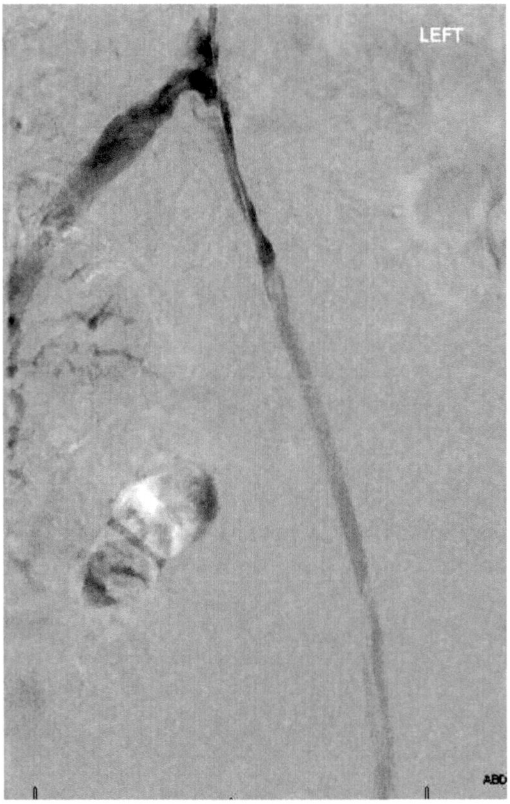

Fig. 28.3 Crossing left common iliac artery occlusion using brachial artery access

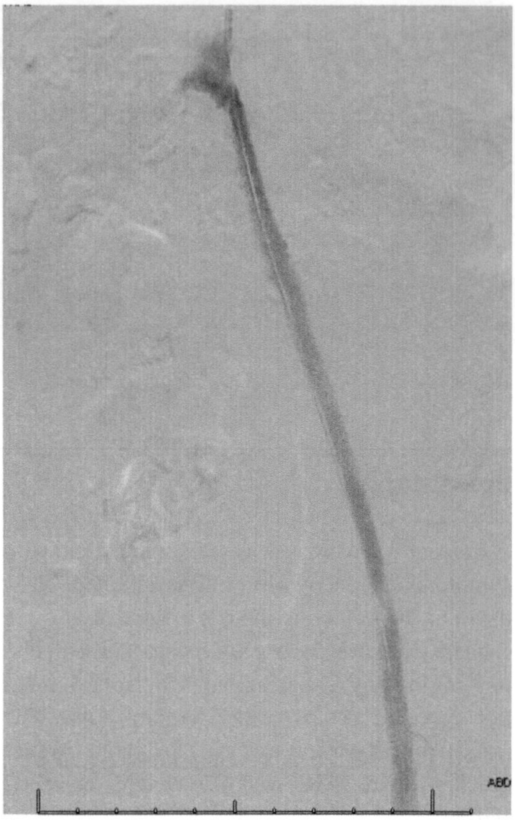

Fig. 28.4 Deployment of left common iliac artery stent

She was evaluated in the vascular clinic in December 2023 with recurrent symptoms of intermittent claudication of the left lower extremity, along with the new onset of symptoms of intermittent claudication of the right lower extremity. Non-invasive Doppler arterial in December 2023, showed an ABI of 0.58 (left) and 0.79 (right). She was taken to the interventional radiology suite for percutaneous intervention. Using ultrasound guidance, bilateral femoral artery access was obtained, and 6F sheaths were inserted on each side. Abdominal aortogram showed distal aortic ectasia with 70% stenosis of the distal aorta at the aortic bifurcation with large lumbar collaterals and 70% stenosis of the proximal right common iliac artery with post stenotic dilatation and in-stent stenosis of the left CIA (Fig. 28.5). Following bilateral iliac angioplasty distal abdominal aorta and both com-

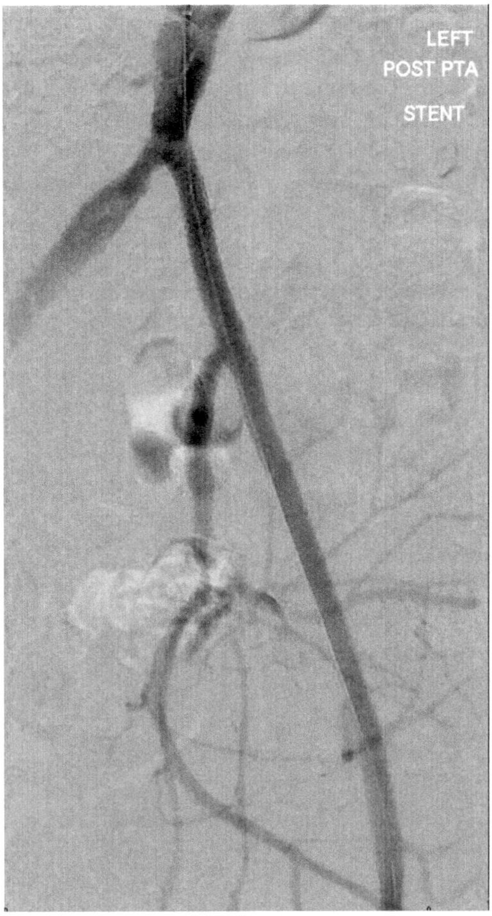

Fig. 28.5 Completion aortogram showing patent left common iliac artery stent with mild stenosis of right common iliac artery

mon iliac arteries were treated with two 7 × 4 Armada balloons. Simultaneously, bilateral kissing stents were deployed in the distal abdominal aorta and extending into both common iliac arteries; an 8 × 39 Omnilink stent on the right and an 8 × 19 Omnilink stent on the left. Completion of aortogram showed satisfactory results (Figs. 28.6 and 28.7). The patient was last seen in May 2025,

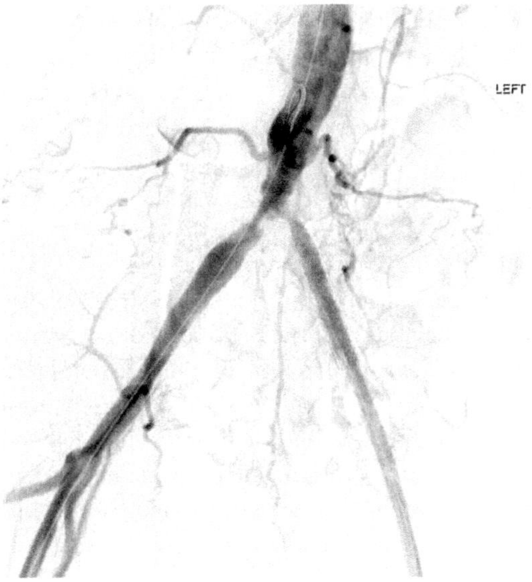

Fig. 28.6 Abdominal and pelvic aortogram 31 months later showing distal abdominal aortic stenosis, progression of right common iliac artery stenosis, and in-stent stenosis in left common iliac artery

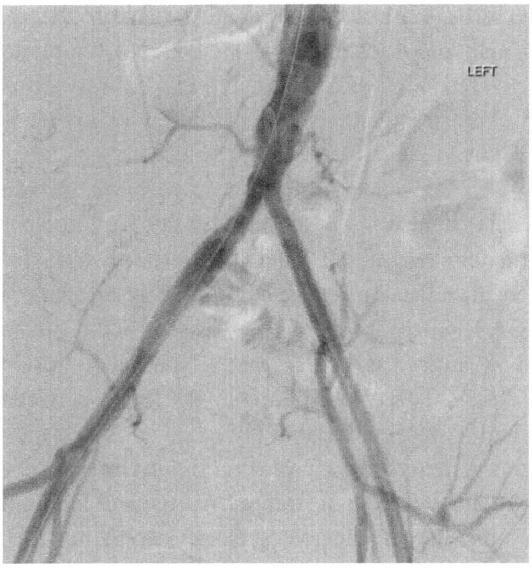

Fig. 28.7 Deployment of bilateral iliac bare metal kissing stents extending into the distal abdominal aorta

with resolution of symptoms of intermittent claudication, and a noninvasive Doppler arterial study showed ABI right (1.0″) and left (1.0″).

Discussion

The advantage of covered stents as compared to bare metal stents in preventing in-stent stenosis is that the graft material provides a direct barrier to tissue ingrowth from neointimal hyperplasia. Angioplasty and stenting result in vessel wall injury with activation of the macrophages and the release of pro-inflammatory mediators that promote growth of neointima, metalloproteinases, cytokines, and other growth factors. Use of covered stents imparts a direct barrier to the ingrowth of neointimal hyperplasia, sealing off the exposed inflammatory surface and thus potentially inhibiting restenosis [1]. On the other hand, restenosis can occur at the edges of the covered stent where injured intima is not covered by the graft material in the covered stent. This type of restenosis at the edges is unique to covered stents as compared to in-stent restenosis in bare metal stents, where the entire lumen is involved [1].

The advantage of covered stent over bare metal stent was not established in a multi-center randomized single-blinded controlled trial for advanced lesions in the common iliac artery, as a greater than 3 cm long stenosis or occlusion in 174 limbs with 87 limbs in each group (2012–2019). No difference was found between the balloon expandable covered stents and bare metal stents after a 2-year follow-up from binary restenosis, freedom from occlusion, and freedom from target lesion revascularization [2]. Squizzarto et al., compared covered versus bare metal kissing stents for TASC C and D lesions and collected data from 336 patients undergoing bilateral iliac kissing stents, 201 receiving covered stents and 135 bare metal stents. They reported similar 3-year patency rates in both groups [3]. However, patients with covered stents showed better outcomes in the presence of moderate to severe calcification, which was protective from iliac rupture and had a greater improvement in ankle-brachial index [3].

Symptomatic iliac artery in-stent restenosis occurs at a frequency of 10% at 1 year and may be more common at a long-term follow-up and in patients with more complex lesions [1]. Longer length, small diameter artery, and patients with diabetes mellitus have an increased risk of restenosis [1].

Multiple Choice Questions

1. Symptomatic iliac artery in-stent restenosis at one year occurs at a frequency of
   A. 5%
   B. 10%
   C. 25%
   D. 20%
2. The most common site of the in-stent stenosis after covered stent placement, as compared to the bare metal stent, is
   A. Superior edge
   B. Inferior edge
   C. Both superior and inferior edge
   D. Entire stent lumen
3. Following angioplasty and stenting, there is activation of
   A. Macrophages
   B. Proinflammatory mediators
   C. Both macrophages and proinflammatory mediators
   D. Platelets with the potential for thrombus formation

Answers: 1(B), 2(C), 3(C)

References

1. Kwa A, Dawson D, Laird J. Covered stents for treating Aortoliliac occlusive disease. Endovasc Today (April). 2011:53–6.
2. Bekken JA, Vroegindeweij D, Vos JA, de Vries JPM, Lardenoije J, Petri BJ, et al. Editor's choice—two-year results of the randomised DISCOVER trial comparing covered versus bare metal stents in the common iliac artery. Eur J Vasc Endovasc Surg. 2023;65(3):359–68. PMID:36336284
3. Squizzato F, Piazza M, Pulli R, Fargion A, Piffaretti G, Pratesi C, et al. Covered versus bare metal kissing stents for reconstruction of the aortic bifurcation in the ILIACS registry. J Vasc Surg. 2021;73(6):1980–1990.e1984. PMID:33253875

29 Iliac Artery Stenting Using Right Brachial Artery Access with Prior Failed Femoral Access

Presentation

A 57-year-old woman was evaluated by another vascular surgeon for symptoms of lifestyle--limiting right thigh and calf intermittent claudication. She had a significantly diminished right femoral pulse and a slightly diminished left femoral pulse. Doppler arterial showed an ankle--brachial index of 0.65 (right) and 0.73 (left). Medical comorbidities included Type II Diabetes Mellitus, hyperlipidemia, seizure disorder, chronic obstructive pulmonary disease, stable coronary artery disease, and gastroesophageal reflux. She was a current smoker with history of smoking 40 pack-years. CT angiography demonstrated complete occlusion of the right common iliac artery. Attempted passage of a guidewire across the proximal right common iliac artery occlusion, following ultrasound-guided puncture of both common femoral arteries, was unsuccessful in March 2019 (Figs. 29.1 and 29.2).

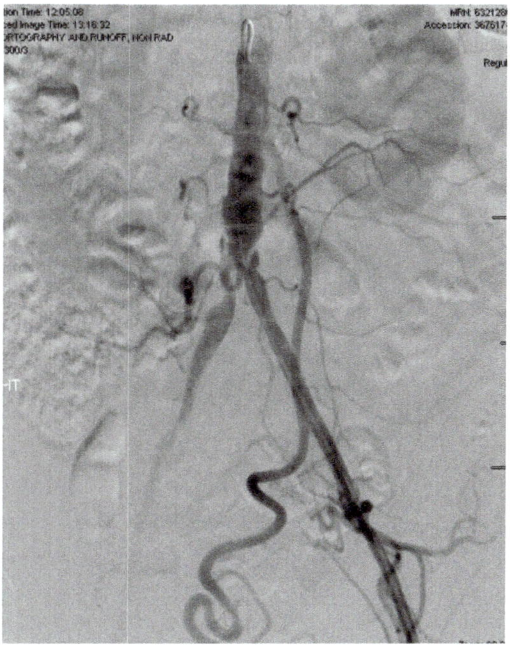

Fig. 29.1 Showing right proximal common iliac artery near occlusion and a moderate left common iliac artery stenosis. There is a large inferior mesenteric artery (IMA)

S. S. Hans, *Secondary and Tertiary Arterial Reconstructions*,
https://doi.org/10.1007/978-3-032-21214-6_29

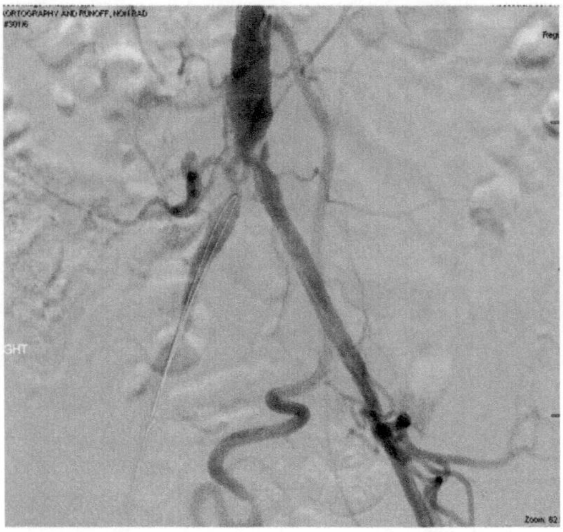

Fig. 29.2 Showing curling of the guide wire in the right common iliac artery

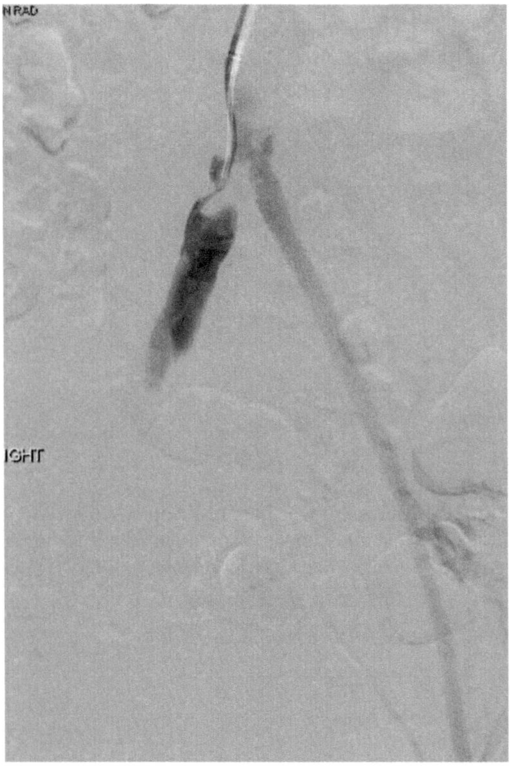

Fig. 29.3 Abdominal and pelvic aortogram using right brachial artery access

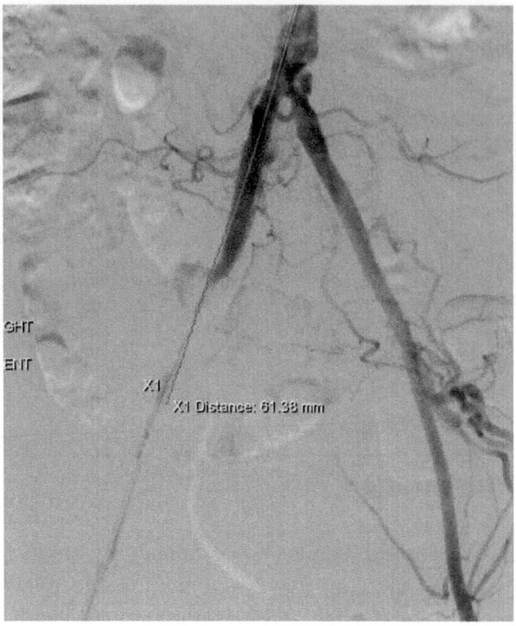

Fig. 29.4 Successful passage of guidewire across common iliac artery occlusion, followed by right common iliac artery angioplasty and stent

On June 17, 2020, right brachial artery access was obtained using ultrasound guidance. Because of a known left subclavian artery occlusion, left brachial access was not attempted. A 90 cm long 6F Pinnacle sheath (Terumo, Somerset, NJ) was advanced, and an exchange length angled stiff 0.035 glide wire (Terumo, Somerset, NJ) was advanced using a 120 cm long 5F vertebral catheter. After a subintimal passage of wire in the common iliac artery, the wire was directed into the lumen of the external iliac artery (Figs. 29.3 and 29.4). Following passage of guidewire across the proximal external iliac artery balloon angioplasty of the common iliac artery with a 6 × 60 mm Armada balloon (Abbott Med, Chicago, IL), an 8 mm × 6 cm Omnilink balloon expandable stent was deployed and a 7 mm × 6 cm right external iliac smart stent deployed to cover the dissection in the external iliac artery (Cordis-Johnson and Johnson, New Brunswick, NJ).

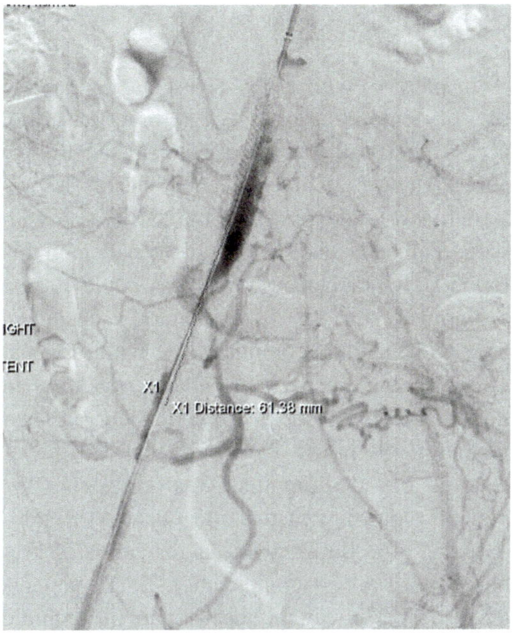

Fig. 29.5 Successful passage of wire into the external iliac artery with non-flow-limiting dissection of the distal common iliac artery, with poor visualization of the external iliac artery

Completion run showed patent right common and external iliac artery without residual stenosis (Figs. 29.5 and 29.6).

Patient subsequently underwent clipping of a symptomatic cerebral aneurysm in May 2021 using right femoral access. In July 2022, the patient underwent left common iliac artery angioplasty and stenting for lifestyle-limiting symptoms of intermittent claudication using left transfemoral access using an 8 × 29 mm Omnilink (Abbott Medical, Abbott Park, Chicago, IL) balloon-expandable stent (Fig. 29.7). Completion aortogram showed resolution of right external iliac artery dissection and satisfactory deployment of left common iliac artery stent. At the completion of the procedure, the patient had a vasovagal episode. She was discharged on the same day. She was last seen in the clinic in June 2024 without any symptoms of intermittent claudication. A noninvasive Doppler arterial study showed an ankle-brachial index 0.98 (right) and 1.01 (left).

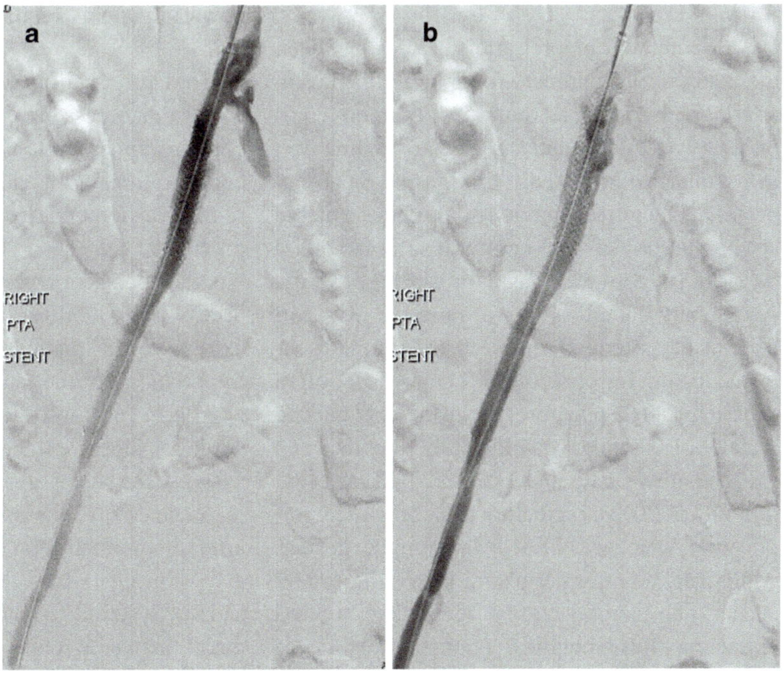

Fig. 29.6 (**a**) Deployment of the right common iliac artery stent and the external iliac stent. (**b**) Patent right external iliac artery stent with satisfactory distal flow

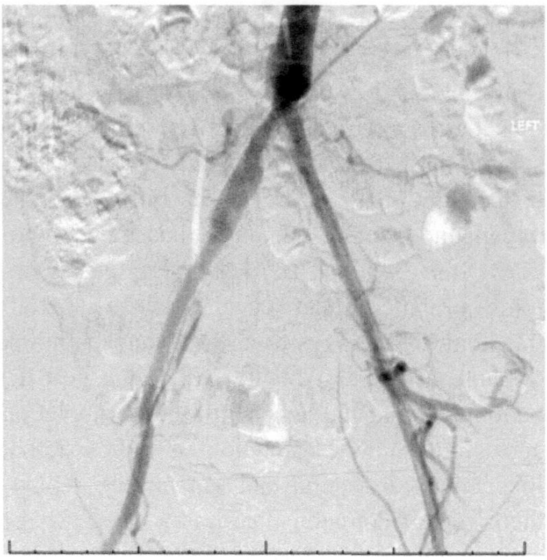

Fig. 29.7 Successful deployment of left common iliac artery stent. Mild ectatia of the distal abdominal aorta. In-stent stenosis of the right common iliac artery stent with remote non-flow limiting dissection in the right mid common iliac artery

Discussion

Use of common femoral artery access has been the mainstay for coronary, peripheral diagnostic arteriography, and interventions. Common femoral artery access is relatively easy to obtain, even in patients with markedly diminished or absent pulses, using ultrasound. It also provides suitable access platforms for successful revascularization of various types of lesions with varying severity. Access site complications occurred in 3.5% of patients like arterial thrombosis, hematoma/pseudoaneurysm, retroperitoneal hemorrhage often caused by high puncture. From a retrospective review of vascular quality initiative data on 22,226 patients who underwent 27,048 intervention (2002–2013), predictors of access site complication were age 77.5 years, female gender, white race, no prior peripheral intervention, >6F sheath, non-femoral arterial access site, arterial dissection, thrombolytics, fluoroscopy time of >30 minutes, urgent indicator nonuse of vascular closure device, non-ambulatory pre procedure status [1].

In patients with failed revascularization, the use of femoral artery access, brachial artery access, and radial artery access are alternative access sites. Left brachial artery access is preferred as it avoids crossing the aortic arch with wires, catheters, and sheaths. In the patient in this report, left brachial artery access could not be performed because of ipsilateral subclavian artery occlusion. Complications with brachial artery access, such as thrombosis resulting in upper extremity ischemia, pseudoaneurysm, and median nerve injury, have been reported. Javier Alvarez-Tostado reported 323 cases in 289 patients requiring brachial artery access for endovascular procedures, with an incidence of brachial artery access complications in 21 patients (6.5%) [1]. Thirteen of those 21 patients required open repair for brachial artery thrombosis and pseudoaneurysm. The complications were more commonly in women (Odds ratio 4:1) and in patients who had a long interventional sheath [1]. Most authors recommend a brachial artery cutdown in patients requiring a 6F or larger sheath [2].

The introduction and widespread usage of transradial access have transformed percutaneous coronary intervention practice, as access site complications are significantly lower than those of the transfemoral access [2]. Transradial access precludes the need for prolonged bed rest. Another benefit of transradial and transbrachial access is the ability to intervene in both lower extremities [3]. Patient selection is of uppermost importance to the success of the transradial approach for lower extremity intervention. In addition, longer catheters, sheaths, and delivery systems for stents are often necessary. Puncture is obtained by ultrasound guidance and intra-arterial administration of calcium channel blockers, nitroglycerine diluted with heparinized saline. Systemic heparin administration with a target activated clotting time of 300 seconds should be adhered to.

Multiple Choice Questions

1. In a 57-year-old woman with multiple medical comorbidities, with symptomatic right common iliac artery occlusion, mild stenosis, including CIA, with unsuccessful attempts to cross the lesion using femoral artery access. The patient has a known left subclavian artery occlusion. The next best option for iliac artery revascularization is
   A. Percutaneous stenting of the left subclavian artery, followed by left brachial access for right iliac stenting
   B. Aortobifemoral graft
   C. Crossover femoral-femoral graft
   D. Right brachial artery access
2. Iliac artery stenting using right brachial artery access, with a 6F sheath, as compared to left brachial artery access results in?
   A. Higher incidence of brachial artery thrombosis
   B. Higher risk of cerebral embolic complications compared to the left
   C. Higher risk of brachial artery pseudoaneurysm
   D. Higher risk of iliac artery dissection/rupture
3. Using brachial artery access for endovascular procedures for lower extremity arterial disease; the incidence of access complications is
   A. 3%
   B. 3.1%–4.5%
   C. 4.6%–6.0%
   D. 6.5%

Answers 1(D), 2(B), 3(D)

References

1. Ortiz D, Jahangir A, Singh M, Allaqaband S, Bajwa TK, Mewissen MW. Access site complications after peripheral vascular interventions: incidence, predictors, and outcomes. Circ Cardiovasc Interv. 2014;7(6):821–8. PMID:25389345
2. Alvarez-Tostado JA, Moise MA, Bena JF, Pavkov ML, Greenberg RK, Clair DG, Kashyap VS. The brachial artery: a critical access for endovascular procedures. J Vasc Surg. 2009;49(2):378–85; discussion 385
3. Parikh SA, Ricotta JJ, Ghamraoui A. The state of transradial access for lower extremity intervention. Endovascular Today. 2021;20(11):76–8.

30 Repeat Iliac Stenting and Simultaneous Right Common Femoral Endarterectomy in a Patient with Multiple Prior Endovascular Interventions and Arterial Bypass

Presentation

A 79-year-old man with a history of severe lower extremity arterial occlusive disease and bilateral carotid endarterectomy. He had coronary artery disease with a history of coronary artery stenting, hyperlipidemia, and type II diabetes mellitus. He was a former smoker with a history of smoking 50 pack-years. He was admitted to the hospital with gangrene of the distal right big toe and ischemic rest pain. He had a history of left common femoral endarterectomy and a simultaneous left femoral-post tibial bypass with reversed great saphenous vein in October 2017 by another vascular surgeon in our hospital. This bypass subsequently occluded, and a left SFA stenting (3 supra stents) was performed for ischemic lower extremity by an interventionalist at an outside hospital using right femoral artery access and snaring the wire with the use of retrograde left pedal access in October 2019. In Dec 2019, the patient underwent shock wave lithotripsy of a totally occluding, severely calcified right SFA occlusive disease with multiple self-expanding stents (Supera stent, Abbott Medical, Abbott Park, IL) placed in the right popliteal and SFA. He also had a history of bilateral iliac stent placement in the remote past.

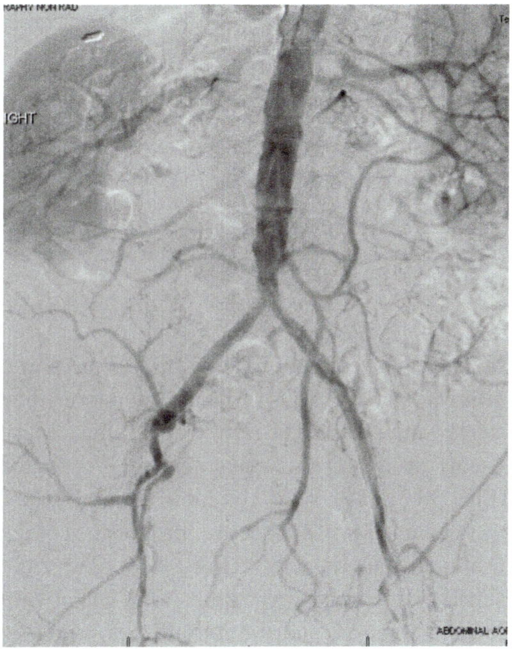

Fig. 30.1 Abdominal aortogram shows a narrow distal abdominal aorta and right external iliac artery occlusion

The patient was taken to the hybrid operating room on May 4, 2022. Utilizing ultrasound guidance, the left common femoral artery was accessed using a micropuncture technique. An abdominal aortogram demonstrated a

S. S. Hans, *Secondary and Tertiary Arterial Reconstructions*,
https://doi.org/10.1007/978-3-032-21214-6_30

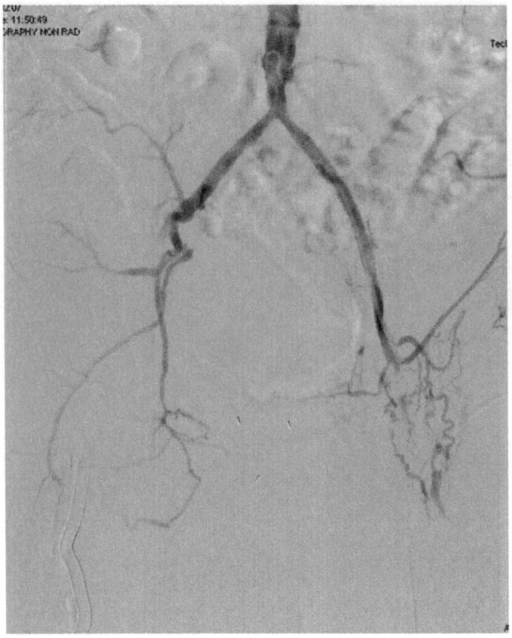

Fig. 30.2 Pelvic arteriogram shows right external iliac artery occlusion and occlusion of bilateral common femoral arteries

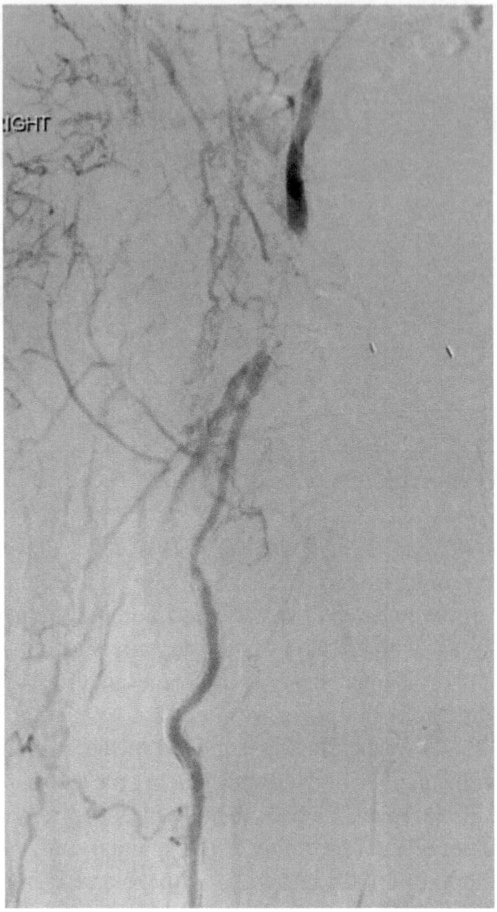

Fig. 30.3 Arteriogram showing right common femoral artery occlusion and visualization of profunda femoris artery branches with numerous collaterals

small-diameter aorta just proximal to the aortic bifurcation (Fig. 30.1). Bilateral common iliac stents were patent. The right external iliac artery (stent) at its origin was completely occluded (Fig. 30.2). The right common femoral artery was occluded, with patency of the branches of the profunda femoris artery (Fig. 30.3). The right superficial femoral artery stents were patent with in-stent stenosis, and the run-off was primarily with the posterior tibial artery (Figs. 30.4 and 30.5). A 5F sheath in the left common femoral artery was exchanged for a 7F, 45 cm Pinnacle sheath and was positioned in the right common iliac artery. For proximal control, a 7 mm × 4 cm Armada balloon was inflated to occlude the right distal common iliac artery, including balloon occlusion of the patent right hypogastric artery. A silastic loop was passed around the distal external iliac artery. A smaller silastic vessel loop wire was passed around the deep epigastric artery and the deep circumflex iliac artery following ligation and division of the deep circumflex iliac vein. The right profunda femoris artery was also looped with a silastic vessel loop. Following systemic heparinization, a longitudinal incision was made in the common femoral artery. A Dacron patch had previously been sutured in the anterior wall of the common femoral artery and was well

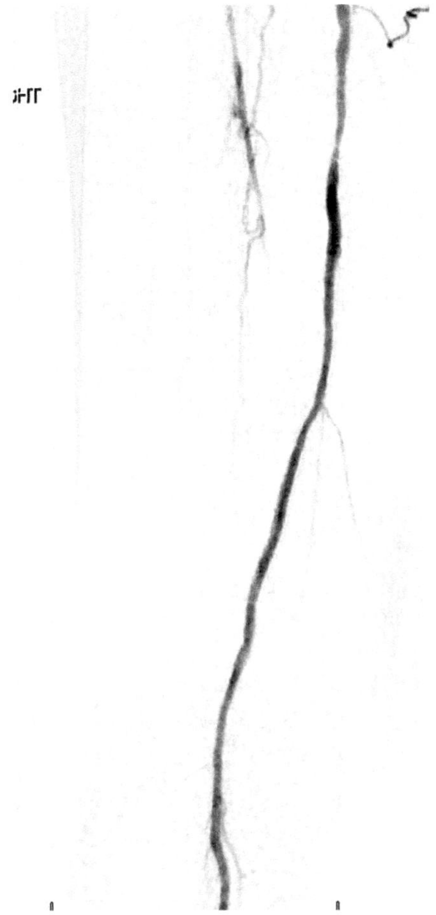

Fig. 30.4 Patent right SFA with in-stent stenosis

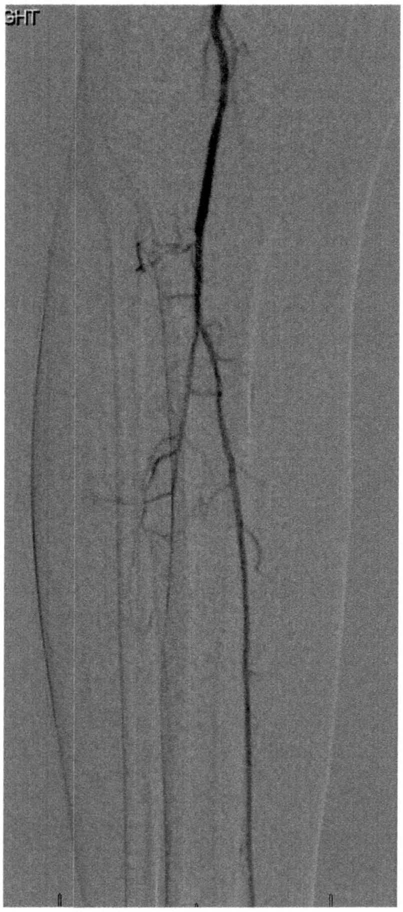

Fig. 30.5 Patency of small diameter right popliteal artery with run off primarily with the posterior tibial artery and diminutive peroneal artery

incorporated. Right common femoral artery endarterectomy and a bovine pericardial patch angioplasty were performed, and the previously placed Dacron patch was removed. Two VBX stents (8 × 39 mm and 8 × 29 mm) were deployed in the right external iliac artery, and the right hypogastric artery patency was preserved (Figs. 30.6 and 30.7). The right superficial femoral artery (SFA) stents showed in-stent stenosis but were not treated at this time (Fig. 30.8). There was satisfactory healing of the right big toe during the subsequent 2 months. Due to severe calcification, ABIs were not accurately obtained, but waveforms showed marked improvement from

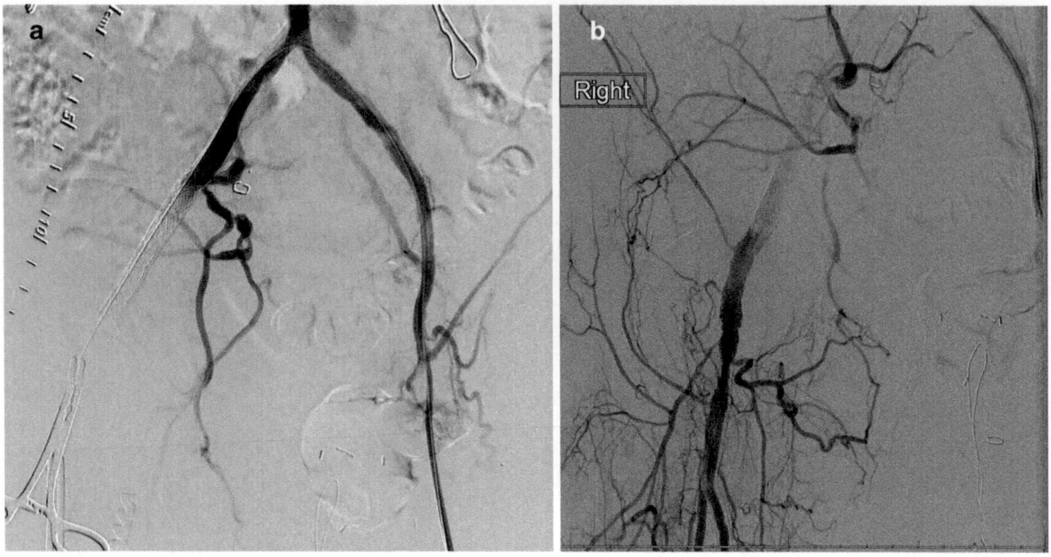

Fig. 30.6 (**a**) Pelvic arteriogram showed occlusion of the right external iliac stent. (**b**) Patent distal external iliac artery with mild stenosis in the proximal common femoral artery at the site of endarterectomy

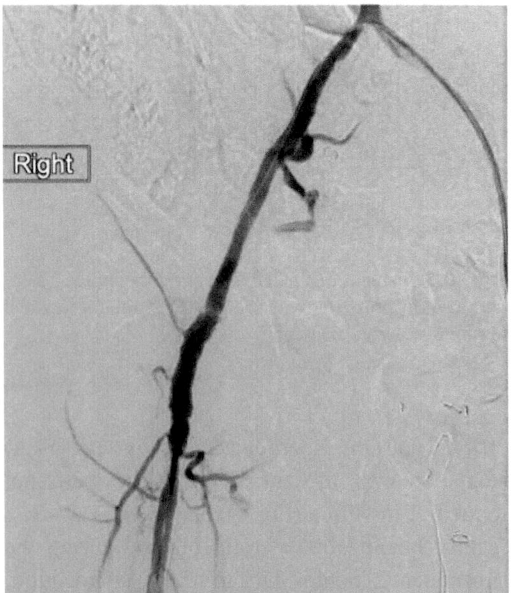

Fig. 30.7 Patency of the right external iliac artery with deployment of two VBX (covered stents). There is 50% stenosis of the proximal common femoral artery

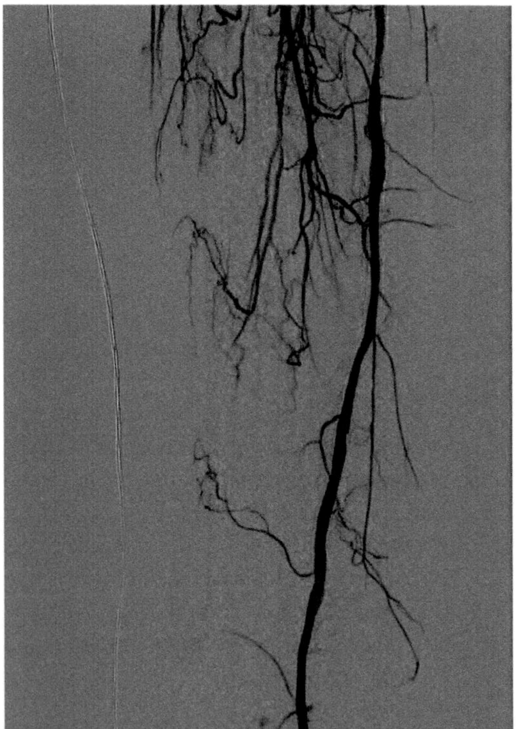

Fig. 30.8 Patent right superficial femoral artery with diffuse in-stent stenoses

preoperative values. The patient underwent left below-knee amputation for infected gangrene of the left foot in April 2024. The patient died in July 2024 from multiple organ failure.

Discussion

Following balloon angioplasty and stenting, an inflammatory response occurs in the host artery, resulting in intimal hyperplasia and tissue ingrowth. Symptomatic iliac artery in-stent stenosis occurs with a frequency of 10% over a 1-year period and is probably more common at a longer follow-up and in more complex lesions [1, 2].

The treatment options for in-stent stenosis include standard balloon angioplasty, cutting balloon angioplasty, or placement of a covered stent. Stent thrombosis tends to occur in longer, more complex lesions, such as occlusions, and in patients with diabetes mellitus and renal failure. Stent under-sizing is also implicated in the etiology of stent thrombosis. Early stent thrombosis can be managed by use of thrombolytic therapy (TPA) and further management by balloon angioplasty and/or placement of a covered stent, depending upon the response to thrombolytic therapy [3, 4]. Late occlusions may be difficult to cross with a wire and often need the use of the mechanical thrombectomy devices to obtain a channel, followed by placement of a balloon expandable covered stent, such as VBX (W.L. Gore, Newark, DE). In some patients with late occlusions of iliac stents with associated symptoms of severe ischemia of the lower extremities, an open aorto-femoral reconstruction should be considered if the patient is an acceptable risk for major arterial reconstruction.

Another often overlooked cause of early thrombosis of TASC C or D lesions is a missed dissection in the distal external iliac artery at the level of the deep epigastric and deep circumflex iliac artery due to coverage of the distal stent/artery junction by the distal portion of the access sheath. Completion arteriogram should be performed after withdrawal of the sheath proximally to visualize the distal end of the stent. In distal lesions close to the junction of the external iliac and common femoral artery, contralateral femoral access or brachial artery access should be considered in order to visualize the distal-most segment of the external iliac artery. Another important cause of late stent occlusion is failure to treat a concomitant common femoral artery disease at the time of iliac stenting. In patients with common iliac artery occlusion and common femoral artery stenosis, the patient should be taken to the hybrid OR. A cut-down in the groin and a common femoral endarterectomy with patch graft angioplasty should be performed at the time of iliac stenting to improve the outflow.

Multiple Choice Questions

1. During external Iliac artery stenting using ipsilateral femoral access, the distal end of the stent and its junction with the distal external iliac artery cannot be clearly seen. The patient should be
   A. Continued on antiplatelet medication and undergo duplex imaging in four weeks
   B. Withdrawal the femoral sheath by a few centimeters and obtain a completion arteriogram
   C. Obtain completion arteriogram via left brachial access
   D. Obtain completion arteriogram using a contralateral femoral access
2. Early stent thrombosis following iliac stenting should be treated with
   A. Lytic therapy and re-stenting/angioplasty
   B. Surgical bypass
   C. Anticoagulation
   D. Open thrombectomy
3. An important cause of late iliac artery stent occlusion is
   A. hypercoagulable state

B. Oversized stents
C. Undetected dissection flap
D. Untreated common femoral artery occlusive disease

Answers 1(B), 2(A), 3(D)

References

1. Kudo T, Chandra FA, Ahn SS. Long-term outcomes and predictors of iliac angioplasty with selective stenting. J Vasc Surg. 2005;42(3):466–75. PMID:16171589
2. Kashyap VS, Pavkov ML, Bena JF, Sarac TP, O'Hara PJ, Lyden SP, Clair DG. The management of severe aortoiliac occlusive disease: endovascular therapy rivals open reconstruction. J Vasc Surg. 2008;48(6):1451–7. 1457.e1451-1453. PMID:18804943
3. Sachwani GR, Hans SS, Khoury MD, King TF, Mitsuya M, Rizk YS, et al. Results of iliac stenting and aortofemoral grafting for iliac artery occlusions. J Vasc Surg. 2013;57(4):1030–7. PMID:23177535
4. Hans SS. Management of Iliac stent thrombosis. In: Hans SS, editor. Challenging arterial reconstructions: 100 clinical cases. Cham: Springer; 2020. p. 399–402.

31 Stent Graft Repair of a Saccular Renal Artery Aneurysm

Presentation

A 68-year-old man was referred to the clinic by his primary care physician for evaluation of a left renal artery aneurysm detected on a CT scan of the abdomen performed in February 2025 for workup of abdominal pain. He denied any flank pain or hematuria. He had a history of well-‐controlled hypertension and coronary artery disease with coronary stent placement in April 2023. Lab data showed a serum creatinine of 0.9 mg/dl and GFR = 93 ml. Computed tomography angiography (CTA) of the abdomen performed in April 2025 showed a 1.4 × 1.2 × 1.9 cm saccular aneurysm of the left renal artery (Fig. 31.1). He had asymptomatic severe stenosis of the celiac axis with a post-stenotic dilatation. He was scheduled for endovascular repair of renal artery aneurysm in the interventional radiology suite.

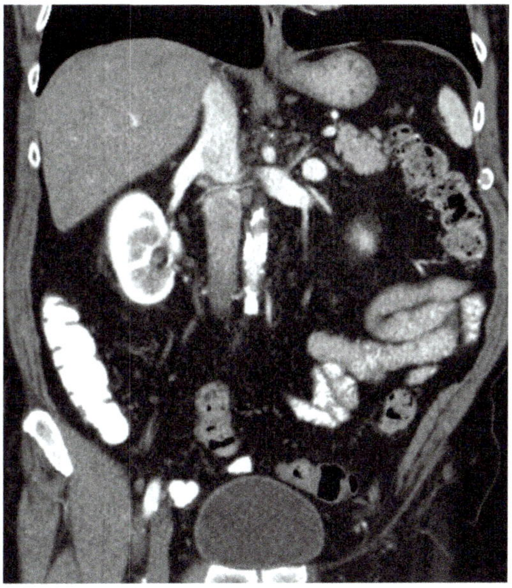

Fig. 31.1 CTA of the abdomen showing saccular aneurysm of the left renal artery

On May 15, 2025, using right femoral artery access, abdominal aortogram and selective left renal arteriogram showed a (19 x16 mm) saccular aneurysm of the superior aspect of the mid-‐segment of the left renal artery (Figs. 31.2 and 31.3). The tip of the Mickaelson catheter (Merit Medical, South Jordan, UT) was placed near the origin of the left renal artery over a glide wire. A lantern delivery microcatheter (Penumbra Inc., Alameda, CA) was placed near the neck of the aneurysm to perform coil embolization. Because of the wide neck of the aneurysm and with the inherent risk of maldeployment of the coils, it was decided to place a covered stent across the neck of the renal artery aneurysm. Mickaelson's catheter was removed, and using a 0.035 Bentson wire, a 6F flexor sheath was advanced. A Cobra 2 catheter (Cook Medicine, Bloomington, IN) was advanced into the left renal artery with tip of flexor sheath advanced for about 1 cm into the proximal renal artery (Fig. 31.4). A 6 × 19 mm VBX covered stent (WL Gore Inc., Newark, DE) was deployed, raised to 12 atmospheric pressures

S. S. Hans, *Secondary and Tertiary Arterial Reconstructions*,
https://doi.org/10.1007/978-3-032-21214-6_31

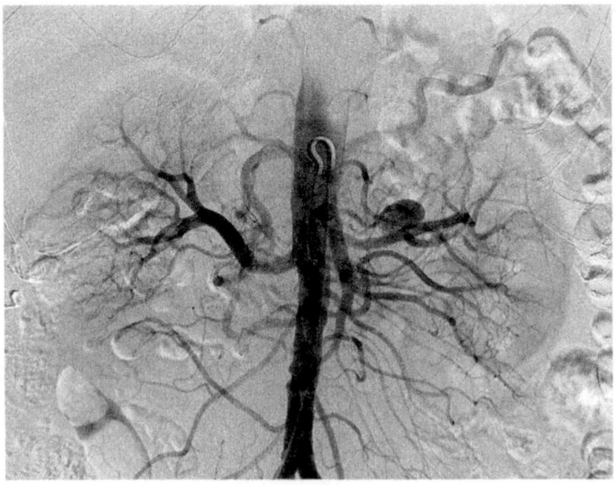

Fig. 31.2 Abdominal aortogram showing a saccular left renal artery aneurysm

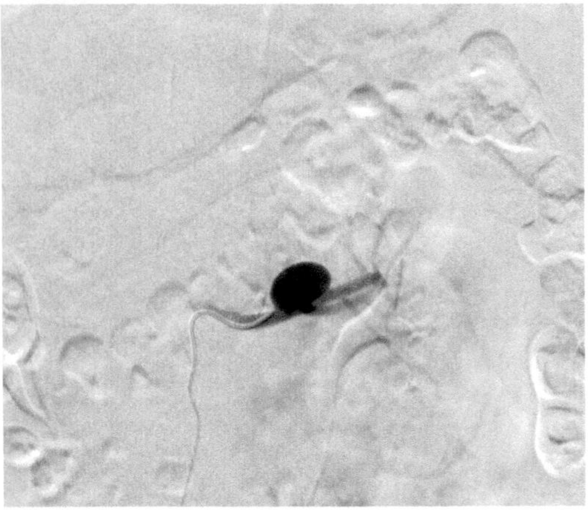

Fig. 31.3 Selective left renal arteriogram showing saccular left renal artery aneurysm just proximal to its bifurcation

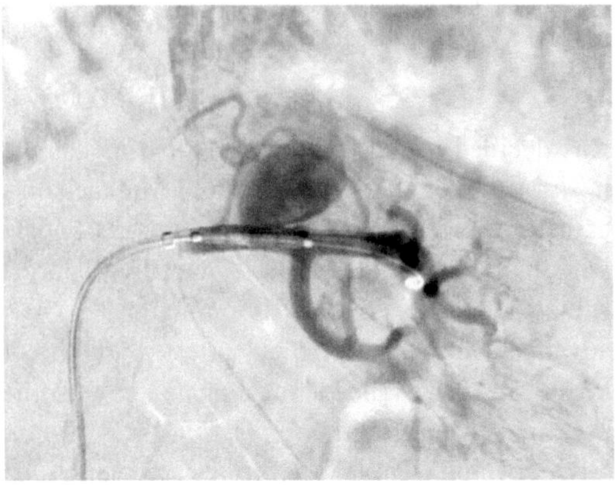

Fig. 31.4 Left renal arteriogram showing tip of the sheath at the origin of the left renal artery with undeployed covered stent at the origin of the saccular aneurysm

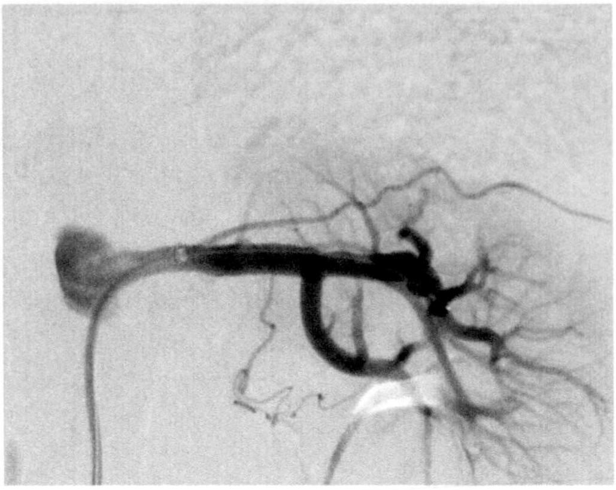

Fig. 31.5 Completion left renal arteriogram showing satisfactory exclusion left renal artery aneurysm

so that the final diameter of the covered stent was 5.9 mm (normal diameter of left renal artery proximal and distal to the aneurysm was 4.9 mm). Completion arteriogram showed satisfactory exclusion of the aneurysm (Fig. 31.5). The patient was discharged on Plavix and aspirin on the same day. The patient was seen in August 2025 in satisfactory condition. A follow-up renal duplex study showed normal flow in the renal arteries with no evidence of stenosis and there was satisfactory exclusion of the renal artery aneurysm.

Discussion

Renal artery aneurysms (RAA's) are the least common of the visceral artery aneurysms. Previously reported studies have recommended that asymptomatic renal artery aneurysms greater than 2 cm in diameter should be repaired [1, 2]. Recent studies suggest that uncomplicated aneurysms equal to or greater than 3 cm should undergo repair, as the growth rate of asymptomatic renal artery aneurysms is slow [3]. Other factors that may necessitate repair of RAA regardless of the size include:- Symptoms such as pain, hematuria, medically refractory hypertension with associated renal artery stenosis, thromboembolism, dissection, and those presenting with rupture [1–3].- Due to increased risk of rupture of the renal artery aneurysm during pregnancy, therapy is recommended for women of childbearing age who might conceive in the future [1, 2]. - Rapid growth, even if the aneurysm is smaller than 2 cm, is an indication for repair.- Saccular aneurysm or any increase in size is also an indication for repair. [1–3]

Open operative repair is recommended as the first line of therapy. Aneurysmectomy and primary or patch graft closure are the most appropriate means of treating most renal artery aneurysms. Solitary aneurysms involving the main renal artery and segmental branch bifurcations may be excised, and the vessel closed primarily in a simple manner. The aneurysm in these cases is resected, leaving a 1–2 mm rim of aneurysmal tissue at the base of the affected artery [1, 2]. Closure of the arterial defect with a simple continuous suture is then performed with a 6′0″ or a 7′0″ cardiovascular polypropylene suture incorporating the rim of aneurysmal tissue. If such a closure is likely to compromise the lumen, then an autologous vein patch closure should be performed [1, 2]. Aneurysmectomy and reimplantation may be appropriate when the aneurysm involves the segmental branches, and its excision necessitates formal arterial reconstruction [1, 2].

In most instances, reimplantation of one artery into the parent vessel is preferred over an arterial bypass. Closed aneurysmorrhaphy of a small renal artery aneurysm (2–3 mm) may be accomplished by plication of the aneurysmal wall and fine polypropylene suture. Aneurysmectomy and aortorenal bypass are preferable where a nearby aneurysm affecting two main proximal or midrenal arteries and distal aneurysms are removed with concomitant renal artery stenosis. In adults, using the great saphenous vein and in children, a segment of the internal iliac artery is a preferred conduit. Perioperative mortality following open aneurysmectomy is rare, but early complications such as acute thrombosis of the reconstructed renal artery or one of its branches may occur in 1–2% of cases. Most large series report post--operative renal artery patency rates over 90% at 10 years.

Wei et al., reported the use of non-covered stent-assisted coil embolization for 28 consecutive wide-based renal artery aneurysms with 100% technical success [4]. A large renal artery aneurysm treated with 5′0″ x 26 mm balloon expandable Jostent GraftMaster stent (Abbott Vascular Instruments, Germany) was reported [5].

Multiple Choice Questions

1. A 32-year-old woman has a 1.5 cm renal artery aneurysm. The best management option is:
   A. Surveillance with imaging studies
   B. Open Repair
   C. Endovascular repair
   D. Open repair when aneurysm reaches 2 cm or is symptomatic
2. A 2.0 cm fusiform aneurysm of mid-renal artery in a 60-year-old man with well controlled hypertension should be managed by:
   A. Surveillance with imaging studies
   B. Aorto renal bypass
   C. Aneurysmorrhaphy
   D. Stent graft
3. The best conduit for the repair of the renal artery aneurysm in a pediatric patient is:
   A. Autologous vein
   B. PTFE graft
   C. Internal iliac artery
   D. Cryovein

Answer: 1 (B), 2 (A), 3 (C)

References

1. Henke PK, Cardneau JD, Welling TH 3rd, Upchurch GR Jr, Wakefield TW, Jacobs LA, et al. Renal artery aneurysms: a 35-year clinical experience with 252 aneurysms in 168 patients. Ann Surg. 2001;234(4):454–62; discussion 462-453. PMID:11573039

2. Klausner JQ, Lawrence PF, Harlander-Locke MP, Coleman DM, Stanley JC, Fujimura N. The contemporary management of renal artery aneurysms. J Vasc Surg. 2015;61(4):978–84. PMID:25537277
3. Chaer RA, Abularrage CJ, Coleman DM, Eslami MH, Kashyap VS, Rockman C, Murad MH. The Society for Vascular Surgery clinical practice guidelines on the management of visceral aneurysms. J Vasc Surg. 2020;72(1s):3s–39s. PMID:32201007
4. Wei X, Sun Y, Wu Y, Li Z, Zhu J, Zhao Z, et al. Management of wide-based renal artery aneurysms using noncovered stent-assisted coil embolization. J Vasc Surg. 2017;66(3):850–7. PMID:28634052
5. Degertekin M, Bayrak F, Mutlu B, Gürses B, Güran S, Demirtas E. Images in cardiovascular medicine. Large renal artery aneurysm treated with stent graft. Circulation. 2006;113(23):e848–9. PMID:16769918

32 Retrograde Superior Mesenteric Artery Stenting for Acute Thrombosis

Presentation

A 69-year-old woman was admitted with supra-umbilical abdominal pain in May 2025. She also complained of generalized weakness. She denied any history of diarrhea or loss of weight. She could not ingest any solid food or liquids for two days prior to admission. She had a history of hypertension and Type II Diabetes mellitus. In 2016, she underwent a total abdominal hysterectomy and bilateral salpingo-oophorectomy with postoperative chemoradiation for carcinoma of the uterus. She was on Apixaban for a history of pulmonary embolism. Vital signs revealed normal blood pressure, but the heart rate was 106/mt. She did not have any history of atrial fibrillation. Lab data showed a WBC count of 18,400. She had E. coli bacteremia and was started on intravenous antibiotics. The CT scan of the abdomen was requested using the pancreas protocol, as the ultrasound was concerning for a pancreatic mass. The CT scan of the abdomen was negative for a pancreatic mass but showed occlusion of the proximal superior mesenteric artery (SMA) with a filling defect suggestive of thromboembolism (Fig. 32.1). She had evidence of significant right renal artery stenosis. She underwent an emergency thrombectomy on May 29, 2025, via midline laparotomy with exposure of the root of the mesentery. A transverse arteriotomy incision was made (Fig. 32.2), and a 1.5 × 0.5 cm greyish red thrombo-embolic material was removed (Fig. 32.3) with the aid of a Fogarty balloon catheter, with the establishment of satisfactory antegrade flow. The small and large bowel appeared to be normal.

Postoperatively, the patient had worsening leukocytosis without any episode of bloody diarrhea. A repeat CTA of the abdomen and pelvis on the third post-operative day showed re-occlusion of the SMA. She underwent abdominal re--exploration on June 1, 2025. The site was reopened with the passage of a Fogarty balloon catheter with the establishment of antegrade flow. The superior mesenteric artery was punctured 3 cm distal to the previous arteriotomy site using the micropuncture technique, and a 6F, 25 cm long sheath was inserted, and a 0.035″ Glide wire advantage (Terumo, Somerset, NJ) was advanced proximally. An aortogram was obtained using an Omniflush catheter. A 7 × 39 mm VBX balloon expandable stent (WL Gore Inc., Newark, DE) was deployed in the proximal SMA. Completion arteriogram (Figs. 32.4, 32.5, and 32.6) showed brisk flow of contrast through the SMA with restoration of satisfactory pulse in the SMA and satisfactory Doppler signals in the periphery of the mesentery.

A small bowel resection of 58 cm length for patchy ischemia of the proximal small intestine was performed with the bowel left in discontinuity. An ABThera (Solventurn, Maplewood, MN) dressing was applied. The patient was kept in the intensive care unit on ventilatory support. She

S. S. Hans, *Secondary and Tertiary Arterial Reconstructions*,
https://doi.org/10.1007/978-3-032-21214-6_32

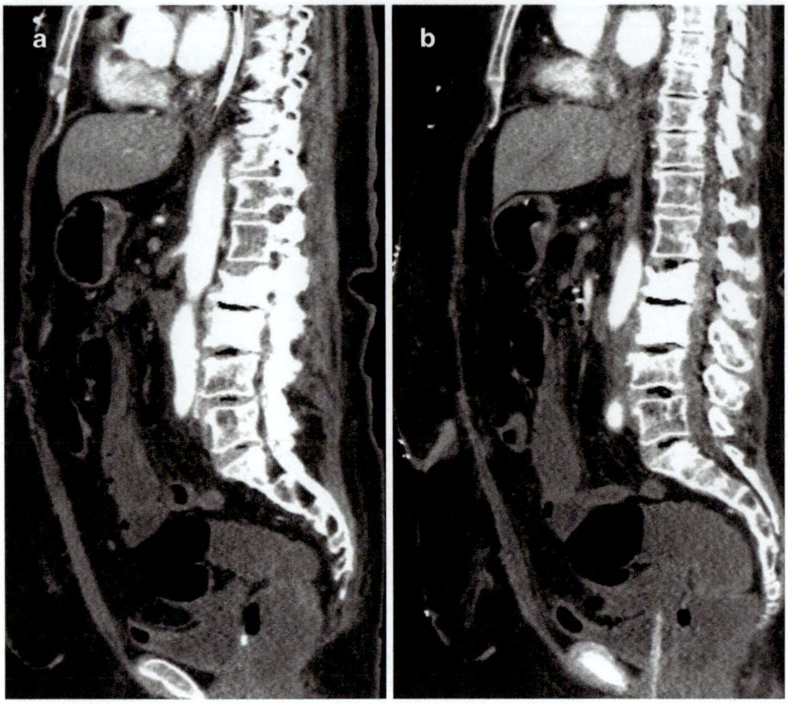

Fig. 32.1 (**a**) CTA sagittal view showing a filling defect at the origin of the SMA. (**b**) CTA showing poor distal filling of the SMA beyond its proximal segmental occlusion

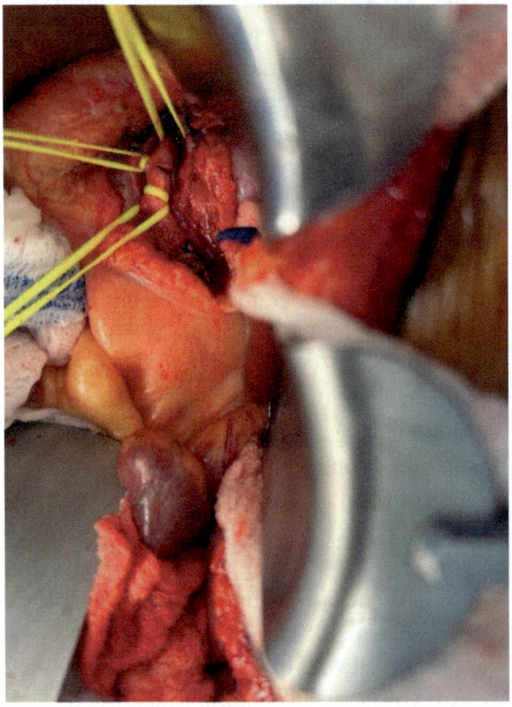

Fig. 32.2 Transverse arteriotomy in the proximal SMA with silastic loops proximally and distally to the arteriotomy site. One loop is around the side branch of the SMA

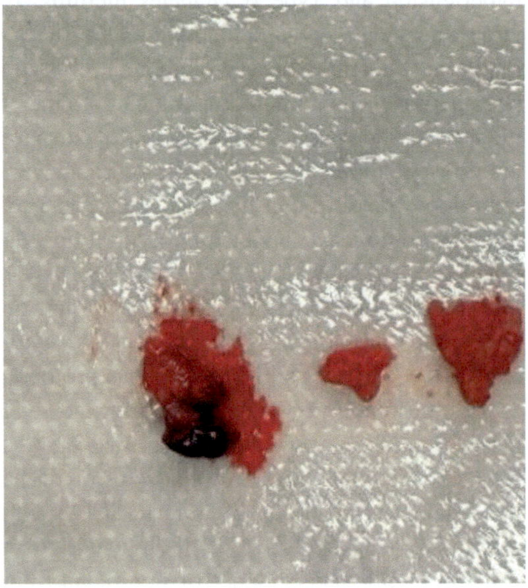

Fig. 32.3 Thromboembolic material removed from the SMA

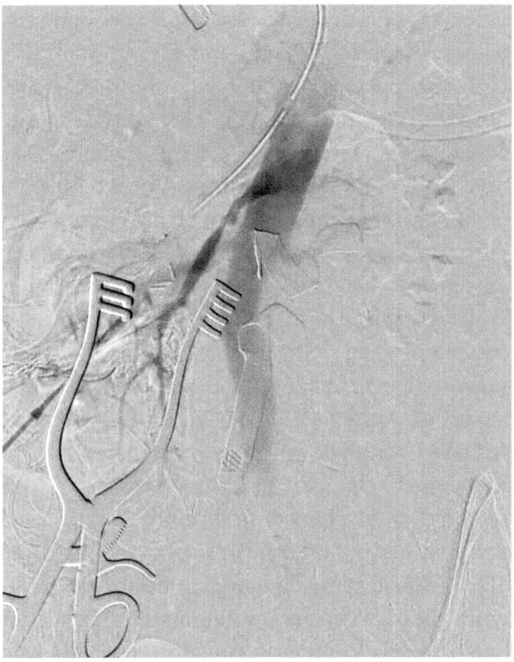

Fig. 32.4 Aortogram showing significant proximal SMA stenosis/residual thrombus

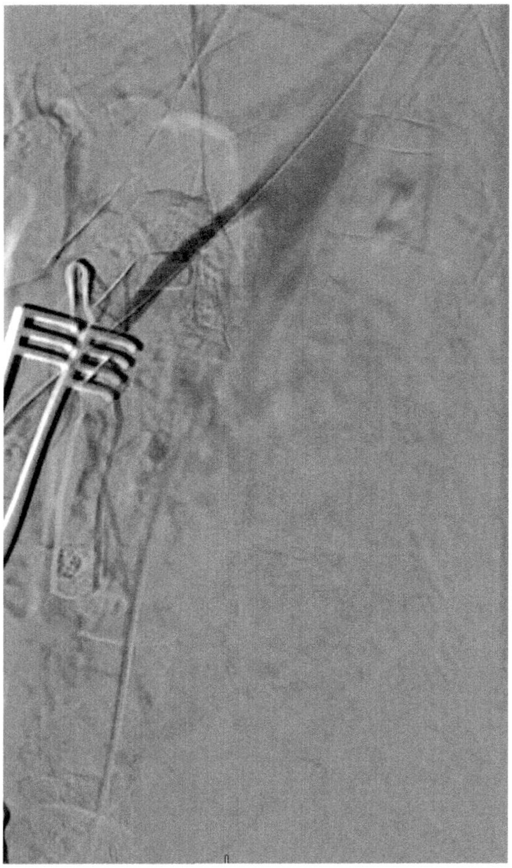

Fig. 32.5 ROMS with guidewire in the proximal abdominal aorta via a 6F sheath distal to the arteriotomy site in the SMA and with a covered stent in the proximal SMA

was reexplored 24 h later and was found to have a viable small and lower intestine. The small bowel anastomosis was performed by general surgery, and the fascial and the remaining abdominal closure were performed. She was kept on nasogastric suction, and the nasogastric tube was discontinued on the fifth postoperative day. She was transferred to the surgical floor after discontinuation of ventilatory support as she continued to show satisfactory progress with gradual return of gastrointestinal function and resolution of leukocytosis. She was discharged after 3 weeks

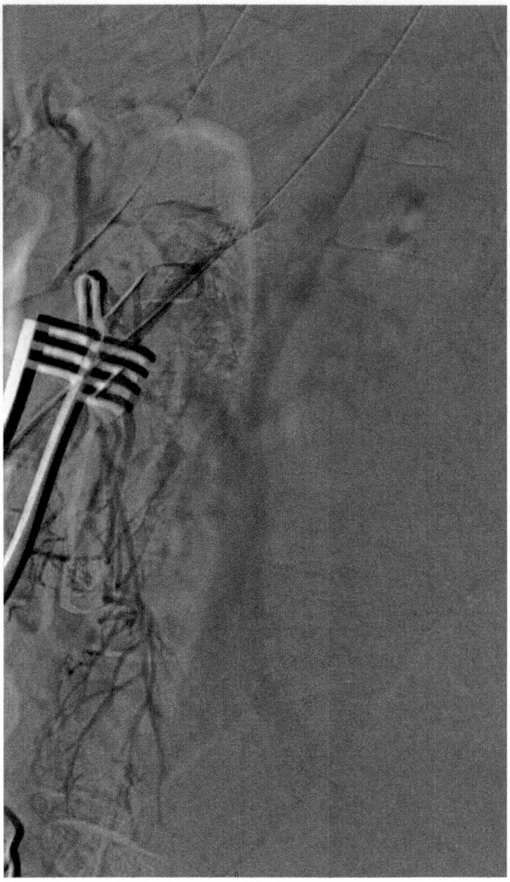

Fig. 32.6 Completion arteriogram showing filling of the distal branches of the SMA

of hospital stay. The patient died of septic shock at an outside hospital on August 10, 2025.

Discussion

Open SMA embolectomy remains the standard treatment for management of acute mesenteric ischemia (AMI), secondary to embolic occlusion. Recently, Penumbra suction thrombectomy has been used successfully in a high-risk elderly patient with a low suspicion of necrotic bowel in a patient with multiple comorbidities [1]. In recent years, an endovascular first approach has become more popular because of lower morbidity and improved 30-day mortality with decreased length of stay. A large analysis from the National Surgery Quality Improvement Program showed a 2.5-fold decrease in the risk of death associated with endovascular as the first-line therapy [2]. The endovascular first approach is best suited for prohibitively high-risk patients without any signs of bowel necrosis (leukocytosis WBC count >10,000, elevated lactate levels >7.0, or free pneumatosis, dilatation of bowel, or intraperitoneal fluid on computed tomography of abdomen) [2]. However, most studies advocating an endovascular approach are either isolated case reports or small case series with retrospective data analysis [3]. In most patients, open SMA thrombo-embolectomy remains the treatment of choice. A multicenter study of retrograde open mesenteric stenting (ROMS) through laparotomy for treatment of acute and chronic mesenteric ischemia was reported in 54 patients from 2001 to 2013, and reported early mortality was 45% for AMI and 10% for subacute-on-chronic mesenteric ischemia [4]. ROMS offers an alternative to bypass or percutaneous stenting in patients with AMI who require abdominal exploration and those who have flush mesenteric occlusions and have failed to respond to or are considered unsuitable for stenting by a percutaneous approach [4]. Despite good technical success, mortality remains high in patients with AMI. Patency rates and freedom from symptom recurrence and reintervention are comparable to the results achieved with percutaneous stenting. Andraska et al. reported the results of ROMS in 34 patients as an alternative to bypass as the initial approach to acute mesenteric ischemia and concluded that, given similar postoperative outcomes to open bypass with a shorter operative time, it should be considered as a first-line option for AMI [5].

Diagnostic algorithms for acute mesenteric ischemia have seen a paradigm shift during the past two decades. In the past, early catheter-based diagnostic arteriography has been supplanted by computed tomographic angiography (CTA) when AMI is suspected. In recent years, mortality after revascularization for AMI has declined from 50% in the 1990s to 30% in the 2000s; however, mortality still remains high in patients with AMI even after successful revascularization. Factors associated with high mortality are renal insufficiency, age older than 70 years, metabolic acidosis, symptom duration, and need for bowel resection during the second-look operation [6].

Multiple Choice Questions

1. A 70-year-old man who after fibrillation presents with abdominal pain of sudden onset, soft abdomen, absent bowel signal, WBC count is 10,000/mm^3 CTA abdomen shows a filling defect at the origin of the SMA. The optimal management is
   A. Percutaneous thrombectomy of the SMA
   B. SMA embolectomy
   C. Anticoagulation
   D. Repeat CBC, lactate every 4 h if normal, perform suction thrombectomy of the SMA followed by laparotomy
2. Compared to open bypass, ROMS has
   A. lower morbidity
   B. lower mortality
   C. lower morbidity and mortality
   D. same morbidity and mortality
3. Compared to open bypass, ROMS has
   A. longer operative time
   B. shorter operative time
   C. better primary patency
   D. better secondary patency

Answers: 1(B), 2(C), 3(B)

References

1. Creisher BA, Palvannan P, Salvatore DM, DiMuzio PJ, Abai B, Nooromid MJ. Penumbra aspiration thrombectomy of the superior mesenteric artery for mesenteric ischemia. J Vasc Surg Cases Innov Tech. 2023;9(4):101278. PMID:37767355
2. Beaulieu RJ, Arnaoutakis KD, Abularrage CJ, Efron DT, Schneider E, Black JH 3rd. Comparison of open and endovascular treatment of acute mesenteric ischemia. J Vasc Surg. 2014;59(1):159–64. PMID:24199769
3. Branco BC, Montero-Baker MF, Aziz H, Taylor Z, Mills JL. Endovascular therapy for acute mesenteric ischemia: an NSQIP analysis. Am Surg. 2015;81(11):1170–6. PMID:26672589
4. Oderich GS, Macedo R, Stone DH, Woo EY, Panneton JM, Resch T, et al. Multicenter study of retrograde open mesenteric artery stenting through laparotomy for treatment of acute and chronic mesenteric ischemia. J Vasc Surg. 2018;68(2):470–480.e471. PMID:29548812
5. Andraska E, Haga L, Li X, Avgerinos E, Singh M, Chaer R, et al. Retrograde open mesenteric stenting should be considered as the initial approach to acute mesenteric ischemia. J Vasc Surg. 2020;72(4):1260–8. PMID:32276014
6. Schermerhorn ML, Giles KA, Hamdan AD, Wyers MC, Pomposelli FB. Mesenteric revascularization: management and outcomes in the United States, 1988-2006. J Vasc Surg. 2009;50(2):341–348.e341. PMID:19372025

33 Crossover Femoral–Femoral Bypass Graft with Lateral Thigh Routing of the Graft

Presentation

A 67-year-old man was seen in the clinic in 2019 with pain in the right lower extremity on walking 25 yards and paresthesia in the right foot. He was a current smoker with a history of smoking 60 pack-years. Medical comorbidities included: coronary artery disease with remote myocardial infarction, seizure disorder, hypertension, chronic back pain, hyperlipidemia, and chronic obstructive pulmonary disease. He had a history of multiple trauma in 1997 as a road worker when a motor vehicle hit him in the lower torso. He sustained a fracture of the pelvis. He developed right femoral artery thrombosis, which was treated with an interposition 8 mm PTFE graft (WL Gore, Newark, DE) from the proximal common femoral artery to its bifurcation. The patient developed a surgical site infection and was treated with local wound care and antibiotics. The groin incision healed by secondary intention. Eight months later, he presented in the clinic with ischemic rest pain with an absent right femoral artery pulse. Non-invasive arterial study revealed an ankle-brachial index ABI on the right 0.38 (RT) and left 1.07 (LT). A catheter based abdominal and pelvic arteriography revealed an occlusion of the femoral interposition graft.

In 1998, the patient underwent repeat arterial reconstruction with explant of the previously placed PTFE graft. A spiral vein graft was constructed by harvesting the great saphenous vein from the entire length of the right lower extremity. The vein was slit along its entire length using Potts scissors and sutured over a 24F chest tube using a continuous 6-0 cardiovascular polypropylene suture (Ethicon, Rariton, NJ) resulting in 8 mm lumen of the spiral vein graft. The spiral vein graft was sutured to the distal right external iliac artery proximally and distally to the common femoral artery at its bifurcation after explant of the PTFE graft. The patient moved out of state after his last follow-up in 2000, which showed a patent spiral vein graft with normal ankle--brachial indices on both sides.

Patient moved back to Michigan in 2019 and presented with symptoms of intermittent claudication and ischemic rest pain associated with paresthesias in the right lower extremity with absent right femoral pulse with ABI on right (0.34) and left (1.07). The patient underwent abdominal and pelvic aortography and run-off study using left femoral access which showed occlusion of the right external, iliac artery, and common femoral artery with stenosis of the proximal superficial femoral artery and the origin of profunda femoris artery with numerous collaterals in the groin and upper thigh. The popliteal artery was patent with run off primarily with anterior tibial artery. The posterior tibial

S. S. Hans, *Secondary and Tertiary Arterial Reconstructions*,
https://doi.org/10.1007/978-3-032-21214-6_33

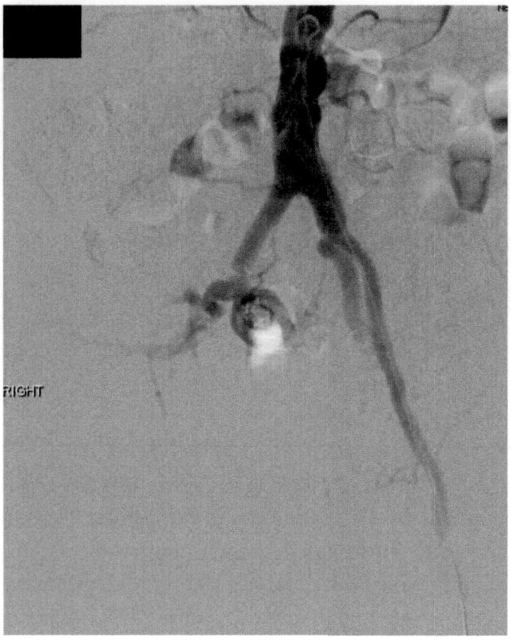

Fig. 33.1 Abdominal aortogram showing occlusion of the right external iliac artery

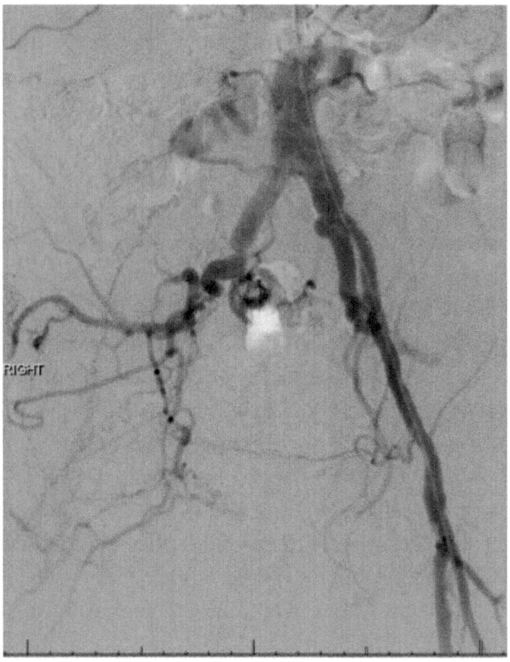

Fig. 33.2 Abdominal and pelvic arteriogram showing occlusion of the right external iliac artery with satisfactory flow in the left common and external iliac and common femoral artery and its proximal superficial femoral and profunda femoris artery

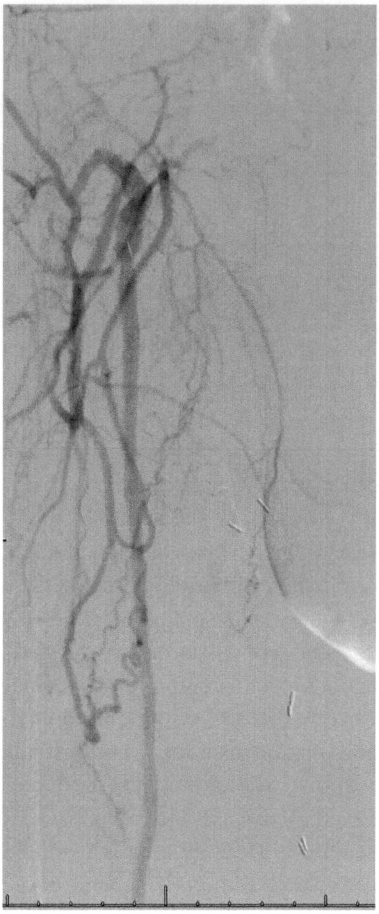

Fig. 33.3 Arteriogram showing right common femoral artery occlusion and patent right superficial femoral artery and distal segment of the profunda femoris artery

artery and the peroneal artery were occluded (Figs. 33.1, 33.2, 33.3, and 33.4).

As the patient had multiple comorbidities with advanced COPD and a hostile right groin, aortofemoral graft was not considered as the best option (Fig. 33.5). A crossover femoral-femoral graft (8 mm) interring PTFE graft (W.L. Gore Inc., Newark, DE) originating from the left common femoral artery using a left groin incision with routing the graft in an anterolateral location in a subcutaneous plane in the lateral thigh and tunneled medially. An incision was made in the right upper lateral thigh, and the lateral border of the sartorius was exposed. The right superficial femoral artery was exposed in the Hunter's

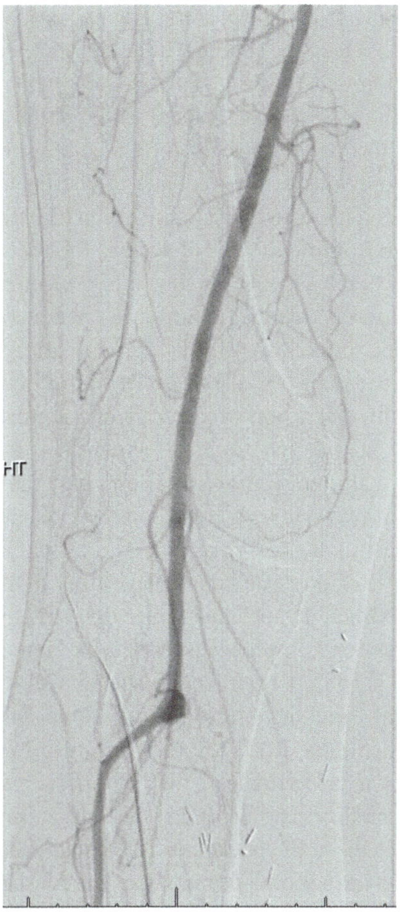

Fig. 33.4 Occlusion of tibio-peroneal trunk and runoff with anterior tibial artery. Posterior tibial artery and peroneal artery are occluded

canal, and the distal anastomosis was performed in an end-to-side manner with a continuous 5′0″ cardiovascular polypropylene suture. Postoperative CTA showed a patent crossover left common to right proximal superficial femoral artery bypass (Fig. 33.6). A follow-up arterial study 7 months later showed ABI on the right (0.89) and left (0.91). However, the crossover femoral-femoral graft occluded 18 months postoperatively, with return of symptoms of mild intermittent claudication with ABI of RT (0.50) and LT (0.98). He was last seen in the clinic in April 2025 with mild stable intermittent claudication involving the right lower extremity.

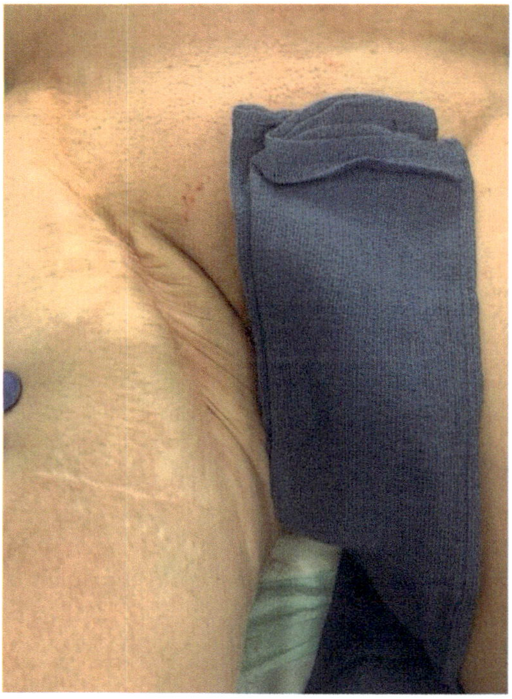

Fig. 33.5 Picture showing significant scarring in the right groin from two prior open femoral artery reconstruction

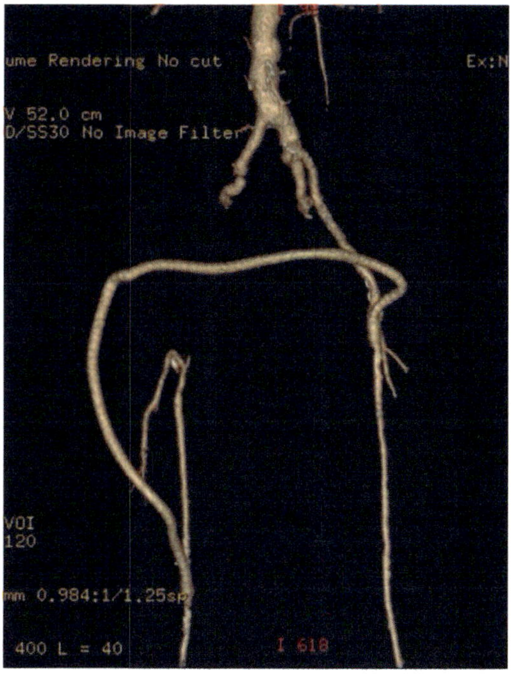

Fig. 33.6 Postoperative CTA showing patent crossover left common femoral artery to right mid SFA bypass graft with lateral routing of the graft. There is mild stenosis at the right curve of the crossover graft

Noninvasive arterial study showed ankle-brachial index RT (0.38) LT (0.85).

Discussion

Crossover femoral–femoral bypass graft is a low-risk arterial reconstruction in the high-risk group of patients, as aortic clamping and laparotomy are avoided. Confirmation of a satisfactory inflow in the donor iliac/femoral artery should be evaluated with thorough clinical examination by an easily palpable pulse and confirmed by duplex imaging, computed tomography angiography, or conventional catheter-based arteriography [1]. The common femoral artery (CFA), superficial femoral artery (SFA), or profunda femoris artery (PFA) can be used as a suitable target for outflow anastomoses [1]. Endarterectomy of the inflow or outflow may also be required as an adjunct procedure. The procedure is performed under general or regional anesthesia, depending upon the anesthetic risk and preference of the surgeon [1]. A vertical or a hockey stick incision in each groin is made. The groin lymphatics are mobilized medially and laterally to avoid transection; larger lymphatics should be individually ligated. A suprapubic tunnel is created in a gentle C-shaped curve. For anastomosis, the common femoral artery immediately adjacent to the inguinal ligament should be avoided because of the tendency of the graft to kink when anastomosed to the proximal segment of the common femoral artery due to abdominal pannus on assuming upright posture. Anastomosis to the distal segments of the common femoral artery, proximal superficial femoral artery or profunda femoris artery is preferable. Anastomosis to the proximal segment of the common femoral artery may result in kinking of the crossover graft.

In a patient with a groin infection or extensive scarring from prior groin exposures or post radiation, lateral routing of the graft is preferable to standard placement because of the risk of skin breakdown with resulting exposure of the superficially placed graft. This patient had two prior femoral arterial interposition grafting procedures, and the index operation resulted in a surgical site infection and healing with secondary intention. Therefore, SFA was selected as the outflow vessel in this patient because of a hostile groin. We have previously reported lateral routing of the graft in patients with groin infection [2]. Routing the graft through the obturator foramen with inflow at the aorta or the iliac artery is often used for arterial reconstructions in patients with mycotic infections of the femoral artery. The exact cause of occlusion of the was not obvious since the occlusion occurred many months after the reconstruction. Intimal hyperplasia, a slight kink in the graft above and lateral to the groin area, progression of distal disease, as demonstrated by one vessel run off at the time of last reconstruction, probably played a significant role. Although not apparent in this patient, the progression of inflow disease in the donor iliac artery is an important factor causing occlusion of the graft. Kinking of the graft at the femoral anastomosis often leads to early occlusion. Graft infection and patient-specific factors such as diabetes mellitus and nicotine abuse may also contribute to graft occlusion. Patients following cross-over femoral–femoral graft reconstruction should undergo serial noninvasive imaging studies, and correction of any donor iliac artery disease, and anastomotic stenosis if present should be repaired prophylactically to prevent graft occlusion. In this the patient occlusion of the spiral vein graft probably resulted from proximal occlusive disease in the right external iliac artery or intimal hyperplasia at the anastomotic sites.

Multiple Choice Questions

1. In a patient with common femoral artery thrombosis secondary to traumatic dissection, the optimal management consists of:
   A. Thrombolysis and placement of a covered stent
   B. Thrombolysis and placement of a self-expanding stent

   C. Open femoral artery thrombectomy, tacking of the intimal flap
   D. Femoral interposition graft
2. The most common cause of graft occlusion 18 months after the repair is:
   A. Progression of distal disease
   B. Technical factors
   C. Myointimal hyperplasia
   D. Kinking of the anastomosis
3. In patients with hostile groin arterial reconstruction with a normal anastomosis to the iliac artery and distal to the superficial femoral artery, the graft should be routed:
   A. Normal anatomical course
   B. Obturator space
   C. Lateral route around the iliac crest
   D. Obturator space or lateral routing of the graft

Answers: 1(D), 2(C), 3(D)

References

1. Mohammad F, Shepard AD. Extra-anatomic reconstruction for aortoiliac occlusive disease. In: Hans SS, Shepard AD, editors. Endovascular and open vascular reconstruction: a practical approach. CRC Press; 2025. p. 274–9.
2. Hans SS. Exposed graft in the groin following crossover femoral-femoral graft and aorto-uniiliac stent graft. In: Hans SS, editor. Challenging arterial reconstructions: 100 clinical cases. Cham: Springer; 2020. p. 287–90.

34 Carotid Interposition Graft in a Patient with Prior Transfemoral Carotid Stenting for Acute Stroke

Presentation

A 67-year-old woman presented to the emergency room of her local rural hospital with right-sided facial droop, difficulty with finding words, and right upper extremity weakness (NIH stroke scale 9) on March 5, 2017. Medical comorbidities included hypertension, type II diabetes mellitus, and nicotine abuse. She has a history of smoking, 50 pack-years. She was transferred to an outside tertiary care center and underwent an unenhanced CT scan of the head and a CT perfusion study. In addition, she underwent a CTA scan of the head and neck, which showed high-grade stenosis (> 90%) of the left internal carotid artery and a moderate stenosis (70%) of the right internal carotid artery. There was complete occlusion of the left M-1 segment at its origin (middle cerebral artery). There were narrowing and lumen irregularities in the left A-1 segment of the anterior cerebral artery.

Patient underwent Trevo embolectomy using femoral artery access of the left middle cerebral artery. The left carotid stent was deployed (Acculink-Abbott) using a distal protection device (Spider X). At the completion of the intervention, the patient had TICI 3 flow. There was evidence of mild stenosis distal to the stent on the completion arteriogram. Neurological deficit completely resolved in the ensuing few weeks. Patient was seen in the clinic in 2019, and a carotid duplex study showed a high-grade stenosis of the left internal carotid artery distal to the stent (80%) and severe in-stent stenosis. A stent was visualized in the distal common carotid artery, and calcific stenosis was present, distal to the stent at the origin of the left internal carotid artery. She underwent CT angiography, which confirmed findings of the carotid duplex study (Fig. 34.1).

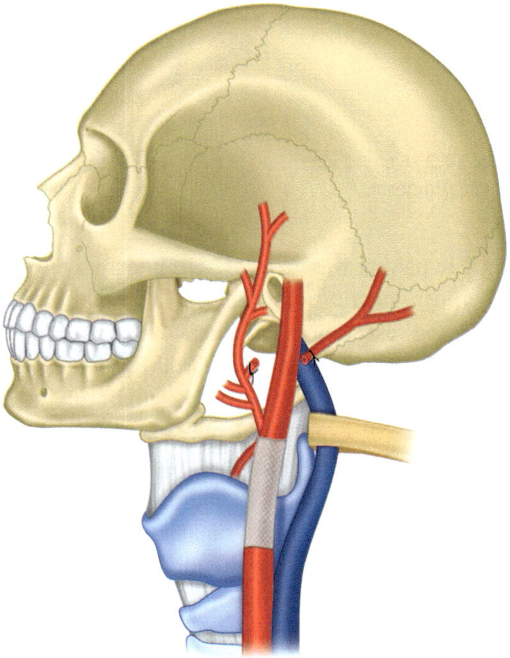

Fig. 34.1 Anatomical relations of the left carotid stent

S. S. Hans, *Secondary and Tertiary Arterial Reconstructions*,
https://doi.org/10.1007/978-3-032-21214-6_34

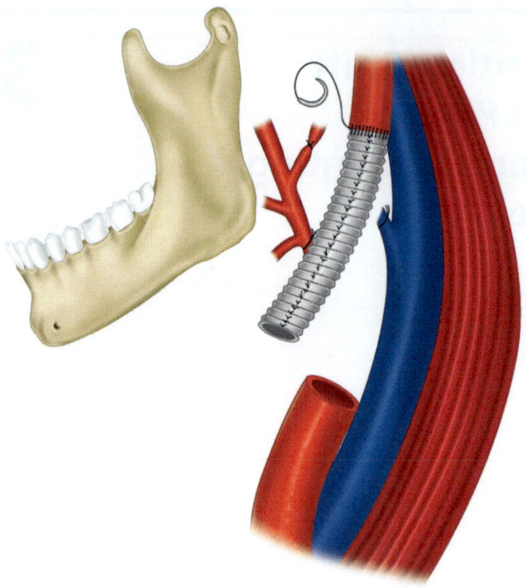

Fig. 34.2 Carotid interposition graft with completed distal anastomosis

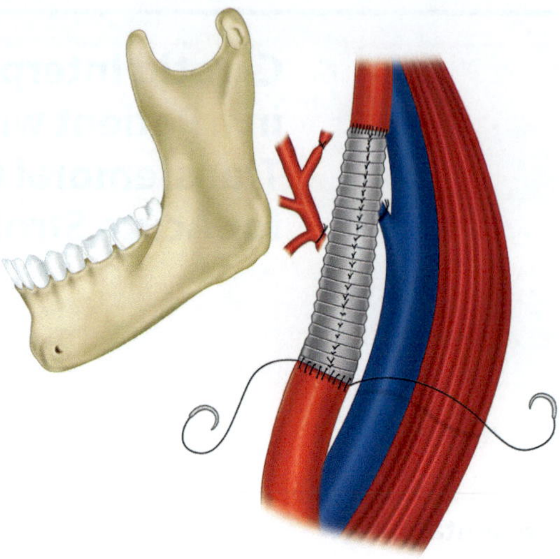

Fig. 34.3 Carotid interposition graft with completed proximal anastomosis

The patient was scheduled to undergo carotid interposition grafting with removal of the carotid stent and resection of the distal common carotid artery and proximal internal carotid artery. Under general anesthesia with EEG monitoring and median nerve evoked potential monitoring, the patient underwent resection of the distal 4 cm of the common carotid artery and proximal 2 cm of the internal carotid artery, and a tapered PTFE graft (7 × 4 mm), which was divided in a spatulated manner that the lumen of the distal end of the graft was 5 mm. This graft was interposed between the divided common carotid artery and the internal carotid artery. The external carotid artery was suture ligated (Figs. 34.2, 34.3, 34.4, and 34.5). Patient was discharged on postoperative day one in satisfactory condition. She was last seen at follow-up in July 2025 with no further neurological symptoms. A carotid duplex study showed 50–69% stenosis in the right internal carotid artery and less than 50% stenosis of the left internal carotid artery.

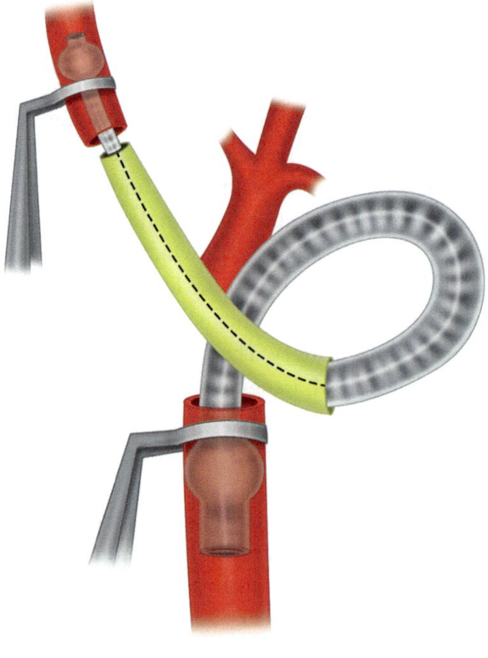

Fig. 34.4 Carotid Interposition graft over the shunt

For carotid in-stent stenosis, repeat endovascular therapy (balloon angioplasty with a drug-eluting balloon or repeat stenting) or carotid endarterectomy with patch graft is the initial treatment option. A patient who fails carotid artery stenting because of a heavy calcific burden, recurrent carotid in-stent stenosis or structural failure of the stent is best managed by the resection of the distal common carotid artery and proximal internal carotid artery, including the

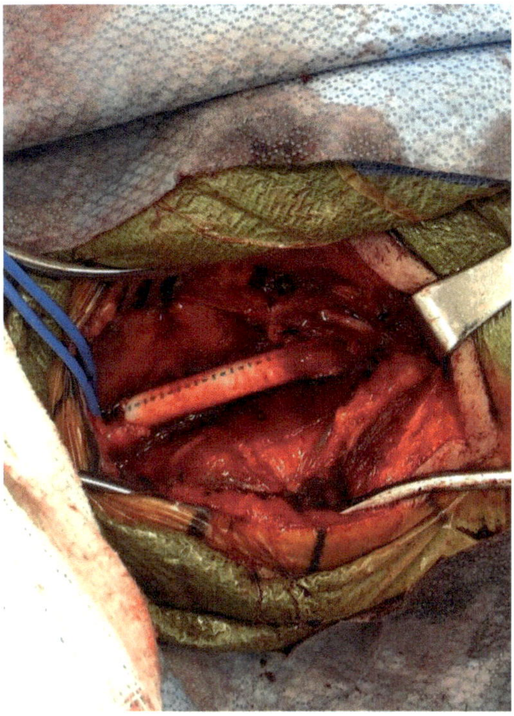

Fig. 34.5 Operative photograph showing an interposition PTFE graft from the common carotid artery to the internal carotid artery

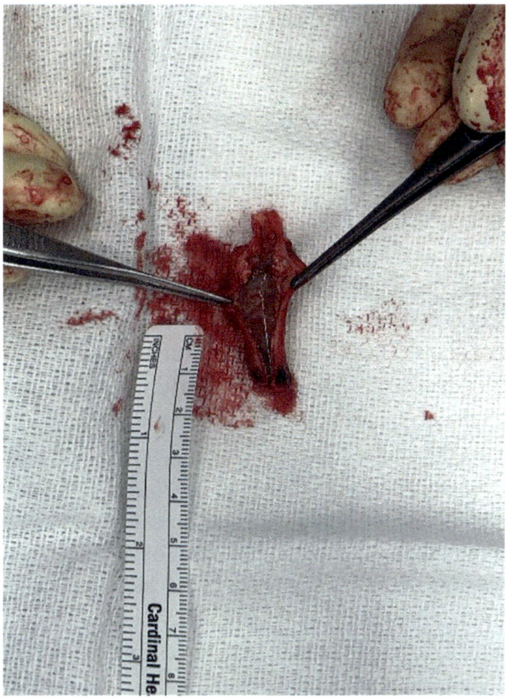

Fig. 34.6 Resected distal common and proximal internal and external carotid artery at its bifurcation with removal of the carotid stent

stent. An interposition graft between the common carotid artery and proximal internal carotid artery is performed [1, 2]. CT angiography of the neck and head should help in determining the cephalad extension of the stent [1]. If the stent extends at or superior to the level of the C2 vertebral body, additional exposure of the distal internal carotid artery in the neck is necessary. Balloon occlusion of the internal carotid artery by placing a small Fogarty catheter 3F over a 0.014 wire is advanced following 7 F sheath placed in the common carotid artery in the proximal common carotid artery. Intraluminal control of the distal internal carotid artery is obtained by inflating the balloon catheter with diluted contrast media.

If EEG and somatosensory median nerve evoked potentials indicate cerebral ischemia or if the stump pressure is below 40 mmHg, in a patient without EEG monitoring, an indwelling shunt is recommended. The distal end of the shunt is first advanced into the divided internal carotid artery; after there is back bleeding from the shunt, the proximal end of the shunt is inserted into the common carotid artery. The interposition graft is subsequently placed over another shunt (second shunt); the first shunt is removed, and the second shunt with the interposition graft around it is inserted. Distal end-to-end anastomosis is performed first, followed by proximal anastomosis to the divided common carotid artery (Fig. 34.6). Before proximal anastomosis is completed, the shunt is removed, and the suturing is completed. In this patient, the carotid stent placement at the index procedure did not treat the site of proximal internal carotid artery stenosis. In stent carotid stenosis and worsening ICA stenosis, resection of the distal CCA and ICA, including the stent, is favored. Various factors that determine the type of secondary intervention include anticipated neck "hostility," site of recurrent lesion in the ICA, patient's overall health status, and anticipated life expectancy. In addition, the open and endovascular skill sets of the treating surgeon need to be considered when determining the best approach for a patient in these circumstances.

If the superior end of the stent is at the lower half of the C2 vertebral body or inferior to that location, balloon occlusion of the distal ICA is not necessary. Distal clamping of the ICA can be performed by careful mobilization. Stump pressure (back pressure) (SP) is recorded with a 21-G needle placed below the proximal end of the stent. The ICA is opened transversely with a No. 15 blade scalpel, a few millimeters inferior to the cephalad end of the stent, and is then separated from the distal ICA with caudal retraction. The origin of the ECA is divided, and the distal end is suture-ligated with a running polypropylene suture; the proximal end of the CCA is divided. In patients with distal balloon occlusion, after the ICA has been circumferentially divided, it is further mobilized cranially. The balloon is deflated and removed, and an atraumatic vascular clamp or clip (Yasargil® aneurysm clip (Aesculap, Inc., Center Valley, PA, USA)) is applied. The specimen, consisting of the distal CCA, proximal ICA, and stent, is removed. A 4 × 7-mm tapered PTFE graft is fashioned from W. L. Gore & Associates, Inc., Flagstaff, AZ, USA, and distal anastomosis is performed with a 6-0 cardiovascular polypropylene suture. After completion of the distal anastomosis, blood is allowed to flow retrograde to remove any debris, the graft is flushed with heparin–saline solution, and the vascular clamp is applied just proximal to the distal anastomosis. Proximal anastomosis is then performed with either a 5-0 or 6-0 cardiovascular polypropylene suture. Appropriate antegrade and retrograde flushing and declamping are performed. The author prefers PTFE as a graft conduit, although reversed great saphenous vein (GSV) harvested from the upper thigh or non-reversed GSV with valve lysis can be used as alternative conduits. Completion arteriogram is performed either with a 5-F sheath inserted into the CCA below the proximal anastomosis. Contrast with 50% dilution in an amount of 5–7 cc is injected to obtain images of the neck and brain.

If the completion arteriogram does not show any abnormalities, the opening in the common carotid artery after removal of the sheath is closed with a 6-0 cardiovascular polypropylene suture. Subcutaneous tissue, including the platysma muscle, is sutured with a 3-0 absorbable suture, and the skin is approximated with 3-0 nylon interrupted sutures and staples.

Discussion

The incidence of cranial nerve injury and myocardial infarction is greater in patients undergoing redo carotid operations [3]. In most patients, cranial nerve palsy is reversible [3]. There is a higher incidence of carotid restenosis after carotid artery stenting as compared to redo carotid endarterectomy or carotid interposition graft at the long-term follow-up.

Multiple Choice Questions

1. A 70-year-old woman presents with severe in-stent stenosis in the distal CCA with >80% stenosis of the proximal ICA superior to the stent. The best management option is
   A. Repeat Carotid Stenting
   B. Balloon Angioplasty
   C. Carotid Endarterectomy
   D. Carotid Interposition Graft
2. Cephalad dissection for exposure of the internal carotid artery superior to the stent in a patient undergoing carotid interposition graft requires division of the posterior belly of the digastric and stylohyoid with removal of the styloid process. The most common nerve injury encountered with such exposure is
   A. Glossopharyngeal
   B. Hypoglossal
   C. Vagus
   D. Loop of Ansa cervicalis
3. Distal control of ICA in a patient with a carotid stent extending cephalad to the superior aspect of C_2 vertebral body is obtained by

A. Distal exposure of ICA at the level of the styloid process
B. Balloon occlusion with a 3F Fogarty balloon catheter of the distal ICA by passage of a 0.014 wire into the ICA up near the base of the skull
C. Clamping of the ICA with a stent using the atraumatic vascular clamp
D. Incision in the distal CCA and proximal ICA, and separating the stent, puncturing the wall of the artery, and clamping the ICA after the stent removal

Answers: 1(D), 2(A), 3(B)

References

1. Hans SS, Gassner M. Carotid interposition grafting. In: Hans SS, Shepard AD, Bove P, Weaver MR, Long GW, editors. Endovascular and open vascular reconstruction: a practical approach. Boca Raton: CRC Press; 2017. p. 152–5.
2. Hans SS. Carotid interposition graft in a patient with prior carotid stenting for acute stroke. In: Hans SS, editor. Challenging arterial reconstructions: 100 clinical cases. Cham: Springer; 2020. p. 181–3.
3. Tu J, Wang S, Huo Z, Wu R, Yao C, Wang S. Repeated carotid endarterectomy versus carotid artery stenting for patients with carotid restenosis after carotid endarterectomy: systematic review and meta-analysis. Surgery. 2015;157(6):1166–73. PMID:25840718

35 Open Repair of Postcarotid Endarterectomy Aneurysm

Presentation

A 68-year-old man presented to the ER with symptoms of depression and a right pulsatile neck mass. A CTA of neck and brain showed a 2.7 × 2.5 cm right distal common carotid artery and proximal internal carotid artery aneurysm with contralateral CCA/ICA occlusion (Figs. 35.1, 35.2, and 35.3). He had a history of right carotid endarterectomy in 2005 and a repeat carotid endarterectomy with a patch graft in 2020 at an outside hospital. Details of the first two operations were not available. Medical comorbidities included hypertension and hyperlipidemia. He had a mitral valve replacement in Jan 2021. A diagnostic carotid and cerebral angiogram showed a large carotid aneurysm (Fig. 35.4). The patient underwent resection of the right common carotid and internal carotid under general anesthesia on April 21, 2025. An extended neck incision beyond the previous scar was made due to two prior carotid endarterectomies. The carotid

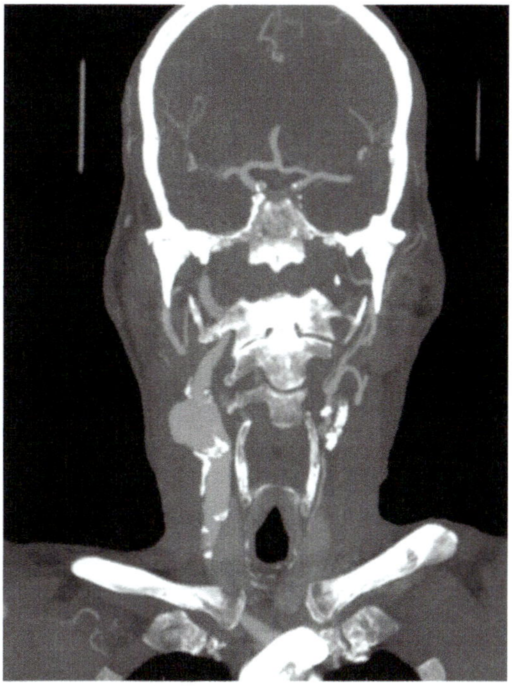

Fig. 35.1 CTA neck and brain (coronal view) showing Rt CCA/ICA aneurysm

S. S. Hans, *Secondary and Tertiary Arterial Reconstructions*,
https://doi.org/10.1007/978-3-032-21214-6_35

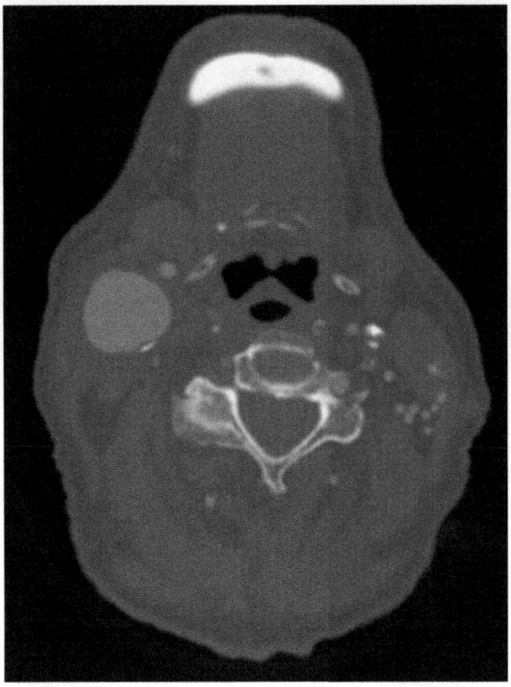

Fig. 35.2 CTA neck and brain-axial view showing Rt carotid aneurysm with contralateral carotid occlusion

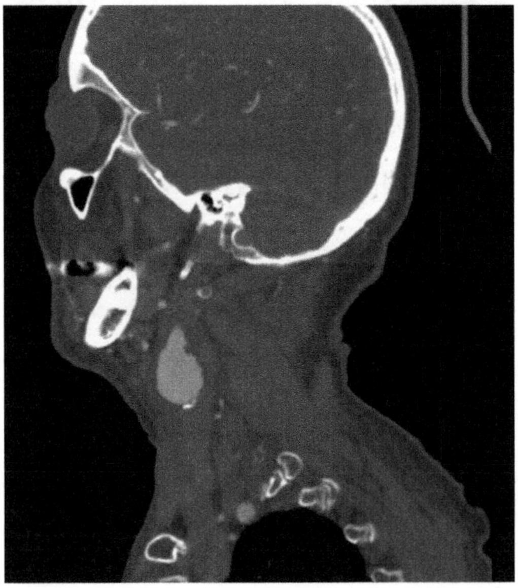

Fig. 35.3 CTA neck and brain-sagittal view showing RT carotid aneurysm

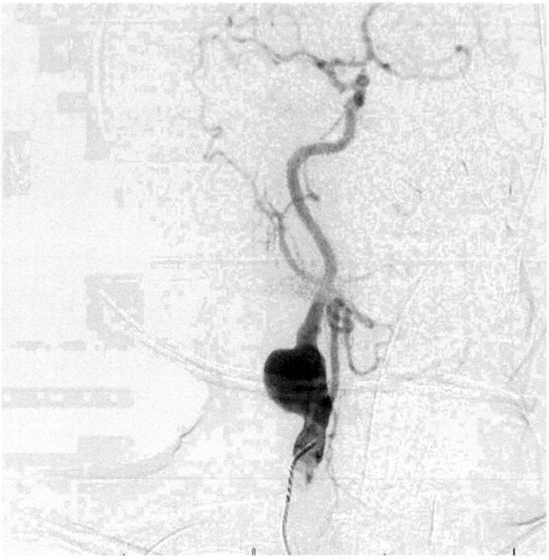

Fig. 35.4 Carotid arteriogram showing proximal right ICA aneurysm

aneurysm was carefully exposed, and a silastic vessel loop was placed near the base of the neck around the proximal common carotid artery. The internal jugular vein was adherent to the wall of the aneurysm and was carefully separated by sharp dissection. The vagus nerve was identified in its anatomical position between the internal jugular vein and the internal/common carotid artery. Cephalad exposure of the internal carotid artery was performed (Fig. 35.5). The hypoglossal nerve was tethered to the internal carotid artery and carefully preserved. Stump (back pressure) was measured by clamping the common carotid artery (CCA) and external carotid artery and inserting the needle into the CCA after systemic heparinization, and measured 72 mmHg. There was no change in the EEG tracings with proximal clamping of the CCA; the indwelling

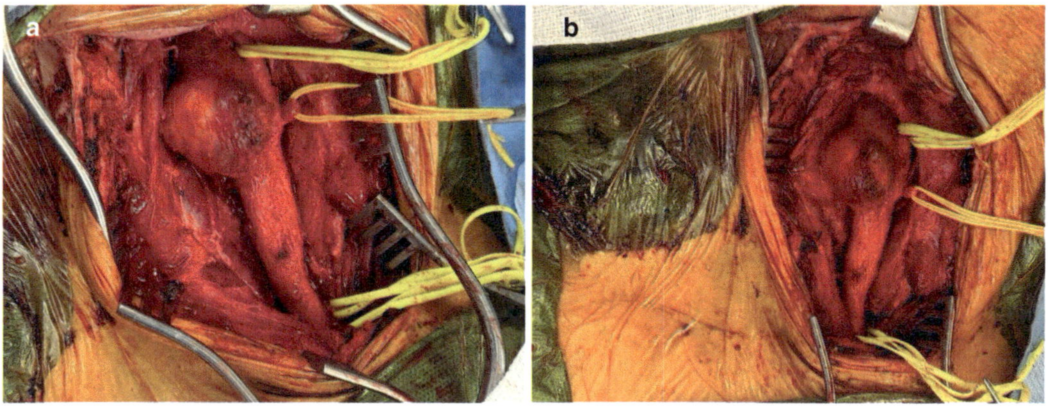

Fig. 35.5 (**a**) Exposed carotid aneurysm with silastic loops around the common carotid artery, superior thyroid artery, and external carotid artery. (**b**) Exposed carotid aneurysm with silastic loops around the common carotid artery, superior thyroid artery, and external carotid artery

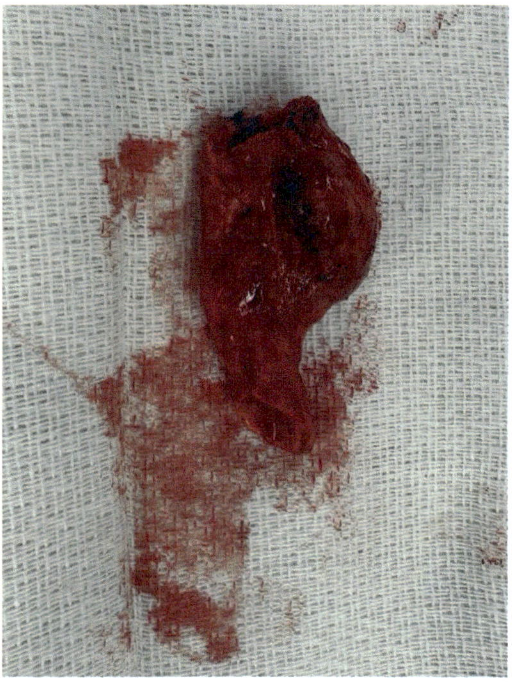

Fig. 35.6 Specimen of excised carotid aneurysm

shunt was not used. The distal CCA and proximal ICA with the aneurysm were resected (Fig. 35.6) external carotid artery (ECA) was suture ligated. An 8 mm PTFE Rifampicin soaked graft was interposed between the CCA and ICA (Fig. 35.7a, b).

The patient had an uneventful course. At the last follow-up, in September 2025, the neck incision had healed well. The patient did not experience any neurological complications. The pathology report showed a degenerative atherosclerotic aneurysmal wall.

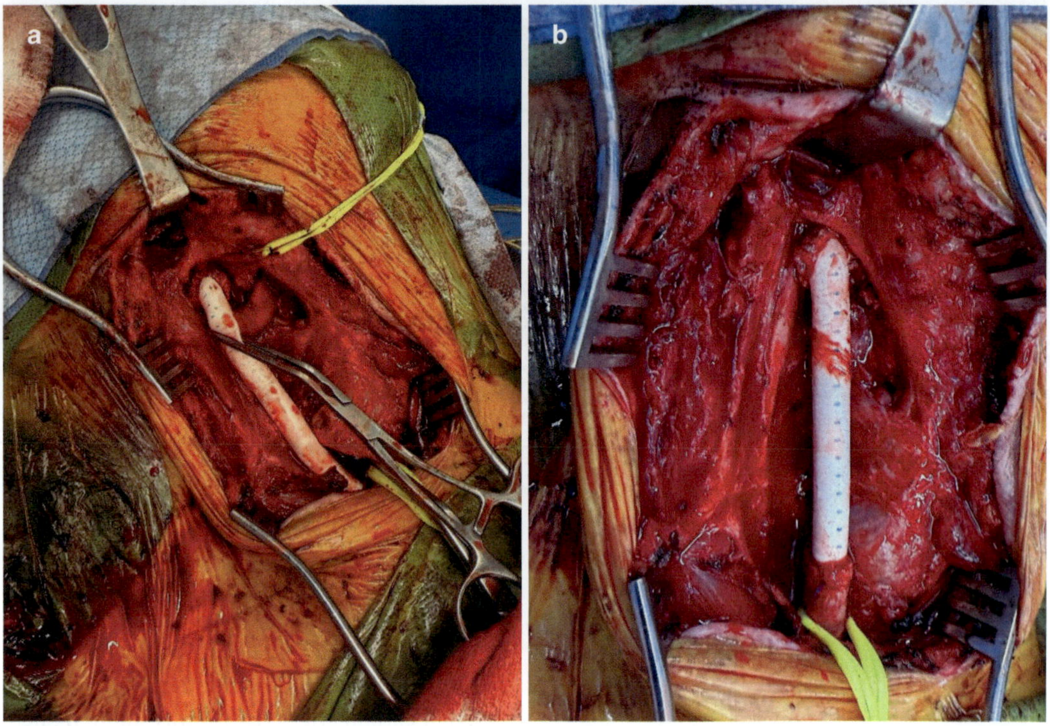

Fig. 35.7 (**a**) Distal anastomosis of the Interposition graft and vascular clamp placed on the interposition graft proximal to the distal anastomosis. (**b**) Interposition graft from ICA to CCA with hypoglossal nerve coursing just distal to the distal anastomosis

Discussion

Extracranial carotid aneurysms are rare, accounting for less than 1% of all arterial aneurysms [1]. Cerebral ischemia in the form of stroke or transient ischemic attack is often the most common presenting symptom [1–4]. True extracranial carotid aneurysm is most commonly atherosclerotic (degenerative) and affects the bifurcation or the proximal internal carotid artery, and the distal internal carotid artery is the next common site. Carotid pseudoaneurysms are usually the result of trauma, patch degeneration, or infection following carotid endarterectomy, and have an incidence of 12–18% of all carotid aneurysms [1, 2]. Carotid duplex study, CTA carotid neck and brain, as well as catheter-based arteriography, aid in the diagnosis and are helpful in planning surgical repair.

Extracranial carotid aneurysms have been classified according to the affected segment, which can be helpful for surgical planning [3]:

Type I—Isolated to the internal carotid artery.
Type II—Involve the internal carotid artery and the bifurcation.
Type III—Aneurysm of the carotid bifurcation.
Type IV—Aneurysm of the internal and common carotid artery.
Type V—Isolated aneurysm of the common carotid artery.

Exposure of the distal internal carotid artery for distal control can be challenging. Retrostyloid exposure of the internal carotid artery can be performed by retracting or dividing the posterior belly of the digastric and stylohyoid muscles and may necessitate excision of the styloid process and taking utmost care to prevent injury to the glossopharyngeal nerve.

For more distal exposure of ICA in the neck, nasotracheal intubation and mandibular subluxation in collaboration with ENT or oral surgeon should be considered.

Ligation of the internal carotid artery in contemporary practice is considered a last option because of the associated high stroke rate and high mortality. In challenging cases with an ICA aneurysm near the base of the skull with difficulty in obtaining distal control, test occlusion of the CCA/ICA can assist in determining the safety of carotid ligation [3]. In patients with a small or focal ICA aneurysms, following resection, can undergo reconstruction with direct end-to-end anastomosis in a continuous or interrupted fashion with polypropylene suture following mobilization in the proximal and distal artery to achieve tension-free anastomosis [3]. Spatulation of both ends of the artery prevents constriction of the suture line. Aneurysmorrhaphy or resection of the aneurysmal wall with either prosthetic or autologous tissue patch angioplasty can be useful in anatomically challenging areas or high lesions [2, 3]. All the debris and aneurysm contents should be removed. Removal of redundant and thin-walled artery permits patch angioplasty in the healthier vessel wall. Interposition grafting with either a synthetic (in the patient described) or an autologous arterial or vein graft, depending upon the vessel size and pathology of the aneurysm [3]. In mycotic aneurysms, autologous venous or arterial conduit is preferable. Because the patency of the synthetic conduits is only slightly inferior to that of autologous vein conduits, and with the easy availability of a synthetic graft, the time taken to harvest an autologous conduit makes synthetic conduits more attractive for use as an interposition graft [3]. Tapered synthetic grafts are more suitable when transitioning from a large CCA to a smaller diameter ICA. Interposition vein grafts are more likely to kink after reestablishment of the flow because of their tendency to elongation [3].

Surgical repair of an extracranial carotid aneurysm is associated with a perioperative stroke rate of 6–9% and a mortality rate of 1–2% [2, 4]. The stroke rate of untreated carotid aneurysms can be greater than 50%. The most common postoperative complication of open carotid aneurysm repair in the neck is cranial nerve injury at 3–17% [2–4].

Multiple Choice Questions

1. What is the incidence of carotid aneurysm among all arterial aneurysms:
   A. Less than 5%
   B. Less than 2%
   C. Less than 1%
   D. Less than 1%
2. The most common complication following resection of an extracranial carotid aneurysm is:
   A. Postoperative stroke
   B. Hematoma neck
   C. Cranial nerve injury
   D. Cardiac complications
3. An extracranial aneurysm has a cephalad extension at the level of C1–C2 vertebral with a tortuous internal carotid artery. A helpful technique in achieving successful exposure includes:
   A. Division of the styloid process and the stylohyoid muscle
   B. Mandibular osteotomy
   C. Caudal traction of the common carotid artery with a silastic loop
   D. Nasotracheal intubation and mandibular subluxation

Answers: 1(D) 2(C) 3(D)

References

1. El-Sabrout R, Cooley DA. Extracranial carotid artery aneurysms: Texas Heart Institute experience. J Vasc Surg. 2000;31(4):702–12. PMID:10753278
2. Srivastava S. Extracranial carotid aneurysm resection. In: Hans S, Shepard A, Weaver M, et al., editors. Endovascular and open vascular reconstruction: a practical approach. Boca Raton: Taylor & Francis Group; 2017. p. 163–6.
3. Attigah N, Külkens S, Zausig N, Hansmann J, Ringleb P, Hakimi M, et al. Surgical therapy of extracranial carotid artery aneurysms: long-term results over a 24-year period. Eur J Vasc Endovasc Surg. 2009;37(2):127–33. PMID:19046645
4. Rosset E, Albertini JN, Magnan PE, Ede B, Thomassin JM, Branchereau A. Surgical treatment of extracranial internal carotid artery aneurysms. J Vasc Surg. 2000;31(4):713–23. PMID:10753279

36 Carotid Endarterectomy in a Patient with a Variant of Ansa Cervicalis

Presentation

A 74-year-old man was seen in the clinic with diminished vision in the left eye secondary to poor retinal flow, diagnosed by his ophthalmologist. Carotid duplex study showed greater than 70% stenosis of the left internal carotid artery (ICA) and less than 50% stenosis of the right ICA. Medical comorbidities included hypertension, aortic valve stenosis with a history of a recent TAVR, type II diabetes mellitus, and hyperlipidemia. He did not have any history of stroke or transient ischemic attack in the past.

CTA of the carotid neck and brain in January 2025 showed 90–95% stenosis with predominantly calcified plaque at the left carotid bulb and involving the proximal ICA (Fig. 36.1). The right vertebral artery was non-dominant and terminated as the posterior inferior cerebellar artery had mild stenosis at its origin.

In May 2025, the patient underwent right carotid endarterectomy under general anesthesia with EEG and median nerve evoked potential monitoring. The back pressure (stump) pressure was 70 mmHg. Carotid clamping did not result in any ischemic changes on EEG; therefore, an indwelling shunt was not used.

During exposure of the common carotid artery (CEA) and ICA, a short loop of ansa cervicalis with a long length of ansa was encountered. The loop was preserved and mobilized medially along with a long length of ansa cervicalis (Fig. 36.2).

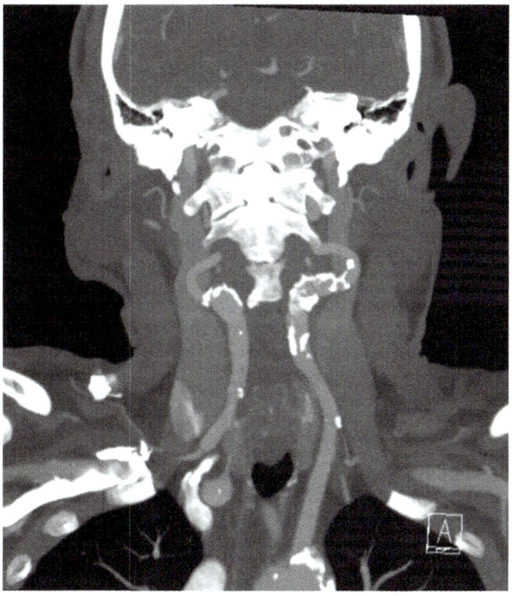

Fig. 36.1 CTA neck and brain showing severe calcific stenosis of the distal left CCA and proximal ICA

A long arteriotomy in the distal CCA and proximal ICA was performed for removal of the plaque; a bovine pericardial patch was sutured over the arteriotomy site with 6′ 0″ cardiovascular polypropylene for CCA and 7′0″ cardiovascular polypropylene ICA, respectively. The patch was brought underneath the loop of the ansa for suturing to be continued in order to preserve the ansa loop.

S. S. Hans, *Secondary and Tertiary Arterial Reconstructions*,
https://doi.org/10.1007/978-3-032-21214-6_36

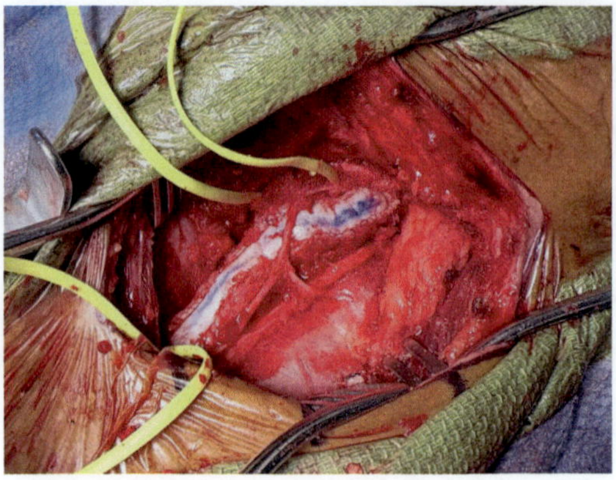

Fig. 36.2 Operative picture of completed left CEA with patch graft with short loop of Ansa at the level of the hyoid bone and the long length of Ansa

The patient had an uneventful course and was discharged on postoperative day one with no neurological or cardiac complications. A follow-up carotid duplex study showed normal left CCA and ICA with minimal intimal thickening.

Discussion

The ansa cervicalis loop is formed by the union of the descending branch of the hypoglossal nerve (superior root) and the inferior root arising from the two ventral cervical rami, most commonly C2 and C3. It is located within the carotid sheath, anterior and medial to the internal jugular vein, and is uniformly encountered during carotid endarterectomy (CEA). The ansa cervicalis innervates all infrahyoid muscles except the thyrohyoid muscle.

Injury to the ansa cervicalis can result in difficulty in swallowing and phonation, especially in patients sustaining bilateral injury. During CEA, three types of loops of ansa and variable lengths are encountered [1, 2]:

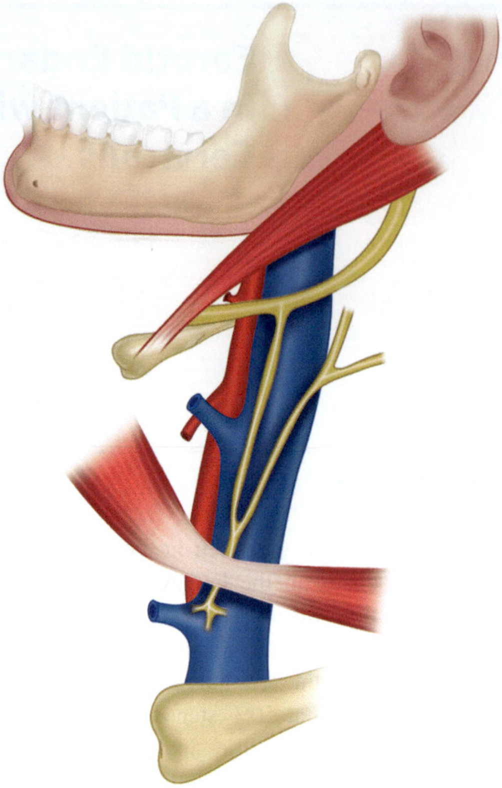

Fig. 36.3 Type A intermediate loop just superior to omohyoid and normal length of ansa

- Type A: Intermediate loop (most common, 90%) just superior to the omohyoid and normal length of the ansa (Fig. 36.3).
- Type B: Long loop (5–6%) inferior to the omohyoid with a short length of the ansa (Fig. 36.4).
- Type C: Short loop (<4%) at the level of the hyoid bone with long length of ansa (Fig. 36.5).

During CEA in patients with intermediate low loop of ansa and a normal loop of ansa, the nerve should be mobilized anteriorly. In patients with a short loop and a long length of ansa cervicalis, mobilization of both roots should be done

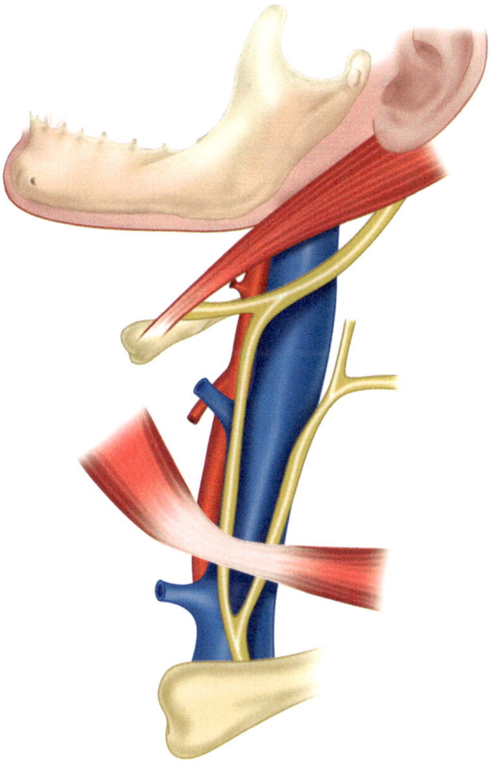

Fig. 36.4 Type B long loop inferior to the omohyoid with short length of ansa

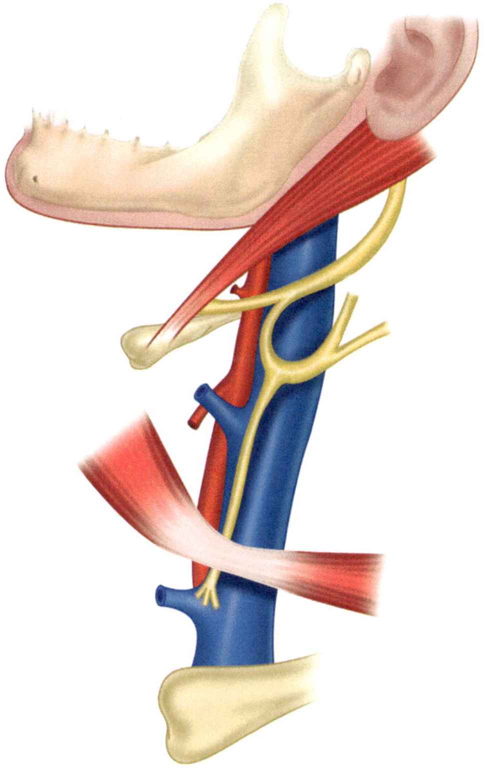

Fig. 36.5 Type C short loop at the level of the hyoid bone with long length of ansa

posteriorly. Abnormal posterior connections of the inferior root to the vagus nerve have been described, and its injury can result in hoarseness. This abnormal connection should be suspected in patients with a larger inferior root, as was present in this case. In this patient with a short loop and a long length of ansa; the patch graft suturing was started at the superior end of the endarterectomy and subsequently the patch was brought under the loop of the ansa as the suturing was continued (Fig. 36.4).

In patients requiring a shunt, preservation of the short loop (Figs. 36.3 and 36.4) can be challenging, and in such instances, sacrificing the nerve is often necessary to facilitate exposure for a safe CEA. However, preservation of the nerve in patients with a short loop and long ansa is feasible in most patients, not requiring a shunt.

Multiple Choice Questions

1. The superior root of the ansa arises from the descending branch of the hypoglossal, and the inferior root arises from the ventral rami, most often from:
   A. C1 and C2
   B. C2 and C3

   C. C3 and C4
   D. C4 and C5
2. Abnormal connection of the inferior root has been described to which cranial nerve?
   A. Vagus
   B. Hypoglossal
   C. Spinal Accessory
   D. Glossopharyngeal
3. The least common variant of Ansa Cervicalis is:
   A. Intermediate loop superior to omohyoid
   B. Long loop inferior to the omohyoid with a short length of the ansa
   C. Short loop at the level of the hyoid bone with a long length of the ansa
   D. No ansa formation

Answers: 1(B), 2(A), 3(C)

References

1. Kumari CK, Udayasree L, Yesupadamu K, Rao SU, Sesi DAVS. Variational anatomy of ansa cervicalis and its clinical implications. Int J Toxicol Pharmacol Res. 2024;14(5):6.
2. Jelev L. Some unusual types of formation of the ansa cervicalis in humans and proposal of a new morphological classification. Clin Anat. 2013;26(8):961–5. PMID:23649553

37 Transcarotid Arterial Revascularization for Recurrent Carotid Stenosis

Presentation

A 67-year-old woman presented with an asymptomatic recurrent left carotid stenosis. She was a current smoker, with a history of smoking 60 pack-years. Her medical comorbidities included hypertension, hyperlipidemia, and hypothyroidism. The patient underwent left carotid endarterectomy in October 2018 for a 90% asymptomatic left internal carotid artery (ICA) stenosis with ulceration and intraplaque hemorrhage. In November 2023, Carotid duplex confirmed 80% recurrent stenosis involving the left ICA with:

- Peak systolic velocity of left ICA =400 cm/s.
- End diastolic velocity 120 cm/s.

CT angiography of the neck in December 2023 showed 80% recurrent stenosis of the left ICA using NASCET criteria. Carotid arteriogram showed 80% irregular left ICA stenosis (Fig. 37.1). The patient underwent left transcarotid arterial revascularization under general anesthesia on Jan 12, 2024 (Fig. 37.2). The right common femoral vein puncture was performed using ultrasound guidance. Silk road venous sheath was introduced and sutured in place.

A 4 cm vertical incision was made on the left neck just above the clavicle between the two heads of the left sternocleidomastoid muscle (SCM). Dissection was carried down to the level of the internal jugular vein with electrocautery. The internal jugular vein was reflected laterally, and the omohyoid muscle was identified at the superior aspect of the field, and the clavicle at its inferior portion. The vagus nerve was identified and protected. Self-retaining retractors were placed; the common carotid was identified, and 5000 U of heparin was administered. The common carotid was circumferentially dissected, and umbilical tape was passed, and a Rommel tourniquet secured. ACT was reported as >250, at this point a 4-0 Prolene Z stitch was placed on the surface of the proximal common carotid artery, and a rubber shod was attached. The Silk Road micro needle was inserted in the center of the Z stitch, the micro wire was inserted to the marker, the needle was removed and exchanged for the micro sheath inserted to 2.5 cm marker. The wire and dilator were removed, and a DSA image was obtained. The carotid bifurcation was marked, and the view was satisfactory (Fig. 37.1). The 0.035″ Silk Road J-wire was then advanced under fluoroscopic guidance in a stop-short fashion, and the sheath was exchanged for the arterial working sheath. The wire and dilator were removed, and the ENROUTE® transcarotid arterial sheath (8F) was exchanged and sewn in place. The ENROUTE® flow reversal system was attached and flushed.

The activated clotting time was ensured above 250, the systolic blood pressure > 160 mmHg, and the patient was pretreated with glycopyrrolate to prevent

S. S. Hans, *Secondary and Tertiary Arterial Reconstructions*,
https://doi.org/10.1007/978-3-032-21214-6_37

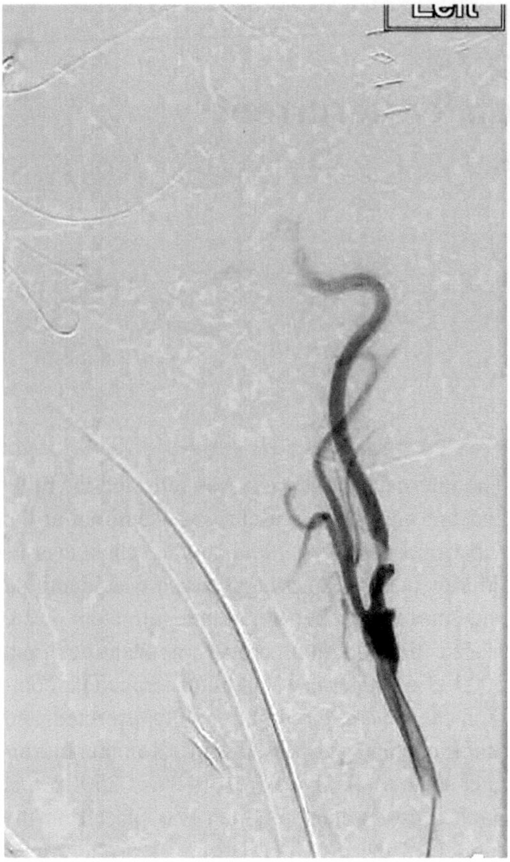

Fig. 37.1 Carotid arteriogram showing recurrent left ICA stenosis

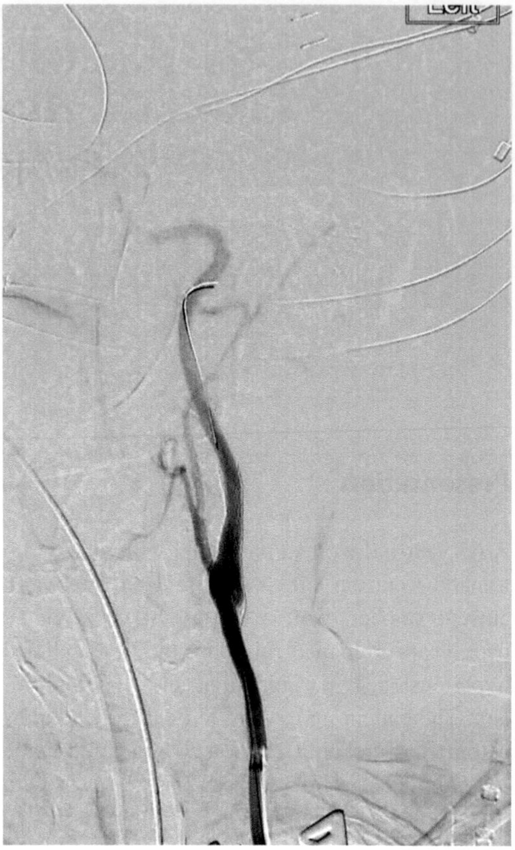

Fig. 37.2 Deployment of left carotid stent with guidewire in the distal ICA in the neck

bradycardia. The common carotid artery was occluded by tightening the Rommel tourniquet, and flow reversal was checked and confirmed. Next the working wire and balloon were introduced, the internal carotid artery lesion crossed, and the distal wire was visualized, making the bend at the petrous ridge. The 5 mm balloon was inflated to profile at 8 mmHg and deflated, then removed, and a 9 × 40 mm self-expanding EnRoute stent was introduced and positioned. The stent was deployed under fluoroscopic guidance, and the delivery system was removed. Two minutes were allowed to elapse, and completion imaging was then obtained. The stent was in good position with <20% residual stenosis and good wall apposition (Fig. 37.2). The wire was removed, and the common carotid artery unclamped; the blood pressure was allowed to normalize, and the arterial sheath unthreaded and removed while the pre-placed 4-0 Prolene was secured. The flow reversal system was unhooked and passed off the field. Hemostasis was achieved in the neck exposure, Flowseal was placed in the wound bed, and the wound was closed in two layers. 25 mg protamine was administered, and the venous sheath was removed with 15 min of manual compression.

The patient tolerated the procedure well and had a normal neurological exam. Follow-up carotid duplex study and CTA of the neck showed 65% stenosis of the right ICA and 50% in-stent stenosis of the left ICA (Fig. 37.3). The patient remained neurologically asymptomatic. Follow-up with the best medical management, surveillance with yearly carotid duplex imaging was planned.

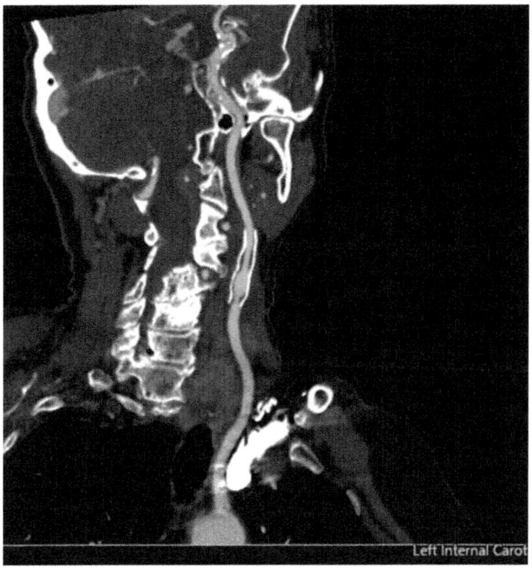

Fig. 37.3 Follow-up CTA neck showing carotid in-stent stenosis

Discussion

Both transfemoral carotid artery stenting (TCAS) and transcervical carotid artery revascularization (TCAR), redo carotid endarterectomy, carotid interposition graft and best medical management are useful modalities in managing carotid restenosis following CEA. The introduction of transcarotid artery revascularization with flow reversal has shown promising results. The subset of patients included in the ROADSTER 2 trial with recurrent stenosis following CEA had low rates of procedural stroke (1.4%), MI, or death within the 30-day postoperative period [1]. There is currently no consensus as to which treatment method provides the safest and best long-term outcomes for the treatment of carotid restenosis.

Preoperative imaging of the lesion should provide information regarding the degree of lesion calcification. Extensive circumferential calcium increases the risk of incomplete stent expansion that ultimately could lead to stent thrombosis and residual stenosis. Bulky circumferential plaque would typically be a better candidate for CEA. ICA diameter, tortuosity, and long lesions requiring multiple stents can be problematic for long-term stent patency and post-procedural stroke as well.

The proximal common carotid artery just above the clavicle must be healthy, free of any disease, and of adequate length to safely place the carotid flow reversal sheath. Extensive plaque and calcium at the access site can increase the risk of dissection during access and lead to difficulty with arteriotomy closure. The distance from the clavicle (access site) to the carotid bifurcation should be ≥5 cm to allow for safe placement of the carotid flow reversal sheath prior to engaging the lesion with the wire. It is also noted that a common carotid artery depth of >4 cm or excessive tortuosity can increase case complexity and subsequently increase the risk of complications. In addition, the common carotid artery diameter of >6 mm and an internal carotid artery diameter of >4 mm are prerequisites for success of the procedure. Hostile necks, including prior surgery or radiation, have also been shown to be safe for TCAR with decreased risk of cranial nerve injury.

TCAR is noted to have decreased operative time and flow reversal time compared to CEA and therefore decreased time under general anesthesia and cerebral ischemic time. This makes patients with significant cardiac and respiratory comorbidities good candidates for TCAR. Diagnoses considered high risk include CHF with an ejection fraction <35%, need for open heart surgery, recent MI, and severe pulmonary dysfunction, which are indications to consider TCAR over CEA. Patients who are unable to tolerate dual antiplatelet for at least three months are contraindicated for TCAR due to risk of stent thrombosis [1].

Data observed from the secondary analysis of the International Carotid Stenting Study (ICSS) concluded that the long-term risk of moderate or higher (≥50%) restenosis or occlusion of the carotid artery was significantly higher after stenting than after endarterectomy [2]. In both the stenting and endarterectomy groups, those with at least moderate (≥50%) restenosis had a significantly increased risk of subsequent ipsilateral stroke compared with those without restenosis. The increase in stroke risk in patients with restenosis was significantly higher after initial treatment with endarterectomy, but not after initial treatment with stenting [3]. Findings from randomized trials have shown that with symptomatic carotid stenosis, stenting is associated with a greater risk of non-disabling procedural stroke than carotid endarterectomy, but the long-term efficacy at preventing stroke is equivalent for each procedure [3]. Older age, female gender, history of CAD (angina), current or former smoking history, non-insulin diabetes mellitus, greater degree of stenosis in the contralateral carotid artery at randomization, higher systolic or diastolic blood pressure at randomization, and higher total serum cholesterol at randomization are independent predictors of restenosis [3]. The risk of severe (≥70%) carotid restenosis or occlusion did not differ between the treatment groups. The reason why the female gender is associated with a higher risk of restenosis is not entirely clear; however, this association might be related to the smaller diameter of the carotid arteries in women as compared to men. In ICSS, most occurrences of restenosis in both treatment groups were diagnosed in the first 2 years, nonetheless restenosis increased the risk of stroke in the CEA group [3].

Multiple Choice Questions

1. The reverse flow used during the carotid artery stenting procedure (ROADSTER 2) trial showed a 30-day stroke rate of:
   A. Less than 1.0%
   B. 1.4%
   C. 1.8%
   D. 2%
2. The risk factors for recurrent carotid stenosis include:
   A. Former or current smoking history, older female gender, higher BP at randomization, hyperlipidemia, Type II DM, coronary artery disease, greater degree of contralateral carotid stenosis
   B. Female gender and diabetes mellitus
   C. Female gender, diabetes mellitus, and hyperlipidemia
   D. Failure to remove fibers of the media at the time of carotid endarterectomy
3. The risk of severe carotid stenosis (70%) or occlusion following carotid endarterectomy and transfemoral carotid stenting is:
   A. Higher or greater after CEA as compared to CAS
   B. Greater after CAS as compared to CEA
   C. Similarities between CEA and CAS
   D. Recurrent stenosis following CAS and CEA is extremely uncommon

Answers: 1(B), 2(A), 3(C)

References

1. Kashyap VS, Schneider PA, Foteh M, Motaganahalli R, Shah R, Eckstein HH, et al. Early outcomes in the ROADSTER 2 study of transcarotid artery revascularization in patients with significant carotid artery disease. Stroke. 2020;51(9):2620–9. PMID:32811386
2. Bonati LH, Gregson J, Dobson J, McCabe DJH, Nederkoorn PJ, van der Worp HB, et al. Restenosis and risk of stroke after stenting or endarterectomy for symptomatic carotid stenosis in the International Carotid Stenting Study (ICSS): secondary analysis of a randomised trial. Lancet Neurol. 2018;17(7):587–96. PMID:29861139
3. de Borst GJ, Zanen P, de Vries JP, van de Pavoordt ED, Ackerstaff RG, Moll FL. Durability of surgery for restenosis after carotid endarterectomy. J Vasc Surg. 2008;47(2):363–71. PMID:18155873

38 Thrombus at the Proximal Anastomosis of the Common Carotid to the Internal Carotid Artery Interposition Graft for Recurrent Carotid Stenosis

Presentation

A 74-year-old woman was seen in the clinic for follow-up clinical evaluation and surveillance carotid duplex imaging in August 2017. She denied any history of focal TIA/stroke. She complained of headaches and occasional dizziness. Medical comorbidities include stable coronary artery disease, hypertension, hypothyroidism, chronic obstructive pulmonary disease (COPD), and depression. She was a current smoker with a history of smoking cigarettes for 60 pack-years.

In March 2005, she underwent right carotid endarterectomy with Hemashield Dacron patch graft (Getinge, Gothenberg, Sweden) for 80% asymptomatic stenosis of the right ICA. During initial follow-up, duplex carotid imaging did not show any recurrent stenosis. There was evidence of reversal of left vertebral artery flow secondary to near occlusion of the proximal left subclavian artery.

However, at 13 months follow-up, carotid duplex imaging showed greater than 70% recurrent stenosis of the right internal carotid artery, confirmed with a CT angiography of the neck. The patient underwent an interposition carotid graft from the mid common carotid artery (CCA) to the proximal internal carotid artery using a 4 × 7 mm PTFE tapered graft (WL Gore Newark, DE) fashioned in a way that a 6 cm length of the graft was required. Its distal end was spatulated in such a manner that its ultimate diameter was 5 mm diameter for its distal anastomosis to the internal carotid artery and 7 mm for the proximal common carotid artery anastomosis. The external carotid artery was ligated.

She was followed in the clinic with carotid duplex imaging every 6 months for one year and then yearly. On August 25, 2017, a carotid duplex study showed a peak systolic velocity of right ICA (49 cm/s), left ICA (104 cm/s), right CCA (21 cm/s), and left CCA (59 cm/s). She had no focal neurological symptoms. CTA of the neck showed high-grade stenosis (90%) at the proximal anastomosis of the CCA-ICA interposition graft (Figs. 38.1 and 38.2). NM myocardial perfusion imaging did not show any evidence of myocardial ischemia.

On October 12, 2017, the patient underwent a third cervical carotid revascularization operation. Using a sharp dissection, the carotid interposition graft and proximal CCA in the base of the neck were carefully exposed, and a silastic vessel loop was passed around the proximal carotid artery just above the base of the neck. The distal anastomosis of the interposition graft to the ICA was exposed carefully, preserving the hypoglossal nerve. The vagus nerve was preserved posterolateral to the CCA as well.

Stump pressure measured 84 mmHg. The shunt was not used. Following systemic heparinization, the proximal CCA and ICA were clamped with a vascular clamp, and a longitudinal incision was made in the proximal position of the well-

S. S. Hans, *Secondary and Tertiary Arterial Reconstructions*,
https://doi.org/10.1007/978-3-032-21214-6_38

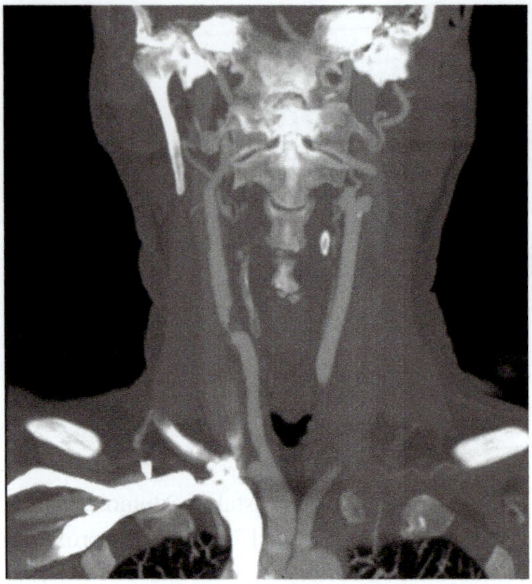

Fig. 38.1 CTA of the neck showing high-grade stenosis of the right internal carotid artery

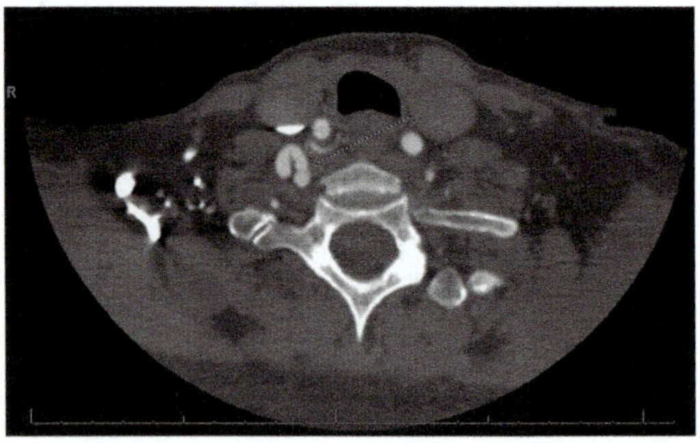

Fig. 38.2 CTA of the neck—axial view showing a filling defect in the proximal common carotid artery

incorporated PTFE graft and the proximal CCA. A thrombus was seen adherent proximal to the suture line with mild stenosis. The plaque was removed from the common carotid artery near the proximal suture line (Figs. 38.3 and 38.4). After thorough irrigation of the interposition graft and the CCA, and removal of any loose debris, a bovine pericardial patch was sutured at the site of longitudinal incision in the graft at the proximal anastomosis and in the common carotid artery. Her post-operative course was uneventful. Follow-up carotid duplex imaging study on September 15, 2020, showed a peak systolic velocity of RT ICA—117 cm/s and of CCA

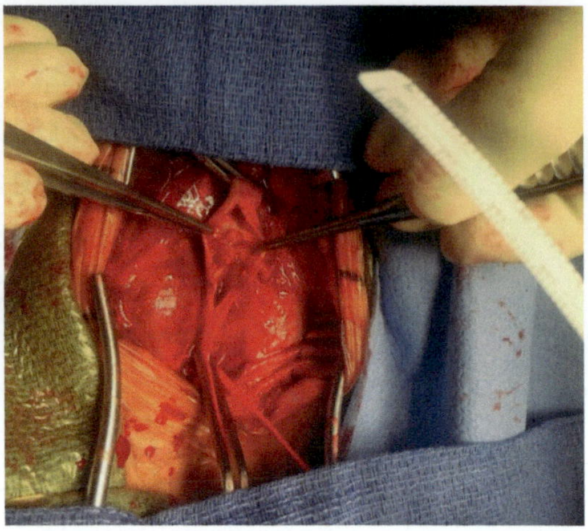

Fig. 38.3 Intraoperative photograph of a thrombus at the proximal suture line with mild stenosis

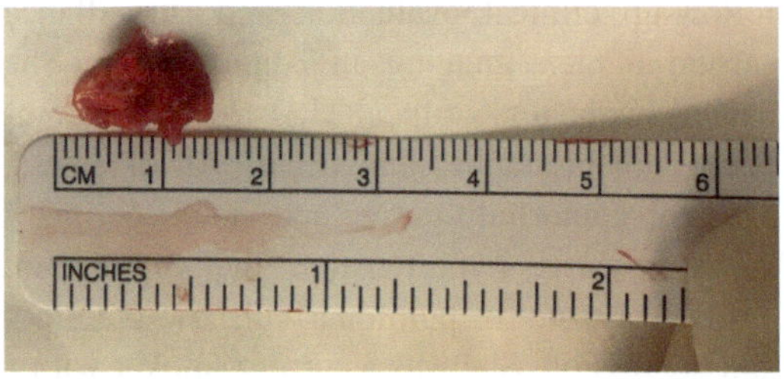

Fig. 38.4 Intraoperative photograph of the plaque and the thrombus removed from the common carotid artery

59 cm/s. She subsequently underwent robotic left upper lobe lobectomy and mediastinal node dissection in August 2019 and expired from metastatic disease under hospice care on October 28, 2021.

Discussion

Extracranial carotid stenosis is responsible for ischemic stroke in 10–20% of all ischemic events. In patients with symptomatic moderate to severe carotid stenosis, carotid endarterectomy (CEA), transfemoral carotid angioplasty, and carotid artery stenting (CAS) have been performed to lower the risk of stroke. Carotid endarterectomy has been found to be superior to the best medical therapy, according to three large randomized controlled trials. Following CEA and CAS, carotid restenosis remains a significant problem.

The incidence of carotid restenosis ranges from 5% to 22% after CEA, and in-stent restenosis (ISR) rates range from 21% to 33%. Transcarotid revascularization (TCAR) is a satisfactory option for the management of carotid restenosis. Carotid restenosis occurring within 2 years of intervention has been associated with myointimal hyperplasia, and stenosis occurring after 2 years is usually caused by recurrent atherosclerotic disease, though there can be some overlap.

Reported risk factors for recurrent carotid stenosis include current smoking, diabetes mellitus, female gender, and the type of stent used for CAS. The major thromboembolic complications appear to be more related to the stability of the plaque rather than the degree of stenosis. The risk of neurological complications in early restenosis due to myointimal hyperplasia is low. Restenosis after CEA was reported in up to 20% of patients in early studies, but subsequent studies report 2–10% at 5 years following CEA. There is a greater risk of restenosis after CAS than after CEA. Carotid occlusion is 2.5 times more common after CAS than after CEA. Results of the SPACE trial reported that the rate of restenosis (≥70%) was 11.1% in the CAS group and 4.6% in the CEA group ($p < 0.0007$).

A systematic review involving 4399 patients with carotid restenosis who had undergone repeated carotid intervention (surgery or stenting) following CEA reported no significant difference in the perioperative (30-day) rates for mortality, stroke, or TIA between CEA and transfemoral CAS. There is a higher incidence of cranial nerve palsy after repeat CEA, even though many such injuries are transient. A similar rate of stroke and death for CAS and CEA (2.7% vs 2.3%, respectively) in patients for restenosis (479 CEA and 653 CAS) has been reported [1].

Coscas et al. reported the results of open surgery for carotid restenosis among 119 patients from 1989 to 2001 with 41% of patients exhibited neurological symptoms. Postoperative (<30 days) combined stroke and death rate was 3.3%, with cranial nerve injury in 4.2% cases. They concluded that despite no prospective randomized trial to compare CAS with CEA, open surgery should remain the first line of therapy when treatment for recurrent carotid stenosis is planned [2]. A case report of recurrent carotid artery stenosis following patch angioplasty and carotid in-stent restenosis after TCAR was treated with drug-coated balloon angioplasty (Paclitaxel-coated) under flow reversal [3].

Multiple Choice Questions

1. The incidence of carotid restenosis after CEA, as reported in recently reported studies, is
   A. 1–2%
   B. 2–10%
   C. 3–12%
   D. 4–14%
2. Results of the SPACE trial showed that the rate of restenosis (≥70%) was
   A. 2.6% in the CEA group and 5.1% in the CAS group
   B. 3.6% in the CEA group and 7.1% in the CAS group
   C. 4.6% in the CEA group and 10.1% in the CAS group
   D. 4.6% in the CEA group and 11.1% in the CAS group
3. The 30-day stroke and death rate for transfemoral CAS and CEA for carotid restenosis is
   A. 2.7% for CAS and 2.3% for CEA
   B. 3.7% for CAS and 3.3% for CEA
   C. 4.7% for CAS and 4.1% for CEA
   D. 4.9% for CAS and 4.5% for CEA

Answers: 1(C), 2(A), 3(A)

References

1. Coscas R, Rhissassi B, Gruet-Coquet N, Couture T, de Tymowski C, et al. Open surgery remains a valid option for the treatment of recurrent carotid stenosis. J Vasc Surg. 2010;51(5):1124–32. https://doi.org/10.1016/j.jvs.2009.12.020. Epub 2010 Mar 19
2. Stilo F, Montelione N, Calandrelli R, Distefano M, Spinelli F, et al. The management of carotid

restenosis: a comprehensive review. Ann Transl Med. 2020;8(19):1272. https://doi.org/10.21037/atm-20-963.
3. Pavlyha M, Farley S, Moore WS. Recurrent carotid artery stenosis was successfully and safely treated with drug-coated balloon angioplasty under flow reversal. J Vasc Surg Cases Innov Tech. 2025;11(2):101728. https://doi.org/10.1016/j.jvscit.2025.101728. PMID: 40008221

Acute Thrombosis of the Popliteal Aneurysm with Severe Ischemia of the Lower Extremity

39

Presentation

A 64-year-old man presented to the Emergency Room with the sudden onset of pain and paresthesia in the right lower extremity with loss of motor function in the distal right lower extremity (Rutherford II B). Medical comorbidities included coronary artery disease, type II Diabetes Mellitus, hypertension, hyperlipidemia, and morbid obesity (BMI 36). On clinical examination, the right femoral pulse was palpable, but no pulse was palpable below that level. He had an easily palpable dorsalis pedis artery (DPA) and posterior tibial artery (PTA) pulse on the left side. A pulsatile mass suggestive of a popliteal aneurysm was palpable on the left side. Doppler arterial study showed absent flow in the right popliteal, DPA, and PTA. Doppler arterial study showed normal arterial flow in the left lower extremity.

Computed tomographic angiography (CTA) showed a small AAA and bilateral large popliteal aneurysms with thrombosis of the right popliteal aneurysm (Fig. 39.1). Because of critical limb threatening ischemia, the patient underwent repair of the large right popliteal aneurysm using a medial approach. The popliteal artery distal to the popliteal aneurysm was opened longitudinally, and the passage of a No. 3 Fogarty catheter did not retrieve any thrombi. There was an absent retrograde flow. The dorsalis pedis artery (DPA) at the ankle was exposed, and arteriotomy in the DPA revealed a small amount of back bleeding.

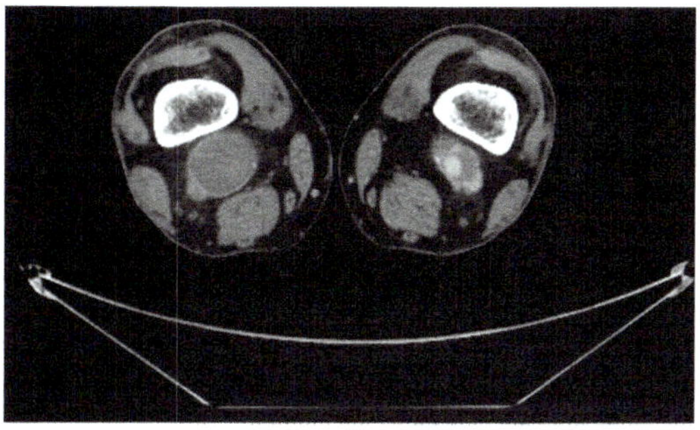

Fig. 39.1 Bilateral large popliteal aneurysms with thrombosis of the right popliteal aneurysm

The patient underwent proximal popliteal artery to a DPA bypass using the translocated right Great Saphenous vein with completion arteriogram (Fig. 39.2). Reperfusion resulted in a marked bulging of the calf muscles; therefore, a four-compartment fasciotomy was performed using medial and lateral calf incisions. The patient subsequently developed interval ischemic necrosis of the medial calf (skin and muscle) and had multiple debridement's and skin grafts despite patent bypass grafts (Fig. 39.3). The patient developed thrombosis of the graft and underwent a thrombectomy of the graft and the graft was rerouted and brought through the interosseous membrane and anastomosed to the DP artery with interposition of a short segment of non-reversed GSV. Despite patency of the bypass graft, the patient required above-knee amputation

S. S. Hans, *Secondary and Tertiary Arterial Reconstructions*,
https://doi.org/10.1007/978-3-032-21214-6_39

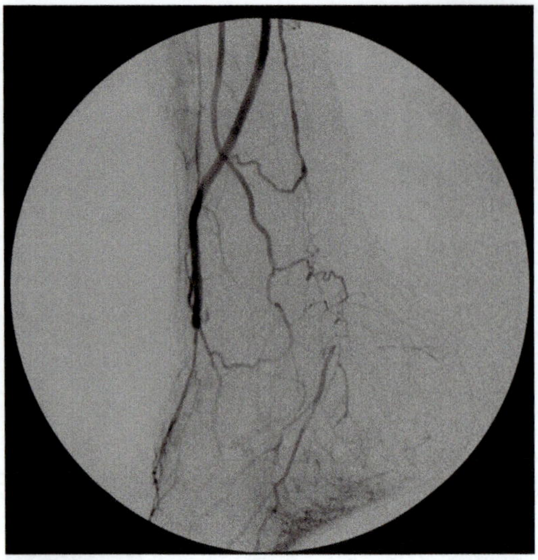

Fig. 39.2 Completion Arteriogram showing patent vein bypass to dorsalis pedis artery following exclusion of thrombosed popliteal aneurysm. The posterior tibial artery is occluded just above the ankle joint

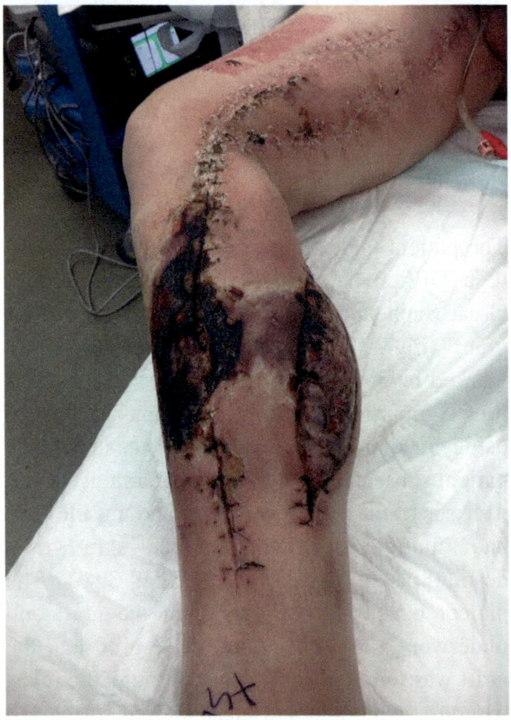

Fig. 39.3 Photograph showing right medial calf ischemic necrosis despite a patent arterial bypass graft

of the leg because of extensive necrosis of the skin and muscles of the calf. The patient died 4 years later due to persistent congestive heart failure.

Discussion

The acute symptoms of thrombosis are manifest in 28% of patients diagnosed with popliteal artery aneurysm (PAA). The manifestation of acute thrombosis is variable. Acute thrombosis may occur in a popliteal aneurysm localized to the knee, or an acute thrombosis may occur in diffusely aneurysmal superficial femoral and popliteal arteries, and the aneurysmal diameter is usually not very large. In several patients, thrombosis of the PAA may only result in symptoms of intermittent claudication, which tend to improve with conservative management. A significant number of patients with thrombosis of PAA present limb threatening ischemia with either no sensory deficits or minimal sensory loss, which in the absence of paralysis, is defined as Rutherford Grade II A, or in the presence of sensory deficit extending to the toes as Grade IIB [1]. Rutherford Grade III limb ischemia presents with associated muscle paralysis of the lower leg, complete sensory loss, and absent doppler signals in the foot. Most patients with thrombosed PAA and Rutherford Grade I ischemia do not need any intervention. Patients with Grade III ischemia most likely will need major amputation (below--knee or above-knee amputation).

Patients with Rutherford Grade II A or B ischemia often present as an emergency with a painful lower extremity associated with paresthesias, motor deficit, and if the ischemia is severe (Rutherford Grade II B), there is often associated thromboembolic occlusion of the runoff vessels.

After obtaining patient history in the ER, a Doppler arterial study is performed, followed by a CTA of the abdominal aorta and a runoff study of the lower extremity. In patients with suspected acute thrombosis of the popliteal aneurysm following clinical examination, duplex imaging with measurement of ankle brachial index, CTA of the abdomen and run-off is obtained. An astute clinician may be able to palpate a pulsatile mass in the contralateral popliteal fossa, as 40–50% popliteal artery aneurysms (PAAs) are bilateral.

The patient should be started on intravenous Heparin drip, and an urgent arteriography should be obtained depending upon the grade of ischemia. A contralateral femoral artery access is preferred. If the aneurysm is thrombosed and run-off vessels are patent, open repair (exclusion) and bypass are performed during the same admission. In the absence of visualization of main outflow arteries (tibial/peroneal) with associated Grade II A ischemia, catheter thrombolysis starts to restore flow into a potential target vessel in the calf. If the limb is immediately threatened (Rutherford Grade IIB), the patient should be emergently taken to the hybrid operating room, and using a medial approach, the distal popliteal artery is exposed. The origin of the soleus muscle is taken down from the soleal line, and the anterior tibial vein crossing the popliteal artery bifurcation is exposed and ligated on each side and divided. A longitudinal arteriotomy incision is made in the distal popliteal artery extending to the proximal tibioperoneal trunk, and a small Fogarty catheter (No. 2 or 3) is passed into each tibial artery to remove any thrombi. Occasionally, no clots can be retrieved due to a very distal embolization or the laminated thrombus adherent to the tibial and peroneal arteries. The author has encountered in some patients that the only run-off artery available for distal reconstruction may be the distal peroneal or distal anterior tibial artery.

Arterial reconstruction is performed with a bypass from the proximal popliteal artery cephalad to the aneurysm and a distal anastomosis to a distal patent target artery. It is important to perform completion arteriography. We have used intraoperative TPA (4 mg) in the target artery as a one-time dose in patients with limited run-off. Following bypass, there is a potential for reperfusion injury, often requiring fasciotomy.

Kropman et al., reported results from eight prospective studies and 25 retrospective studies, including 895 patients with a diagnosis of PAA presenting with acute ischemia from 1990 to 2008; the mortality rate after surgical repair was 3.2% [2]. Thrombolysis before surgery did not result in a significant reduction in the number of amputations compared with surgery (thrombectomy or bypass) alone. The mean primary patency rates of the bypasses at one, three, and five years were 79%, 77%, and 74%, respectively, in the thrombolysis group and 71% ($P = 0.026$), 54% ($P = 0.164$), and 45% ($P = 0.249$) in the thrombectomy group. From a Swedish Vascular registry of 717 primary operations for PAAs in 571 patients, who were registered prospectively from 1987 to 2002, 235 legs presented with acute ischemia [3]. Immediate surgery was performed on 135 legs, including intraoperative thrombolysis in 32 cases (immediate surgery group). Preoperative thrombolysis was performed on 100 legs, in acute cases (less than 24 h) on 41 legs; elective surgery was performed on 59 legs (delayed surgery group). The delayed surgery group had a smaller size PAA (27 versus 37, $P < 0.001$) and were younger (67 versus 72 years, $P < 0.001$) [3]. Run-off was worse in the delayed surgery group than in the immediate surgery group ($P < 0.001$) and improved in 87% after thrombolysis. The amputation rate was 27% in the immediate surgery group and 7% in the delayed surgery group ($P < 0.0001$). The immediate surgery group required fasciotomy in 30% compared to 11% in the delayed surgery group ($P = 0.0001$) [3].

Multiple Choice Questions

1. Acute thrombosis of the popliteal aneurysm occurs in
   A. 40% of all popliteal aneurysms
   B. 30–39% of all popliteal aneurysms
   C. 25–29% of all popliteal aneurysms
   D. 15–18% of all popliteal aneurysms

2. For patients with Rutherford Grade III ischemia due to a thrombosed popliteal aneurysm who present 24 h after the onset of symptoms, the best management strategy is
   A. Arteriography and thrombolysis
   B. Operative arteriogram, bypass to any patent infrapopliteal artery
   C. Endovascular repair
   D. Primary below-knee or above-knee amputation
3. The mortality rate following open repair of a thrombosed popliteal aneurysm presenting with acute ischemia is
   A. 2.2%
   B. 3.2%
   C. 4.2%
   D. 5.2%

Answers: 1(C), 2(D), 3(B)

References

1. Rutherford RB. Clinical staging of acute limb ischemia as the basis for choice of revascularization method: when and how to intervene. Semin Vasc Surg. 2009;22(1):5–9.
2. Kropman RH, Schrijver AM, Kelder JC, Moll FL, de Vries JP. Clinical outcome of acute leg ischaemia due to thrombosed popliteal artery aneurysm: systematic review of 895 cases. Eur J Vasc Endovasc Surg. 2010;39(4):452–7. PMID:20153667
3. Ravn H, Björck M. Popliteal artery aneurysm with acute ischemia in 229 patients. Outcome after thrombolytic and surgical therapy. Eur J Vasc Endovasc Surg. 2007;33(6):690–5. PMID:17275362

40 Open Repair of a Giant Recurrent Popliteal Artery Aneurysm

Presentation

A 74-year-old man presented to the clinic with a pulsatile mass in the right medial thigh above the knee. The patient was a former smoker with a history of smoking 50 pack-years. He also had a history of hypertension. Past surgical history included a right knee arthroplasty, an exclusion of a left popliteal aneurysm with bypass, which failed, resulting in above-knee amputation in 1996 at an outside hospital. At the same hospital, the patient underwent right popliteal aneurysm exclusion and bypass (saphenous vein) in 1997. The medical records from the outside hospital were not available.

Color flow duplex imaging revealed 6 × 7 cm popliteal aneurysm in the right lower thigh (Fig. 40.1). CT angiography showed a 5.7 × 8.1 cm aneurysm above the knee with a large amount of laminated thrombus (Fig. 40.2). Abdominal aortogram and right lower extremity arteriogram showed large aneurysm at the junction of the distal SFA and proximal popliteal artery and a patent bypass just distal to a tortuous proximal popliteal and distal SFA aneurysm (Fig. 40.3).

The patient underwent open repair of a large distal SFA/popliteal aneurysm under general anesthesia. A longitudinal incision was made in the right mid-thigh, and mid-SFA was exposed in the Hunter's Canal. The saphenous nerve was

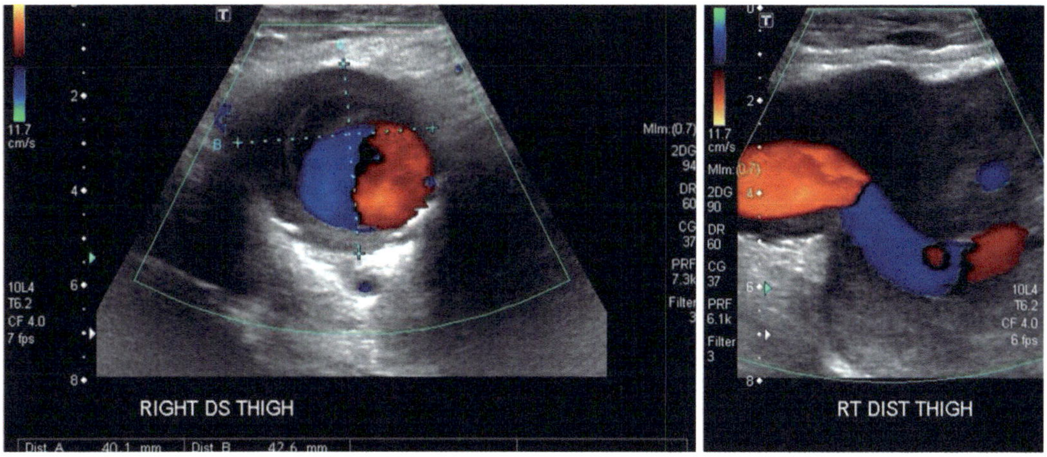

Fig. 40.1 Duplex ultrasound of the popliteal fossa showing a large popliteal aneurysm

S. S. Hans, *Secondary and Tertiary Arterial Reconstructions*,
https://doi.org/10.1007/978-3-032-21214-6_40

preserved, and the femoral vein was carefully dissected free from the superficial femoral artery. A skip longitudinal incision was made in the lower thigh, knee, and upper medial leg. The anterior border of the Sartorius muscle was mobilized posteriorly. After entering the fascial sheath posterior to the medial intermuscular septum, the aneurysm was exposed, and the femoral bypass (vein) was mobilized (Fig. 40.4). Another oblique incision was made in the right upper thigh from the groin crease to harvest the great saphenous vein, which was dissected from the saphenofemoral junction to the upper and mid-thigh junction.

Heparin was administered intravenously by the anesthesia team, and ACT was kept between 250 and 300 s. An arteriotomy incision was made longitudinally in the mid SFA between the two

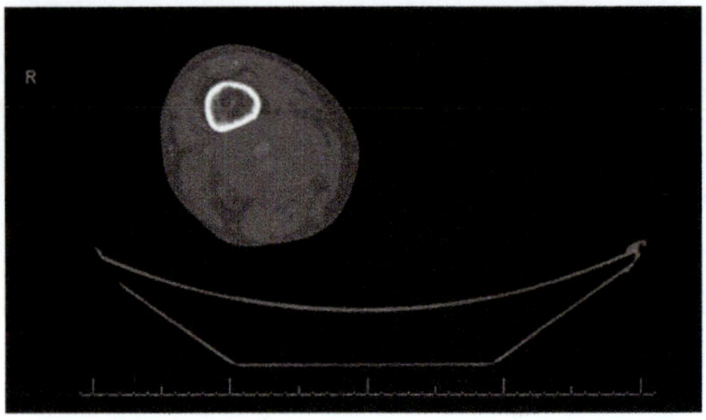

Fig. 40.2 CTA showing a large popliteal aneurysm in the distal thigh with a large amount of laminated thrombus

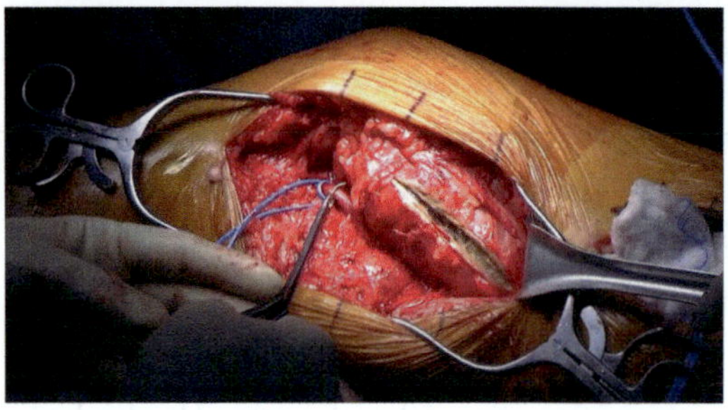

Fig. 40.4 Showing large popliteal aneurysm with a longitudinal incision and a clip inferior to the aneurysm, just proximal to the remote interposition vein graft

Fig. 40.3 Arteriography showing proximal popliteal artery aneurysm with a patent remote interposition vein graft (index operation) inferior to the aneurysm

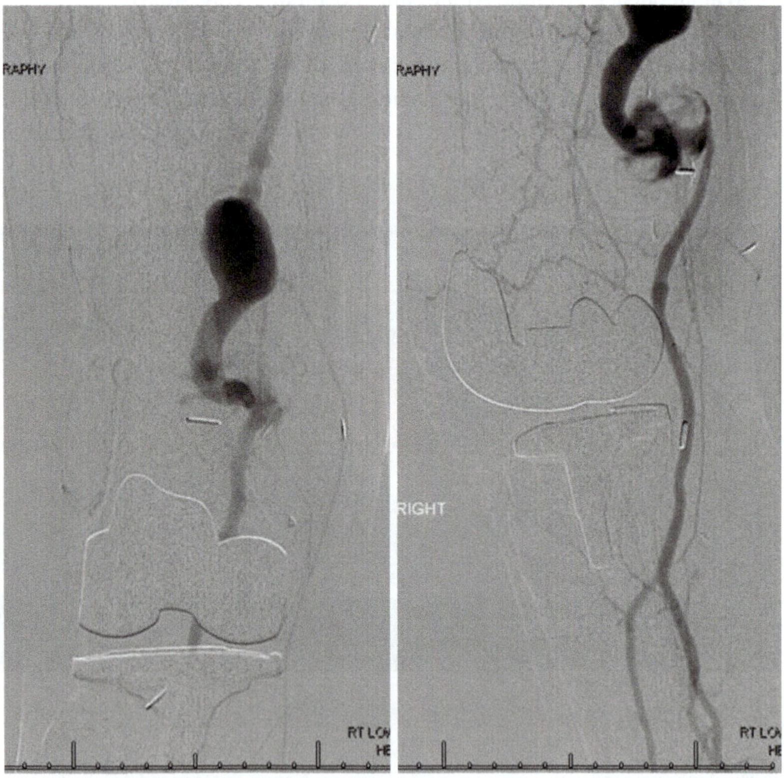

vascular clamps, and a non-reversed GSV was anastomosed to the SFA in an end-to-side fashion after excising the valve leaflet at the proximal end of the GSV. The suturing was done using a continuous 6′-0″ CV polypropylene suture. (Ethicon Cincinnati, OH).

Valve leaflets were incised using a modified Mills (Leather) retrograde valvulotome passed from the inferior end of the vein, and a pulsatile flow was obtained. The vein graft was anastomosed distally in an end-to-end fashion to the remote vein graft, which was transected just distal to the origin of the graft (remote proximal anastomosis) using a continuous 6′-0″ CV polypropylene suture. The patient had a satisfactory perfusion of the lower extremity. The postoperative course was complicated by a surgical site infection with growth of Enterococcus on wound culture. With wound care and appropriate intravenous antibiotics, the incision site healed in the subsequent 3 weeks.

CTA of the abdominal aorta and right lower extremity 2 years following the exclusion and bypass of the recurrent aneurysm showed patency of both (remote and recent) vein bypass graft (Fig. 40.5). Proximal to the site selected for the proximal anastomosis of the graft at the time of index operation may subsequently become aneurysmal in patients with ectatic arteries with aneurysmal disease. The patient was last seen in May 2025 with patent popliteal artery bypass on duplex imaging. The patient was ambulatory with the help of a left above-knee prosthesis. He was experiencing breathing difficulty due to advanced COPD.

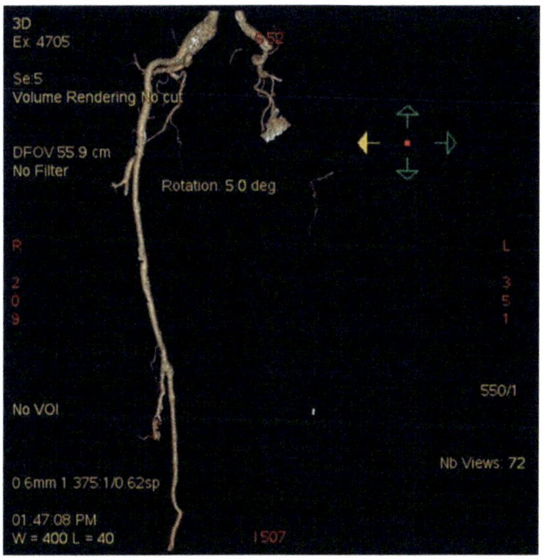

Fig. 40.5 Postoperative CTA showing patient vein bypass graft with right common iliac aneurysm

Discussion

Although rare, popliteal artery aneurysms (PAA's) are the most common peripheral artery aneurysms (70%) with a male-to-female ratio of 20:1. Forty percent of patients have a concurrent abdominal aortic aneurysm, and 39–54% of PAA's are bilateral. Unlike abdominal aortic aneurysm, the incidence of rupture is extremely uncommon (1–4%). Most patients present with an asymptomatic pulsatile mass behind the knee, and clinical examination may reveal a prominent popliteal pulse. More than two-thirds of patients will develop limb ischemia to a varying degree during a 5-year surveillance. Severe limb ischemia due to aneurysm thrombosis or due to distal embolization may be the first presentation of a popliteal artery aneurysm. Due to the high prevalence of ischemic complications leading to a heightened risk of limb loss (30–40%), an intensified approach for the repair of these aneurysms has been recommended. Most vascular specialists recommend a 2 cm threshold for elective repair. In patients with extensive mural thrombus within the aneurysm sac, even a slightly smaller-sized aneurysm should be considered for repair.

The traditional approach to PAA repair consists of exclusion of the aneurysm and simultaneous revascularization with an autologous vein, if available, otherwise with a PTFE graft. Advances in technology during the last two decades have created endografts that support the advantages of a minimal invasive approach with a shorter length of stay and a faster recovery. While PAA's repairs are durable, recurrent aneurysms may occur from the progression of the disease of the artery proximally or distally to the excluded segment of the aneurysmal artery.

Despite the increasing use of endovascular repair of popliteal artery aneurysms during the past two decades, the exclusion and bypass of PAA has remained a durable option. Open repair has better patency than endovascular repair, particularly in patients presenting with acute ischemia due to thrombosis of the popliteal aneurysm. From a Swedish vascular registry, Cervin et al. [2], reported a series of 592 procedures performed for treatment of PAA's. From the analysis of their data, they concluded that open repair is superior to endovascular repair. A more recent Italian multicenter study of endovascular repair of PAA's reported a total of 48 endovascular treatments of PAA's. Short-term and long-term follow-up treated a total of 48 aneurysms, deploying a total of 71 endografts [3]. At a mean follow-up of 25 months, a total of 21 grafts thrombosed (25%), requiring thrombolysis followed by angioplasty. They also reported a slightly higher tendency of graft thrombosis and reduced patency in patients with fewer run-off vessels. Migration and endoleak are known complications of endovascular repair. The main advantage of endovascular is its minimally invasive technology with shorter hospital stay and shorter recovery time.

Jung et al., reported the results of real-world data of popliteal artery aneurysm treatment. Analysis of the POPART registry [4]. From 2014 to 2019, 794 cases were recorded in the POPART registry with open repair in 662 patients and endovascular repair in 106 patients; 23 patients had been treated conservatively. The overall patency for the open and endovascular groups after 12 and 24 months were 83.2% and 44.7% ($p < 0.0005$) and 74.2% and 29.1% ($p < 0.005$), respectively. The outcomes with a prosthetic graft versus an autologous vein were significantly poorer in the open repair group (primary patency 71.4% versus 88.1% at 12 months, respectively. Though the patency in the endovascular group was lower than that of open repair, it has the advantage of shorter hospital stay, and results are satisfactory in patients with good onflow vessels who are asymptomatic [4].

Risk of developing a new aneurysm following open repair of popliteal aneurysms was reported in a study of 571 patients [1]. Among 28 patients who had an isolated PAA at the index operation, 23 of those patients were older ($p = 0.004$). The incidence of graft aneurysm was 4.3% treated by venous bypass graft at the time of re-examination. They concluded that lifelong surveillance may be warranted as the development of new aneurysms was common in patients with PAA. Lifelong surveillance is warranted in patients following repair of popliteal aneurysms, as bilateral popliteal aneurysms are associated with the development of AAA even if not present at the time of index operation for PAA.

Late development of aneurysm in the SFA/popliteal artery proximal to the bypass and exclusion of the aneurysm at the index operation, as demonstrated in this case, or development of aneurysmal changes in the vein graft should be pursued by noninvasive color flow duplex imaging studies serially (6 months to yearly) for the life of the patient. In addition, yearly surveillance using abdominal ultrasound should be performed because of the late development of aortic/iliac aneurysm.

Multiple Choice Questions

1. A 74-year-old man presents with a 5.0 cm recurrent (asymptomatic) right popliteal aneurysm proximal to anastomosis of the interposition graft extending proximally in the middle/lower thigh. The optimal management consists of:
   A. Repair with an interposition vein graft using the posterior approach
   B. Repair using an interposition vein graft following resection of the aneurysm using a medial approach
   C. Repair with interposition of PTFE bypass graft
   D. Surveillance with duplex ultrasound and repair only if the aneurysm becomes symptomatic
2. A 60-year-old man undergoes open repair of the popliteal aneurysm with interposition of a GSV graft, followed by repair of the contralateral popliteal aneurysm 6 months later. At

the time of the popliteal aneurysm repair, there is no evidence of AAA. Which statement regarding surveillance accurately reflects the follow-up:
   A. Patient should undergo yearly arteriography
   B. Yearly duplex ultrasound of the femoral arteries, and if there is no evidence of femoral artery aneurysm, there is no need for further surveillance
   C. Lifelong surveillance with yearly aortic ultrasound, as AAA may develop many years following popliteal aneurysm repair
   D. Patients should have a yearly CTA chest for the detection of the descending thoracic aortic aneurysm
3. The incidence of lower extremity ischemic complications in patients with popliteal artery aneurysm is:
   A. Less than 10%
   B. 10–20%
   C. 21–30%
   D. 30% or greater
4. The reported 5-year primary patency of vein graft following PAA repair is:
   A. 60–70%
   B. 71–75%
   C. 77–90%
   D. 95–100%
5. The reported 5-year primary patency for synthetic grafts following PAA repair is:
   A. 20–25%
   B. 26–30%
   C. 29–74%
   D. 75–90%

Answers: 1(B), 2(C), 3(D), 4(C), 5(C)

References

1. Ravn H, Wanhainen A, Björck M. Risk of new aneurysms after surgery for popliteal artery aneurysm. Br J Surg. 2008;95(5):571–5. https://doi.org/10.1002/bjs.6074.
2. Cervin A, Tjärnström J, Ravn H, Acosta S, Hultgren R, Welander M, Björck M. Treatment of popliteal aneurysm by open and endovascular surgery: a contemporary study of 592 procedures in Sweden. Eur J Vasc Endovasc Surg. 2015;50(3):342–50. https://doi.org/10.1016/j.ejvs.2015.03.026.
3. Guzzardi G, Natrella M, Del Sette B, Petullà M, Fanelli G, Porta C, Carriero A, Laganà D. Endovascular repair of popliteal artery aneurysms: an Italian multicenter study. Radiol Med. 2019;124(1):79–85. https://doi.org/10.1007/s11547-018-0941-0.
4. Jung G, Leinweber ME, Karl T, Geisbüsch P, Balzer K, Schmandra T, et al. Real-world data of popliteal artery aneurysm treatment: analysis of the POPART registry. J Vasc Surg. 2022;75(5):1707–1717.e1702. PMID:35066058

41 Impending Rupture of a Right Popliteal Artery Aneurysm in a Patient with a Prior Femoral–Popliteal Bypass

Presentation

A 59-year-old man presented to the clinic in January 2024 with worsening pain behind the right knee with associated swelling. He was sent to the ER, and computed tomographic arteriography (CTA) of the abdomen and pelvis, as well as the lower extremities, showed a large popliteal artery aneurysm (PAA). He was a current smoker with a history of smoking 45 pack-years. His BMI was 26.6. He had a history of atrial fibrillation (on Apixaban), deep vein thrombosis, hypertension, hyperlipidemia, and a bleeding duodenal ulcer. In 2012, the patient underwent right common femoral artery to above-knee popliteal artery bypass using a non-reversed great saphenous vein. The patient was lost to follow-up for 10 years due to a lack of medical insurance.

In 2023, the patient underwent exploratory laparotomy, duodenotomy, suture ligation of bleeding duodenal ulcer, jejunal serosal patch, and gastrojejunostomy.

The patient also underwent percutaneous cholecystostomy. CTA abdomen and run off showed a large popliteal artery aneurysm (Figs. 41.1, 41.2, and 41.3) measuring 9.1 cm (AP) × 10.2 cm (Tr) 11.4 cm (cranio-caudal). There was aneurysmal dilatation of the distal common femoral artery measuring 2 cm and a fusiform dilatation of the right common iliac artery measuring 2 cm in transverse diameter.

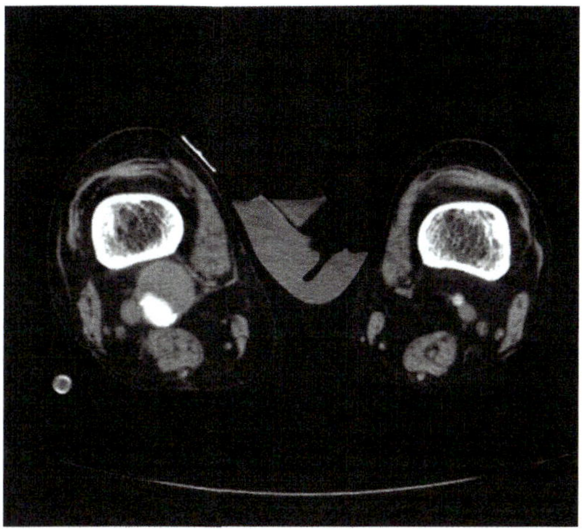

Fig. 41.1 CTA Axial view showing a large right popliteal artery aneurysm

The patient was taken to the operating room emergently, and a posterior approach was selected for repair with the patient in the prone position. A "lazy S" shaped incision was started from the lower medial thigh across the popliteal fossa and curving longitudinally in the upper calf slightly lateral to the midline. The previously placed femoral–popliteal bypass was mobilized and encircled with a silastic vessel loop (Fig. 41.4). The hamstring muscles were separated along with the separation of the two heads of gastrocnemius following division of its fascia. The below-knee popliteal artery was identified and encircled with

S. S. Hans, *Secondary and Tertiary Arterial Reconstructions*,
https://doi.org/10.1007/978-3-032-21214-6_41

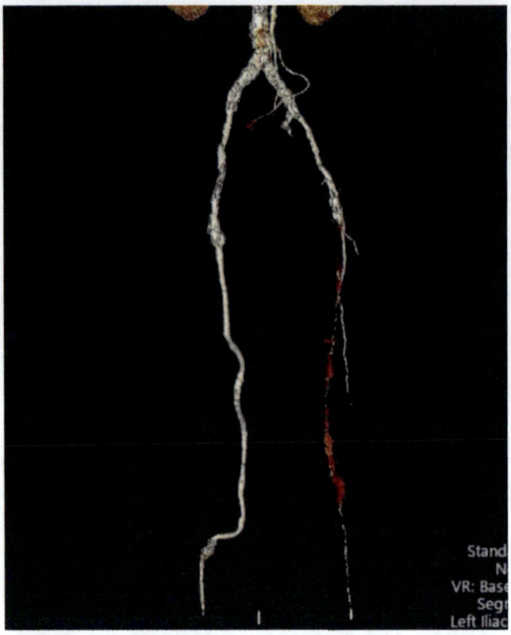

Fig. 41.2 CTA with run off showing a small right common femoral artery aneurysm. Patent right femoral—popliteal artery bypass and a proximal popliteal artery aneurysm

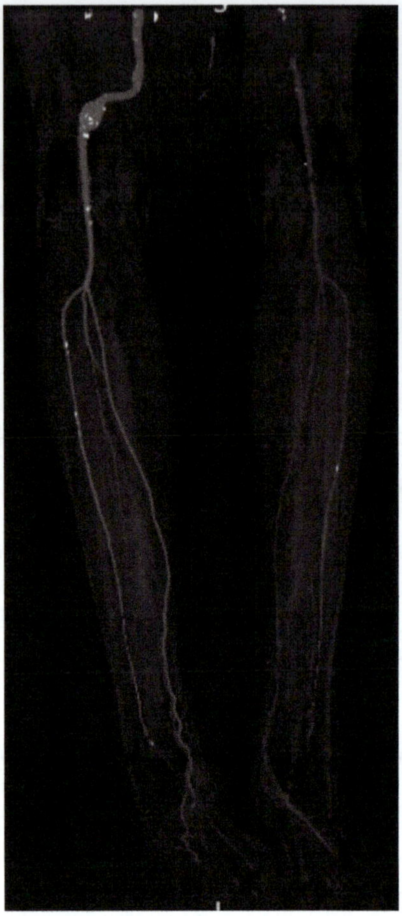

Fig. 41.3 CTA with run off showing right popliteal artery aneurysm with patent femoral–popliteal bypass with patency of infrapopliteal arteries

a silastic vessel loop. Following systemic heparinization and proximal and distal clamping, the large aneurysm sac was opened with an 11-blade scalpel, and a large amount of thrombus was removed. There were no identifiable feeding genicular arteries into the aneurysm. The distal segments of the vein bypass were ligated with “0” silk suture and divided. A 7 mm externally supported ring PTFE graft (W.L. Gore Inc., Newark, DE) was fashioned to fit the spatulated vein graft in an anastomosed end-to-end fashion proximally with a 5″0′ cardiovascular polypropylene suture (Fig. 41.5).

The distal anastomosis was performed subsequently in a similar fashion after tunneling the graft in the midline of the popliteal fossa and anastomosed to the transected distal popliteal artery. A large flat drain was placed in the popliteal fossa and brought out through a separate stab incision. An incisional wound VAC was placed. The patient had an uneventful postoperative course and was discharged home with physical therapy.

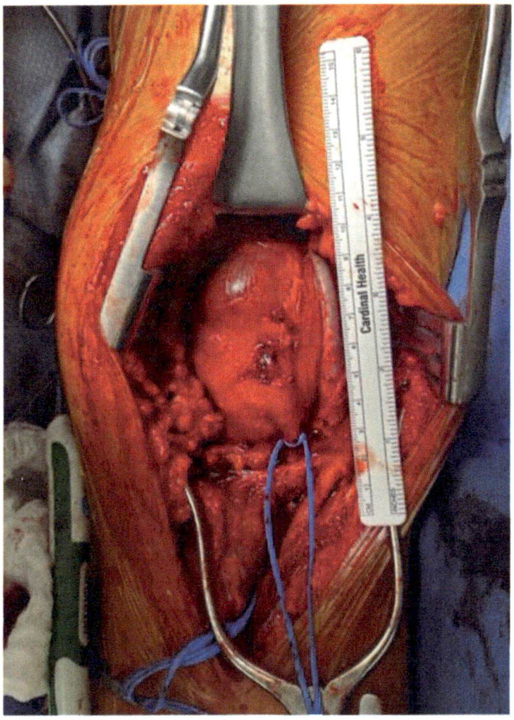

Fig. 41.4 Posterior exposure of popliteal artery aneurysm and silastic vessel loop around the distal popliteal artery

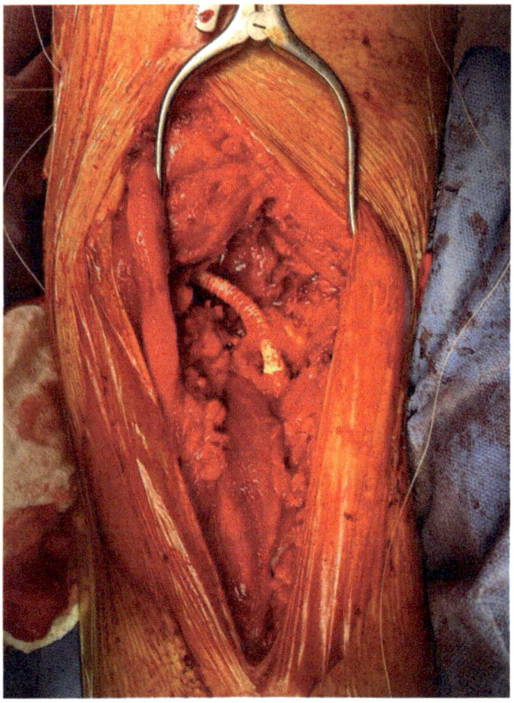

Fig. 41.5 Operative picture showing distal end-to-end anastomosis of a 7 mm ringed PTFE graft to the popliteal artery

Discussion

Although not completely certain, it appears that the large PAA was a true degenerative aneurysm and not an anastomotic aneurysm in this patient.

Popliteal anastomotic aneurysms following vein bypass are extremely uncommon. The presence of a small common iliac artery aneurysm in this patient is also suggestive of degenerative arterial pathology for a popliteal artery aneurysm.

Rupture of the PAA is relatively uncommon; approximately 3–7% of patients with PAA present with rupture [1–3]. Most ruptures occur in patients with very large-sized aneurysms, and rupture is usually contained [2, 3]. In the reported literature, ruptured PAA are either small case series or isolated case reports. As a result, short--term and long-term results are not well defined. Patients with a contained rupture present with a painful, tender, pulsatile mass behind the knee with associated skin ecchymosis in some cases. The risk of amputation is much higher in patients presenting with rupture and acute ischemia as compared to repair of the popliteal aneurysm in patients with symptoms of chronic ischemia or in those without symptoms. Initial clinical presentation may be non-specific, and thus the possibility of a contained leak should be entertained in an elderly man presenting with a painful pulsatile mass in the lower medial thigh or at the posterior aspect of the knee. A free rupture of a popliteal aneurysm is extremely rare. Rupture of a popliteal aneurysm in a patient with previous exclusion and bypass of the aneurysm has not been reported. Most patients should undergo open repair either using a medial or a posterior approach, depending upon the location of the aneurysm and the familiarity of the surgeon.

Following resection of the interposition of a PTFE graft or great saphenous vein as an arterial conduit depends upon the availability of a satisfactory great saphenous vein as an arterial conduit and the medical status of the patient. Endovascular repair is only possible a small number of patients with a leaking popliteal aneurysm because of extreme tortuosity of the artery proximal and distal to the aneurysm.

Multiple Choice Questions

1. Rupture of the popliteal aneurysm occurs in what percentage of popliteal artery aneurysms?
   A. 1–2%
   B. 2–3%
   C. 3–7%
   D. 7–8%
2. Repair of a contained rupture of a popliteal aneurysm present in the lower medial thigh is best performed by:
   A. Open repair using the posterior approach
   B. Open repair using medial approach
   C. Endovascular repair with stent graft
   D. Thrombin or glue injection into the aneurysm sac
3. Distal anastomosis of a large leaking popliteal aneurysm extending below the knee joint line should be performed
   A. Just distal to the aneurysm at the level of the knee joint, even if the artery is slightly dilated
   B. Distal anastomosis should be performed to the popliteal artery just above its bifurcation, following ligation and division of the anterior tibial vein, preferably in an end-to-end fashion
   C. To the posterior tibial/peroneal artery
   D. To the anterior tibial artery by routing the graft through the interosseous membrane

Answers: 1(C), 2(B), 3(B)

References

1. Pulli R, Dorigo W, Troisi N, Innocenti AA, Pratesi G, Azas L, Pratesi C. Surgical management of popliteal artery aneurysms: which factors affect outcomes? J Vasc Surg. 2006;43(3):481–7. PMID:16520159
2. Sie RB, Dawson I, van Baalen JM, Schultze Kool LJ, van Bockel JH. Ruptured popliteal artery aneurysm. An insidious complication. Eur J Vasc Endovasc Surg. 1997;13(5):432–8. PMID:9166264
3. Hans SS. Open repair of contained rupture of right popliteal aneurysm. In: Hans SS, editor. Challenging arterial reconstructions: 100 clinical cases. Cham: Springer; 2020. p. 107–10.

42 Deep Vein Arterialization for Severe Infrapopliteal Artery Occlusive Disease with Foot Gangrene

Presentation

A 67-year-old man was seen in the clinic with gangrene of the right great toe. He had a history of left below-knee amputation in 2008, parathyroidectomy, and coronary artery bypass graft (CABG). Comorbidities included diabetes mellitus, hypertension, ESRD on hemodialysis program, and hyperlipidemia.

The patient was seen in the clinic in August 2022 for a gangrene of the distal tip of the right second toe. He underwent arteriography, which showed near occlusion of the proximal popliteal artery just inferior to the adductor canal. The peroneal artery could not be visualized and likely was occluded. The posterior tibial artery was occluded 5 cm from its origin. The foot was primarily supplied by the anterior tibial artery with an incomplete plantar arch. He underwent successful popliteal artery angioplasty with a 5 mm × 10 mm Armada balloon over a 0.018 nitinol wire. The wire crossing was aided by a 0.018 quick cross catheter. The popliteal artery was stented using the Supera stent. The right second toe healed in 6 weeks with loss of the toenail.

The patient was admitted with dry gangrene of the right great toe in October 2024. Catheter--based arteriography showed severe infrapopliteal occlusive disease with anterior tibial artery run-off and abrupt occlusion of the dorsalis pedis artery (Figs. 42.1 and 42.2). The posterior tibial and peroneal arteries were occluded. There was no filling of the plantar or digital arteries (Figs. 42.3, 42.4, and 42.5). The popliteal artery

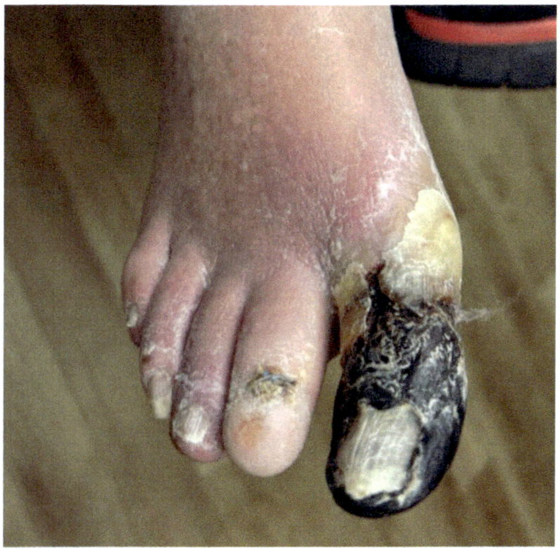

Fig. 42.1 Gangrene right big toe extending to the metatarsophalangeal joint (Dorsal aspect)

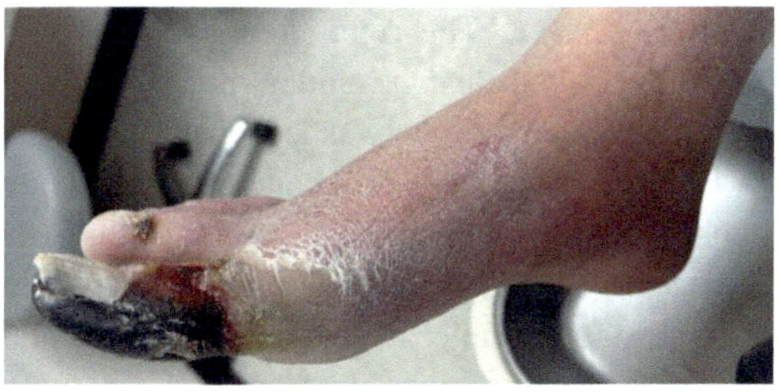

Fig. 42.2 Gangrene of the right big toe (Medial aspect)

S. S. Hans, *Secondary and Tertiary Arterial Reconstructions*,
https://doi.org/10.1007/978-3-032-21214-6_42

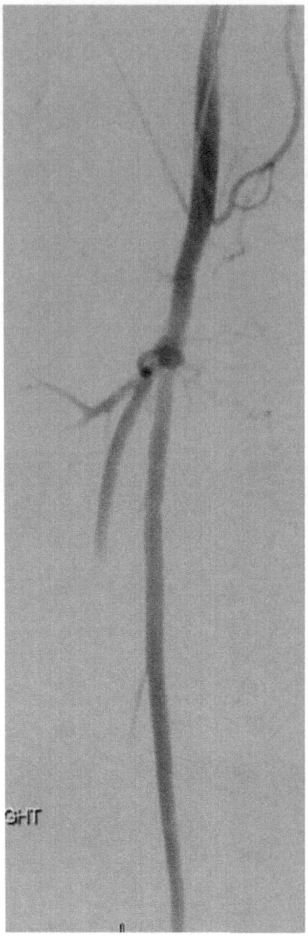

Fig. 42.3 Arteriogram showing patent right common proximal profunda femoris artery and superficial femoral artery in the proximal and in mid segment

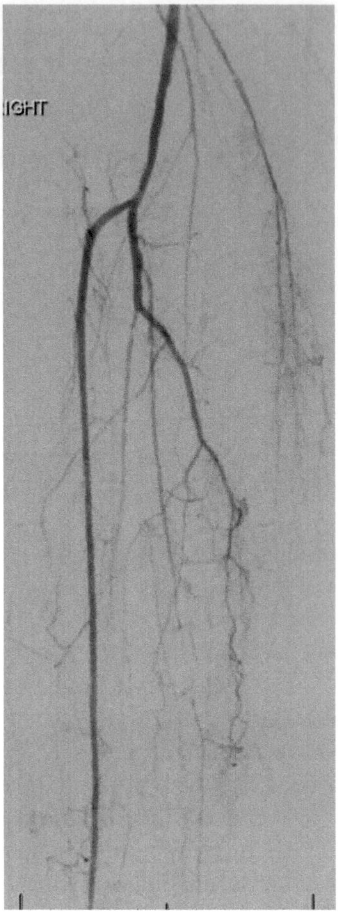

Fig. 42.4 Patent right popliteal artery angioplasty. Runoff with the anterior tibial artery is demonstrated. Tibioperoneal trunk is patent, the post-tibial and peroneal arteries are occluded

stent was patent. The right great toe gangrene became infected, and he underwent right great toe open ray amputation was left open.

Because he was not a candidate for open bypass or further conventional percutaneous therapies, he was evaluated for possible deep vein arterialization. Duplex pedal vein mapping and review of his infrapopliteal arterial anatomy showed that he was a satisfactory candidate for DVA. The lateral plantar vein (LPV) measured 3.2 mm in diameter. The posterior tibial artery was deemed a satisfactory donor artery, without disturbing the native anterior tibial runoff to the foot.

He underwent deep vein arterialization in November 2024. Ultrasound-guided access to the LPV with ascending venography and insertion of a 5F sheath was performed. Antegrade puncture of the common femoral artery using ultrasound guidance, with insertion of a 6F sheath, with arteriography, and detailed imaging of the foot vasculature was obtained. The posterior tibial artery was targeted as the donor vessel for DVA using the LimFlow system.

The 6F short sheath in the common femoral artery was exchanged over a Glidewire Advantage wire (0.035) for a 7 mm × 45 cm Terumo Destination sheath positioned at the level of the popliteal artery. The patient was anticoagulated with 10,000 units of heparin (3000 units at the time of insertion of the plantar venous sheath and

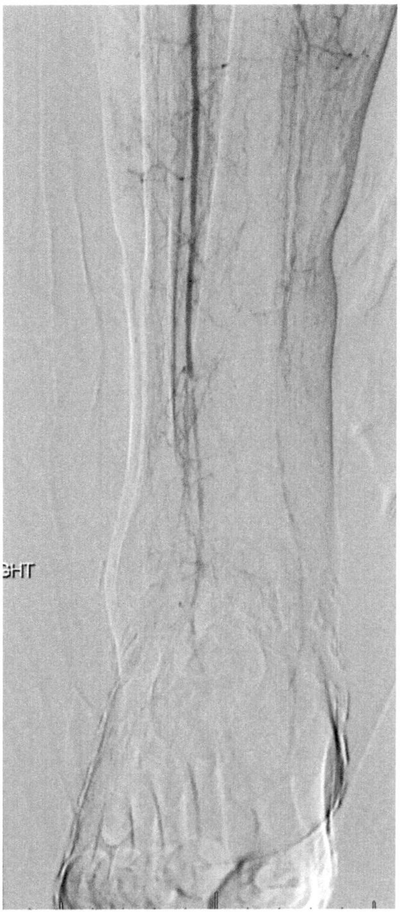

Fig. 42.5 Anterior tibial artery occludes distally near the ankle

7000 units after the 7F arterial destination sheath was placed) to keep the ACT over 250. The Glidewire Advantage was exchanged for a 0.014 Asahi Miraclebros guidewire. This wire was used to cross the stenotic segment in the posterior tibial artery (PTA) and facilitate balloon angioplasty of the proximal 3–4 cm segment of PTA with a 3.5 mm balloon. The Asahi wire (0.014) was exchanged for a stiffer 0.014 Spartacore wire and used to deliver the (ARC) arteriovenous crossing catheter. The crossing catheter was positioned 2 cm beyond the origin of the PTA, and a retrieval basket (V-Ceiver) was delivered retrograde to the adjacent posterior tibial vein through the LPV over an 0.014 wire. The basket and the entry catheter were aligned, the crossing needle was fired from the ARC into the V-Ceiver basket

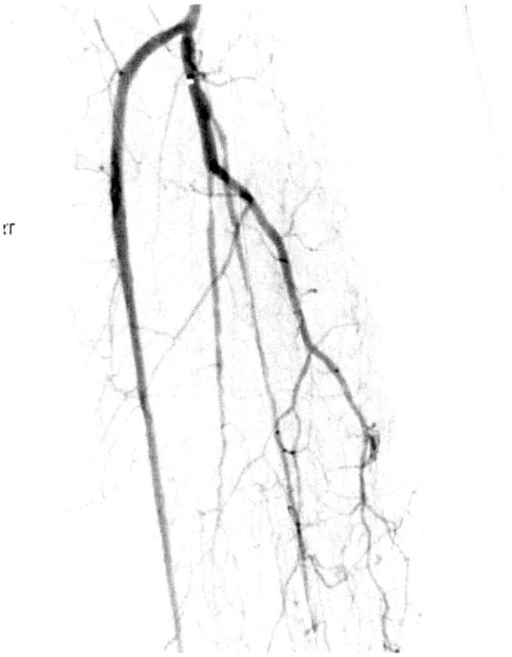

Fig. 42.6 Arteriography showing steps of deep vein arterialization with the catheter tip in the tibioperoneal trunk

with delivery of a 0.018 nitrex wire from the posterior tibial artery to the vein, allowing for through-and-through access from the LPV sheath to the common femoral artery sheath. Balloon angioplasty of the crossing point using a 3.5 mm balloon to expand the new arteriovenous fistulous connection was performed. The LimFlow over-the-wire "push-valvulotome" (Vector) was used to disrupt the posterior tibial venous valves by advancing it distally from the crossover point to the LPV in an antegrade manner. At the level of the mid-calcaneus, a resistant valve required the use of a 4 mm Wolverine cutting balloon (Boston Scientific Marlborough, MA).

The LimFlow overlapping stent grafts were then delivered from distal to proximal, measuring 5 mm × 200 mm, 5 mm × 150 mm, with a proximal 5.5 mm to 3.5 mm tapering-covered stents extending into the posterior tibial artery. These were post-dilated with a 5.5 mm and a 3.5 mm balloon (Figs. 42.6, 42.7, 42.8, 42.9, 42.10, and 42.11). The LPV and venous pedal loop were then accessed with a Command 0.014 using an antegrade approach and the pedal loop was bal-

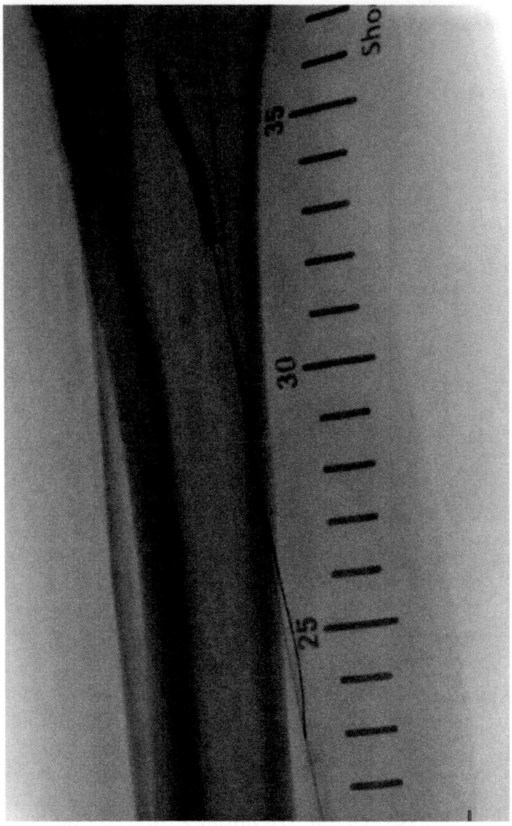

Fig. 42.7 Arteriography showing steps of deep vein arterialization with balloon angioplasty of proximal post tibial artery passage of 0.014 wire into the post tibial artery, in order to facilitate delivery of ARC

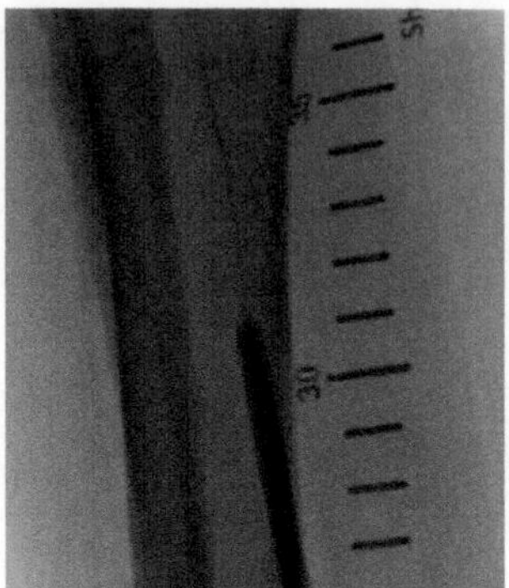

Fig. 42.8 Arteriography showing steps of deep vein arterialization with balloon angioplasty of a long segment of posterior tibial vein after ARC crossing and through-and-through access from posterior tibial artery to vein

looned using a 3 mm balloon to ensure maximal outflow for the stents into the forefoot veins. A 5 mm balloon was used to achieve hemostasis at the plantar access site once the plantar venous sheath was removed. Completion arteriography suggested that the stent and the plantar and pedal outflow were widely patent. There was recoil of the posterior tibial artery donor vessel proximal to the LimFlow stent, and a 3.5 × 28 mm drug-eluting coronary stent was then deployed overlapping with a LimFlow stent to maximize the inflow.

Over the next several weeks, he developed expected progressive venous congestion and ischemic changes in the adjacent toes, common and anticipated early following DVA. The patient underwent open transmetatarsal amputation in January 2025 with excellent bleeding. Negative pressure wound therapy was applied. The wound continued to show significant improvement (Fig. 42.12) with progressive granulation.

A stent duplex study in December 2024 showed acceptable volume flow in the stent (150–350 cc/min), but findings concerning proximal in-stent stenosis were noted. Angiography did not identify any stent-patency-threatening problem. Because of subsequent decreased flow volumes and similar concerns for in-flow stenosis, the patient was taken for angiography again in February 2025 via left (contralateral) femoral artery access under ultrasound guidance. The angiogram showed that the flow within the deep

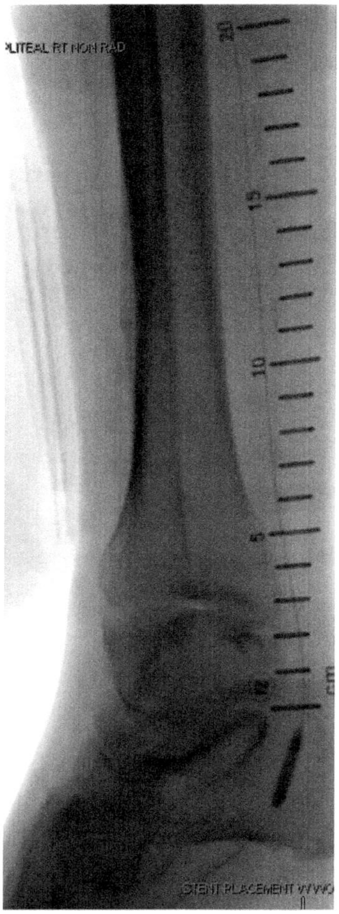

Fig. 42.9 Arteriography showing balloon angiopladty of the LPV at the ankle to facilitate valve lysis and LimFlow stent delivery

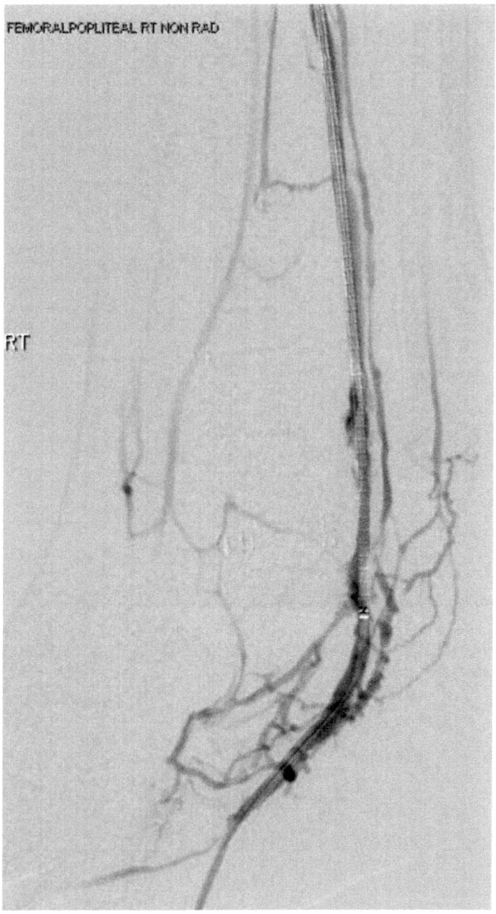

Fig. 42.10 Delivery of LimFlow Stent to LPV (pre-deployment)

vein arterialization was satisfactory, but there was moderate in-stent stenosis involving most of the inflow stent on magnified view. A second drug-coated 3.5 × 28 mm stent was placed to treat this stenosis, extending coverage to the tibioperoneal trunk. This resulted in marked improvement in the flow as well as satisfactory tacking of the inflow stent (Figs. 42.13 and 42.14). In July 2025, the stent acutely occluded, and because of deterioration in the TMA wound, a percutaneous thrombectomy was performed successfully, revealing a new below-knee popliteal artery stenosis compromising inflow again. This required treatment with a 4 mm drug-coated stent as well. His wound granulation and closure resumed progress.

At the last follow-up in December 2025, duplex revealed recurrent thrombosis of the LimFlow stent. Despite this, the dorsalis pedis and the anterior tibial doppler signals were significantly improved, with progressive granulation tissue formation with complete healing of the transmetatarsal amputation site (Figs. 42.15 and 42.16). This suggested successful DVA with successful maintenance of forefoot perfusion and neovascularization, as had been documented on serial arteriography. No further intervention was

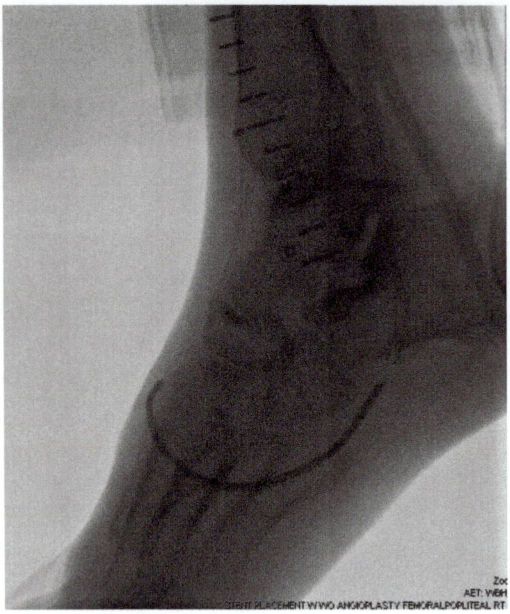

Fig. 42.11 Angioplasty of the transverse pedal venous arch

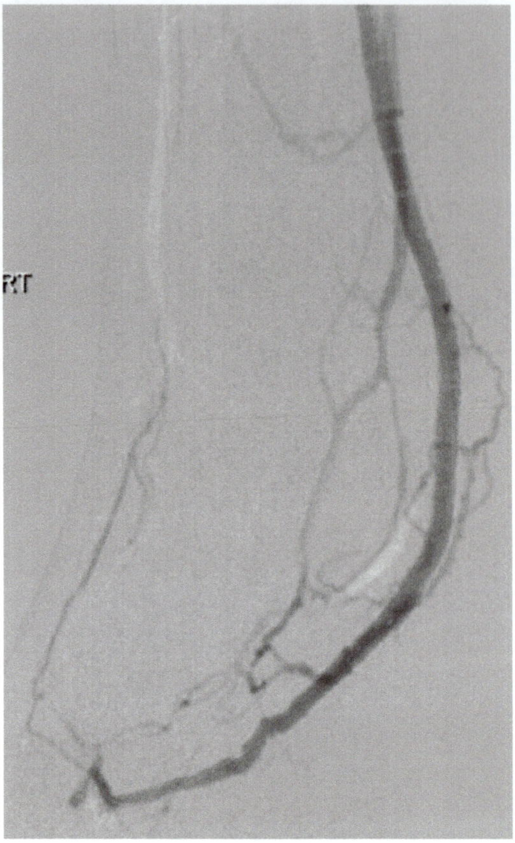

Fig. 42.13 Completion angiogram revealing patent LimFlow stent filling LPV and early filling of pedal venous loop

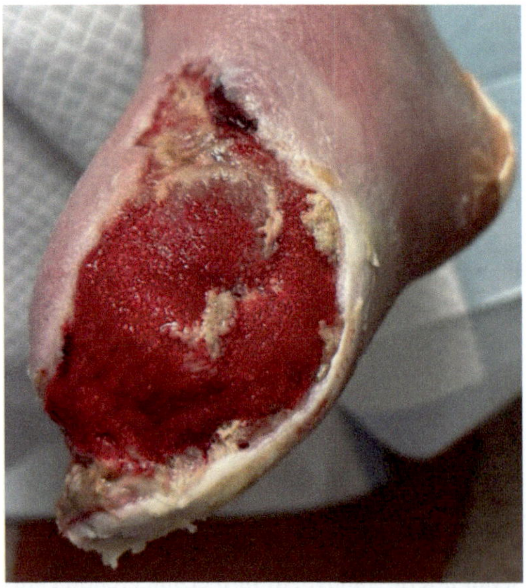

Fig. 42.12 Granulation at the site of transmetatarsal amputation

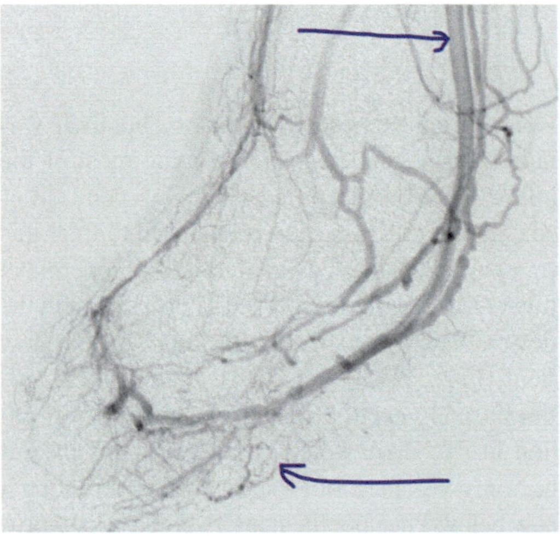

Fig. 42.14 Follow-up angiogram with excellent flow through LimFlow stent into LPV and loop with signs of neovascularization

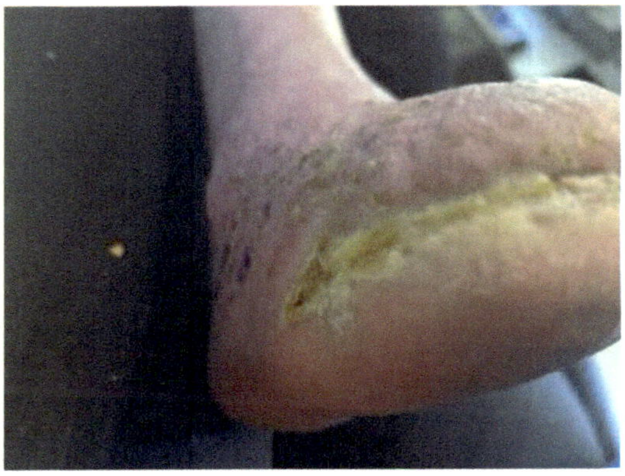

Fig. 42.15 Satisfactory healing at the transmetatarsal amputation site (Front view) December 2025

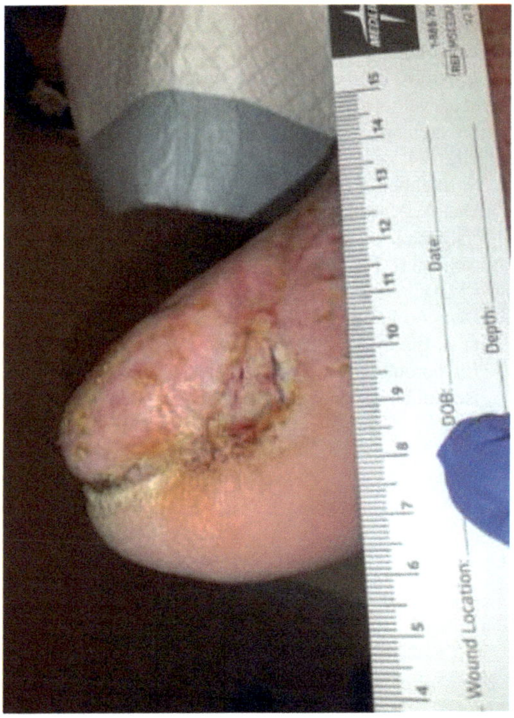

Fig. 42.16 Satisfactory healing at the transmetarsal amputation site (Medial view) December 2025

deemed necessary, and he went on to heal the TMA completely as of December 2025 (approximately 1 year post-index DVA).

Discussion

It has been reported that up to 20% of patients with chronic limb-threatening ischemia are ineligible or have exhausted all conventional treatment options for revascularization, deemed to have "no-option." Such patients face major lower extremity amputation and death. In an effort to improve limb salvage and mortality, Clair et al., reported 6 and 12-month outcomes of the PROMISE I early feasibility study compromising 32 patients for treatment of "no-option" chronic limb-threatening ischemia (CLTI) with percutaneous deep vein arterialization (pDVA) using the LimFlow system [1]. They reported 97% (31 patients) technical success. The 30-day, 6-month, and 12-month amputation-free survival rates were 91%, 74%, and 70%, respectively. The wound healing status of either fully healed or progressive healing was 67% at 6 months and 75% at 12 months. Reinterventions were performed in 16 patients (52%), and 88% of the maintenance reinterventions occurred within the first 3 months. The majority of reintervention (12 patients, 75%) involved the arterial inflow tract proximal to the stented LimFlow circuit, and in-stent stenosis was not determined to have been the cause of reintervention.

From the results of the PROMISE II trial (Prospective single-group, multicenter) among 105 patients with chronic limb-threatening ischemia (CLTI) with a median age of 70 years, 33% women, and 42% were Black, Hispanic or Latino, the study reported a technical success rate of deep vein arterialization in 104 patients (99%). At 6 months, 66% had amputation-free survival. Limb salvage was attained in 67 patients (76%). Wounds showed complete healing in 25% and healing in progress in 51%. The authors concluded that the introduction of transcatheter deep vein arterialization provides the possibility of revascularization in patients with no option for either conventional endovascular or open arterial reconstruction in patients with chronic limb-threatening ischemia, where major amputation was the only treatment option for their care [2]. From a meta-analysis of 27 studies of pedal vein arterialization, comparing surgical with percutaneous techniques, the pooled limb salvage rate at 6 and 12 months was 78% and 74% in the surgical group and 81.7% and 78.6% in the percutaneous group [2]. The study concluded that pedal vein arterialization in CLTI patients showed promising results [2]. In high risk patients, percutaneous deep vein arterialization is a feasible option with favorable limb salvage and wound healing rates [1–3].

Acknowledgement Following popliteal artery intervention by the editor, the LimFlow procedure and follow-up care were provided by Dr. Tamer Boules, MD, Senior Vascular Surgeon and Section Chief, Henry Ford, West Bloomfield, MI 48322.

Multiple Choice Questions

1. The number of patients with CLTI chronic limb-threatening ischemia with no-option revascularization options is:
   A. 10%
   B. 15%
   C. 20%
   D. 25%
2. Results of transcatheter arterialization of deep veins in CLTI in PROMISE II study resulted in limb salvage of:
   A. 60%
   B. 66%
   C. 70%
   D. 76%
3. Complete healing of the wounds in the PROMISE II trial occurred in:
   A. 20%
   B. 25%
   C. 30%
   D. 40%

Answers: Q1 (C), Q2 (D), Q3 (B)

References

1. Clair DG, Mustapha JA, Shishehbor MH, Schneider PA, Henao S, et al. PROMISE I: early feasibility study of the LimFlow system for percutaneous deep vein arterialization in no-option chronic limb--threatening ischemia: 12-month results. J Vasc Surg. 2021;74(5):1626–35. PMID:34019990
2. Shishehbor MH, Powell RJ, Montero-Baker MF, Dua A, Martínez-Trabal JL, et al. Transcatheter arterialization of deep veins in chronic limb-threatening ischemia. N Engl J Med. 2023;388(13):1171–80. PMID:36988592
3. Ucci A, Perini P, Freyrie A, Schreve MA, Ünlü Ç, et al. Endovascular and surgical venous arterialization for no-option patients with chronic limb-threatening ischemia: a systematic review and meta-analysis. J Endovasc Ther. 2025;32(5):1301–16. PMID:38009322

43 A Spliced Femoral–Anterior Tibial Vein Bypass Following Failed Multiple Arterial Reconstructions

Presentation

A 56-year-old man was seen in the clinic in March 2022 with ischemic rest pain in the left foot and paresthesia in the left foot for the previous 9 months. He was a current smoker with a history of smoking 60 pack years. He also had a history of excessive alcohol abuse. Medical comorbidities included hyperlipidemia, peripheral neuropathy, paroxysmal atrial fibrillation, and a 4.5 cm ascending aortic aneurysm. He had undergone multiple arterial reconstructions at an outside hospital. An attempted left iliac angioplasty/stent was apparently unsuccessful. Subsequently, the patient underwent a crossover femoral–femoral graft at an outside hospital. A follow-up CTA showed a patent crossover femoral–femoral graft, left popliteal artery occlusion with one vessel runoff. Because of symptoms of ischemic rest pain and ulceration in the foot, he was scheduled to undergo left femoral to posterior tibial bypass using the great saphenous vein in August 2022. Review of the OR dictation revealed that the exposed posterior tibial artery (PTA) in the lower third of the leg and an arteriotomy in the PTA showed poor back bleeding and was diminutive in size. The reconstruction was abandoned, and the wound was closed in layers. In August 2022, the patient underwent left femoral to posterior tibial artery bypass graft using Cryovein by another vascular surgeon. The graft occluded 9 months later with worsening symptoms of ischemia in the left foot.

After clinical evaluation with a duplex arterial study, the patient underwent arteriography using ultrasound-guided left brachial artery access in March 2023. The findings were a patent crossover femoral–femoral graft, 50% stenosis of the left superficial femoral artery, 3 cm from its origin. Occlusion of the distal superficial femoral artery at the popliteal artery. There was an occlusion of the entire length of the popliteal artery. The runoff was with the anterior tibial artery. The post-tibial artery was patent but stenotic 3 cm above the ankle joint and distally beyond the segment of stenosis. PTA was patent with an incomplete plantar arch (Figs. 43.1, 43.2, 43.3, and 43.4). Vein mapping was performed. The left GSV has been previously harvested, and the right GSV was of adequate caliber from the upper thigh to the knee. It was of inadequate caliber below the knee. Both cephalic and basilic veins in the left arm were adequate in caliber. Following cardiac assessment, the patient underwent left proximal SFA to mid anterior artery bypass using spliced vein: three venous segments of the (1) basilic vein, (2) contralateral GSV below the knee, and (3) cephalic vein anastomosed as veno venostomies in May 2023.

The valves were lysed with a retrograde valvulotome and a non-reversed spliced vein graft bypass to the mid-anterior tibial artery brought through the interosseous membrane between the tendons of tibialis anterior and extensor hallucis longus with establishment of a satisfactory dorsa-

S. S. Hans, *Secondary and Tertiary Arterial Reconstructions*,
https://doi.org/10.1007/978-3-032-21214-6_43

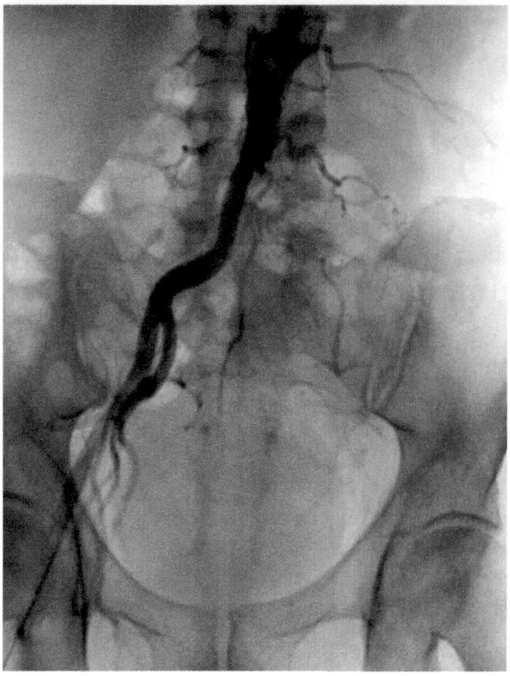

Fig. 43.1 Abdominal aortogram showing left common and external iliac artery occlusion

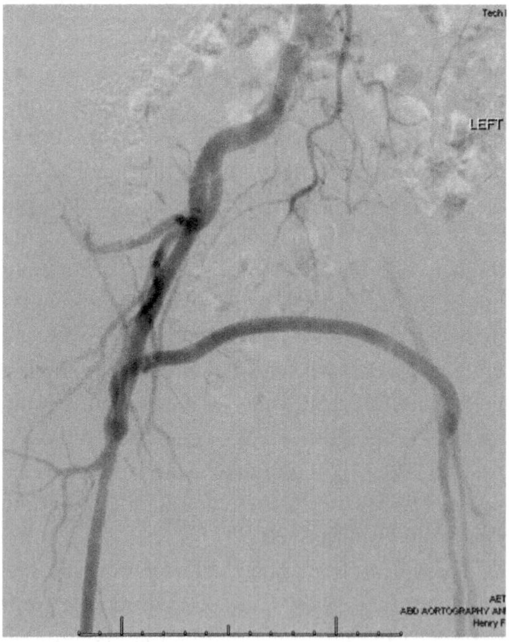

Fig. 43.2 Arteriography showing patent crossover femoral-femoral graft with stenosis of the proximal superficial femoral artery

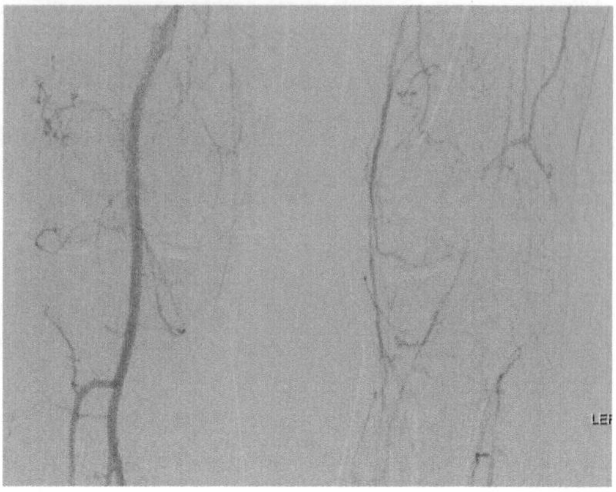

Fig. 43.3 Arteriography shows left popliteal artery occlusion of proximal trifurcation arteries with collaterals

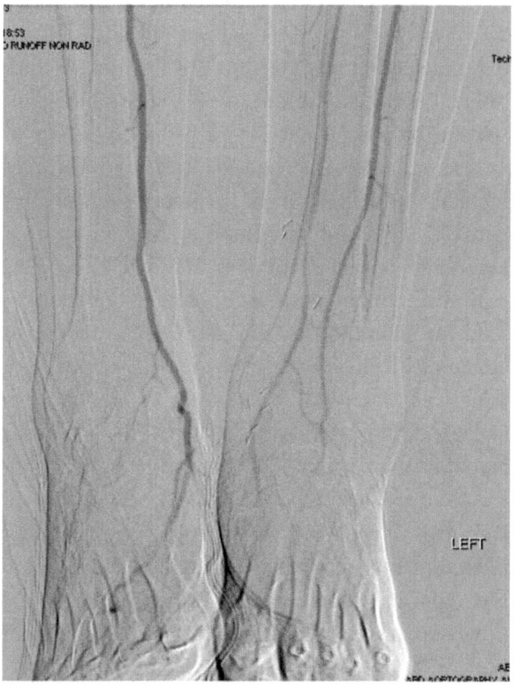

Fig. 43.4 Run off primarily with the anterior tibial artery. The posterior tibial artery shows diffuse narrowing

lis pedis pulse. The patient was discharged on the 5th postoperative day.

Six weeks later, a follow-up duplex arterial study showed an ABI 1 (R) 0.89 (L) in October 2024. The patient had relief of ischemic symp-

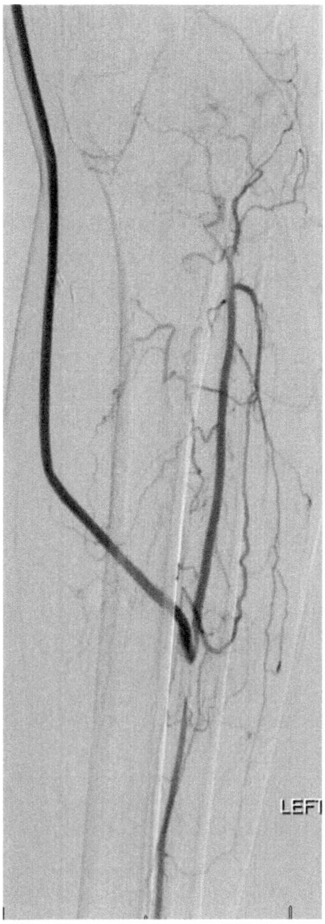

Fig. 43.5 Arteriography showing distal anastomotic stenosis at the level of the mid-anterior tibial artery tunneled through the interosseous membrane

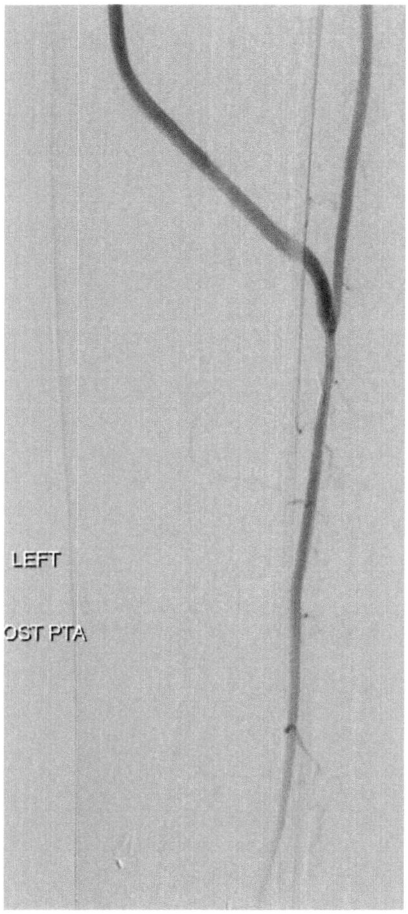

Fig. 43.6 Satisfactory balloon angioplasty of the distal anastomotic stenosis using antegrade left femoral access

toms for 6 months before the symptoms recurred, with duplex imaging showing distal anastomotic stenosis. Using left femoral antegrade access, the patient underwent angioplasty with a 2.5 cm Armada balloon followed by 3 × 4 cm with less than 10% residual stenosis (Figs. 43.5, 43.6, and 43.7). After a follow-up of 6 more months, symptoms returned, and he underwent balloon angioplasty for recurrent distal anastomotic stenosis using ultrasound-guided left femoral antegrade access with easily palpable DP in the left foot.

He was seen in the clinic in April 2025, ABI was 1.0 (right) and 0.89 (left), with TBI 0.85 (right) and 0.45 (left), with relief of ischemic symptoms but with persistent symptoms of peripheral neuropathy. In October 2025, the patient was seen in the clinic with pain and paresthesia in the left leg and stable claudication. Duplex imaging of the graft showed occlusion of the graft about 30 months after the spliced vein bypass. The ankle-brachial index on the left side was 0.41. The patient was admitted to the hospital in November 2025 with epigastric pain, nausea, and vomiting secondary to alcohol consumption and was discharged after a 3-day stay in the hospital. There was no progression of the symptoms of lower extremity ischemia.

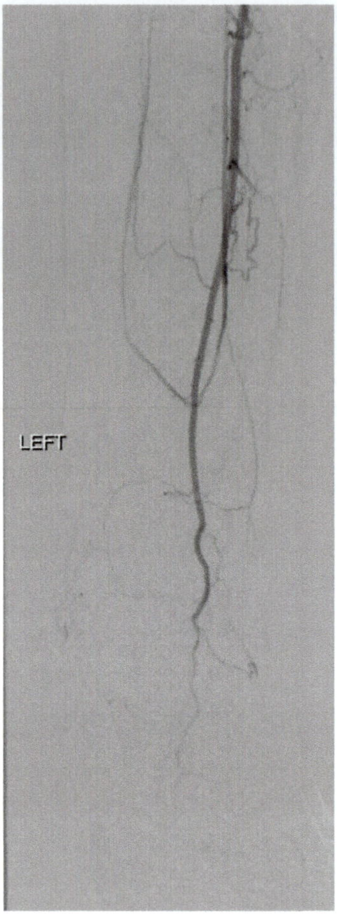

Fig. 43.7 Arteriography post angioplasty showing satisfactory run off with the anterior tibial artery and a small diameter peroneal artery

Discussion

The greater saphenous vein (GSV) is the conduit of choice for femoral–infrapopliteal artery bypass because of its length, size, compatibility, and durability. The GSV is inadequate in 20% of patients. The best alternative conduit for lower extremity revascularization for this group of patients is an issue of ongoing debate. The prosthetic grafts are inferior in patency to autologous vein conduit and should be rarely used. Chew et al. [1], reported 226 infragenicular reconstructions (in 203 patients) with autologous veins taken from the contralateral GSV in 31%, single--segment arm vein 19%, single-segment lesser saphenous vein 5%, and autologous composite vein 48% in the absence of adequate ipsilateral GSV. Bypasses were performed to the tibial and pedal arteries in 84% of cases. The 30-day mortality and occlusion rates were 1% and 9%, respectively. Postoperative morbidity rate was 24%, with a 7% rate of major complications. The 5-year primary patency rates were significantly better for contralateral GSV compared with autogenous composite vein grafts (61% ± 7% vs 39% ± 6%, $p < 0.009$). However, secondary patency and limb salvage rates did not differ between groups (Table 43.1).

Table 43.1 Outcomes by conduit group

Outcome	Contralateral GSV	SSV	AV
Secondary patency	75% (95% CI: 66–83)	75% (95% CI: 66–83)	65% (CI 57–73)
Limb salvage	73% (95% CI: 65–81)	>79% (95% CI: 69–89)	74% (95% CI: 68–80)
Survival (5 years)	89% (95% CI: 82–95)	87% (95% CI: 79–95)	83% (95% CI: 77–89)

Nierdich et al., [2] reported the results of 2642 consecutive infra-popliteal arterial bypasses (1998–2018) using contralateral GSV, short saphenous vein (SSV), arm veins (AV), 1933 procedures using ipsilateral GSV, 644 using contralateral GSV, 101 short saphenous veins, 334 using arm veins, and 61 prosthetic grafts. The median follow-up was 2.3 years. Thirty-day mortality was 1.9% for the entire group and was similar between the three groups. Primary and secondary patency rates after 5 years were comparable between the groups: ($p = 0.46$).

They concluded that all three types of alternative autogenous bypass vein grafts (in the absence of ipsilateral GSV) are equal regarding outcome parameters.

Kreinberg et al., conducted a prospective randomized trial of spliced vein versus polytetrafluoroethylene (PTFE) graft with a distal cuff for limb-threatening ischemia from 1996 to 2000, comprising 39 bypass grafting procedures in 36 patients randomized to either spliced vein bypass grafting (n 19) or PTFE grafting with a distal vein cuff (n 20). The primary patency rate at 2 years 44% for the spliced group and 49% for the PTFE grafting with a distal vein cuff. All patients with PTFE graft and distal cuff underwent anticoagulation with warfarin sodium. In the spliced group, 7 of 19 bypass grafts underwent revision in the follow-up period, and two of the 20 cuffed bypass grafts were revised successfully. The secondary patency rate was 87% and 59% ($p < 0.05$), respectively, with limb salvage rates of 94% and 85% for spliced and cuff groups, respectively. They concluded that both spliced and PTFE with a vein cuff produce acceptable limb salvage rates. The secondary patency of spliced veins is better, but these grafts often need revision [3].

Pascarella et al., reported a retrospective study of 34 bypass operations using a conduit containing at least one arm vein segment and one or more splices for critical limb ischemia. They reported a 1-year patency of 100% and 85% at 2 years [4].

Multiple Choice Questions

1. The GSV is inadequate in how many percent of patients?
   A. 10%
   B. 15%
   C. 20%
   D. 25%
2. A 70-year-old man with an ischemic ulcer requiring femoral–posterior tibial bypass. Left GSV has been removed for CABG. The next best option is:
   A. Arm vein
   B. Short saphenous vein
   C. Cryovein
   D. Contralateral GSV
3. Of all alternative autogenous vein grafts (contralateral GSV, SSV, AV) in the absence of ipsilateral GSV, which one is superior in terms of limb salvage and survival?
   A. Contralateral GSV
   B. SSV
   C. AV
   D. Contralateral GSV, SSV, and AV are similar

Answers: 1(C), 2(D), 3(D)

References

1. Chew DK, Owens CD, Belkin M, Donaldson MC, Whittemore AD, et al. Bypass in the absence of ipsilateral greater saphenous vein: safety and superiority of the contralateral greater saphenous vein. J Vasc Surg. 2002;35(6):1085–92. PMID:12042718
2. Nierlich P, Enzmann FK, Metzger P, Dabernig W, Aspalter M, et al. Alternative venous conduits for below knee bypass in the absence of ipsilateral great saphenous vein. Eur J Vasc Endovasc Surg. 2020;60(3):403–9. PMID:32768278
3. Kreienberg PB, Darling RC 3rd, Chang BB, Champagne BJ, Paty PS, et al. Early results of a prospective randomized trial of spliced vein versus polytetrafluoroethylene graft with a distal vein cuff for limb-threatening ischemia. J Vasc Surg. 2002;35(2):299–306. PMID:11854728
4. McGinigle KL, Pascarella L, Shortell CK, Cox MW, McCann RL, et al. Spliced arm vein grafts are a durable conduit for lower extremity bypass. Ann Vasc Surg. 2015;29(4):716–21. PMID:25638725

44 Left Superficial Femoral Artery Endarterectomy and Left Femoral–Popliteal Bypass in a Patient with a Prior Thrombosed Femoral Artery Stent

Presentation

A 61-year-old woman was seen in the clinic in November 2024 with ischemic rest pain and paresthesia in the left foot for the past 3 months. She was a current smoker with a history of smoking 50 pack-years. Medical comorbidities included chronic obstructive pulmonary disease (COPD), hypertension, and hyperlipidemia. In June 2024, a CT angiography with runoff study performed at an outside facility revealed thrombosis of the left superficial femoral artery (SFA) stent. Review of records from an outside facility revealed that the left SFA stent was performed for symptoms of intermittent claudication. Noninvasive arterial Doppler study performed at the clinic showed:

- ABI: 1.19 (right), 0.44 (left).
- TBI: 0.62 (right), 0 (left).

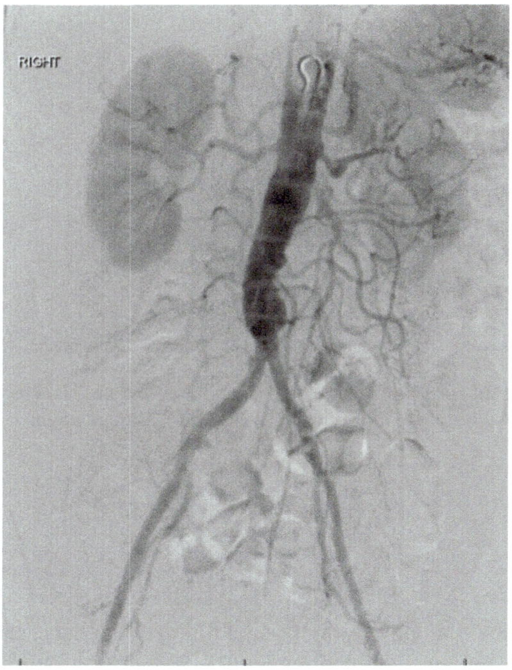

Fig. 44.1 Abdominal and pelvic arteriogram showing a small distal abdominal aortic aneurysm small diameter common iliac and external iliac arteries

In December 2024, the patient underwent abdominal aortogram and runoff study using contralateral right femoral artery access under ultrasound guidance. The arteriography revealed a 2.7 cm saccular infrarenal abdominal aortic aneurysm, a small-diameter left external iliac artery without any stenosis. It also showed occlusion of the left superficial femoral artery, 2 cm from its origin, with stent thrombosis. There was reconstitution of a small diameter above-knee left popliteal artery with runoff primarily via the peroneal artery. The anterior tibial artery was patent but was of a small caliber with two separate areas of 70% stenosis. The posterior tibial artery was occluded. The plantar arch was incomplete (Figs. 44.1, 44.2, 44.3, and 44.4).

On venous mapping of lower extremities, the left GSV was inadequate in size (2.5 mm), and the right GSV measured 3.5 mm proximally,

S. S. Hans, *Secondary and Tertiary Arterial Reconstructions*,
https://doi.org/10.1007/978-3-032-21214-6_44

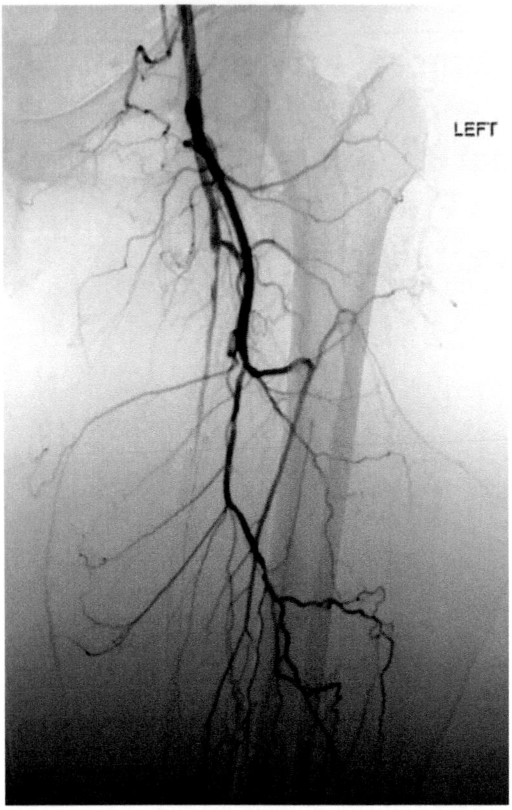

Fig. 44.2 Left lower extremity arteriogram showing occlusion of left SFA a few centimeters from its origin

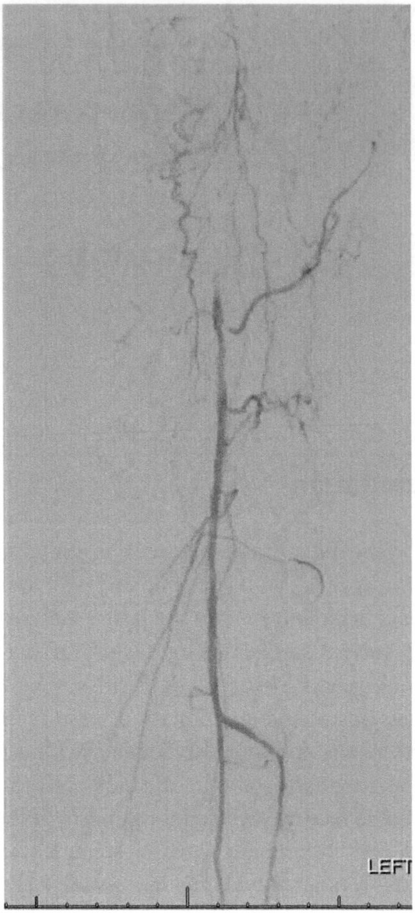

Fig. 44.3 Left lower extremity arteriogram showing occlusion of the left SFA and reconstitution of a small diameter proximal popliteal artery

3.2 mm in mid-thigh, and 2.9 mm at the knee. In January 2025, the patient underwent harvesting of the right GSV as a conduit for the left femoral–popliteal (FP) bypass, but the length of the GSV was inadequate for the above-knee left femoral–popliteal bypass. A long segment left common femoral and superficial femoral endarterectomy was performed and a long calcific atherosclerotic plaque was removed (Fig. 44.5). A 12 cm long and 6 mm wide bovine pericardial patch was sutured at the site of endarterectomy (Fig. 44.6). In the distal portion of the bovine pericardial patch; a 2-cm long incision was made for proximal anastomosis of the left superficial femoral to the popliteal artery just proximal to the knee joint was performed (Fig. 44.7). The vein graft was used as a non-reversed conduit with lysis of the valves following completion of the proximal anastomosis using a retrograde valvulotome. The distal anastomosis, passed from its distal cut end to above the knee, the popliteal artery was performed in an end-to-side manner using continuous 6′0″ cardiovascular polypropylene suture.

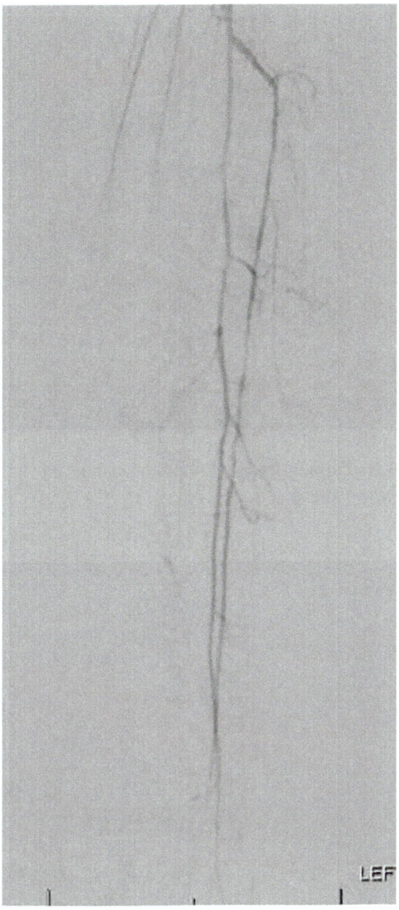

Fig. 44.4 Arteriogram showing runoff with the peroneal artery and a diffusely narrowed anterior tibial artery. The distal anterior tibial artery shows occlusion

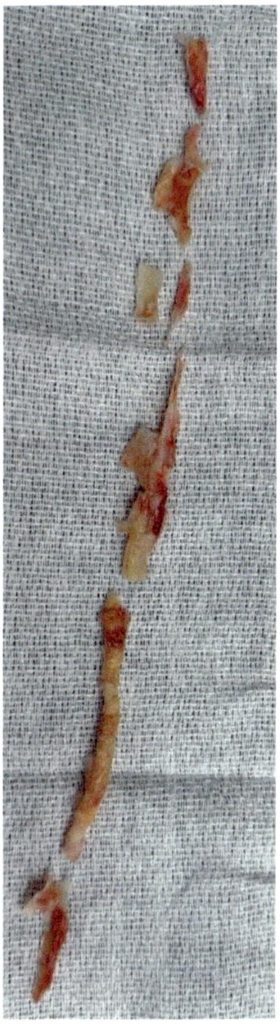

Fig. 44.5 Operative specimen of a long atherosclerotic plaque removed from a long segment left SFA endarterectomy

The patient had a satisfactory postoperative course but developed surgical site infection (SSI) in the left groin and upper thigh, which was treated with wound care, debridement, and antibiotics. Wound culture showed *Staphylococcus aureus* (methicillin-sensitive), and she was treated with oral cephalosporin. The incision healed in 6 weeks with secondary intention.

A follow-up duplex image of the bypass graft in May 2025 showed no evidence of hemodynamically significant stenosis in the proximal SFA endarterectomy and femoropopliteal bypass graft (Figs. 44.8, 44.9, and 44.10). Ankle-brachial

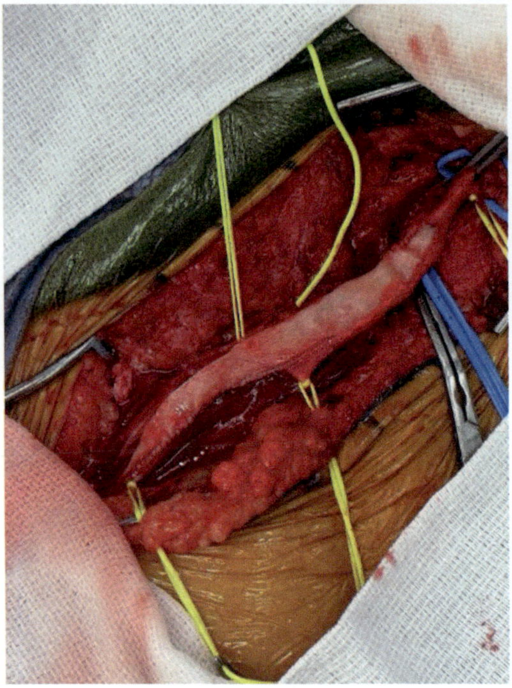

Fig. 44.6 Bovine pericardial patch sutured over a long segment endarterectomy of the left SFA

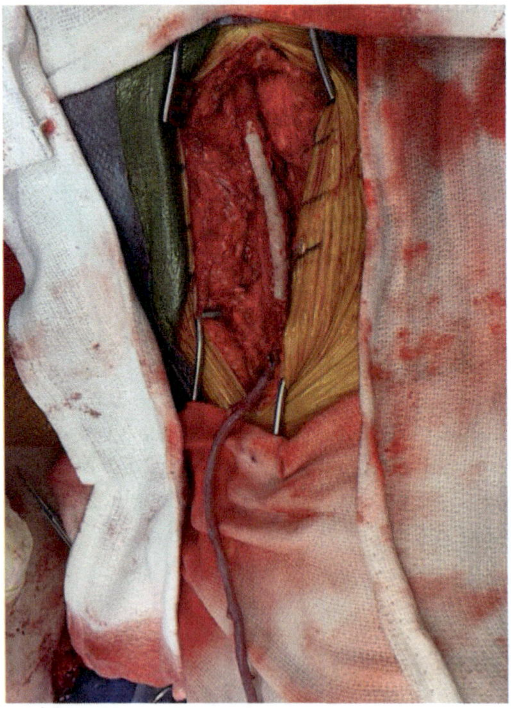

Fig. 44.7 Translocated non-reversed GSV from the contralateral leg anastomosed proximally to the SFA endarterectomy with the bovine pericardial patch. The valves have been lysed with retrograde valvulotome

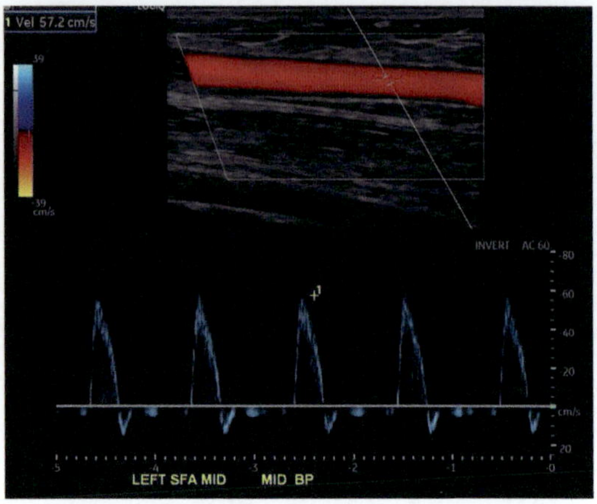

Fig. 44.8 Duplex imaging showing patent left SFA endarterectomy site

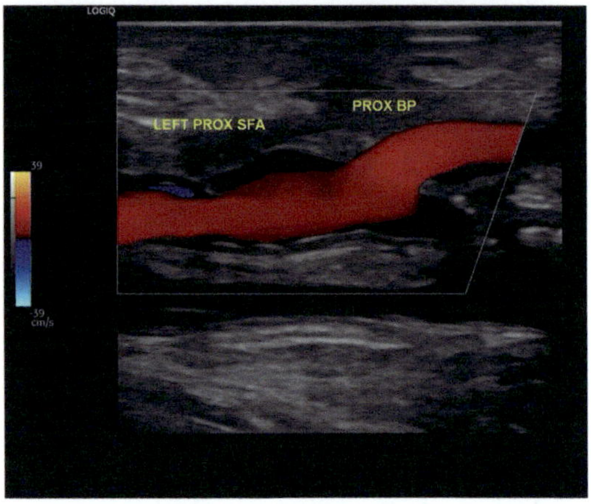

Fig. 44.9 Duplex imaging showing patent proximal segment of the left femoral–popliteal bypass

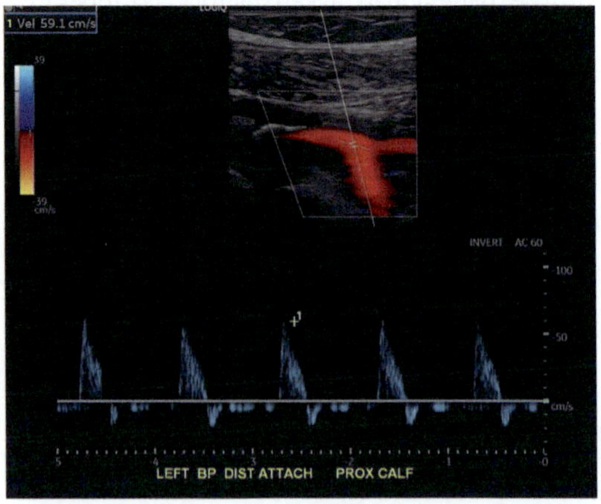

Fig. 44.10 Duplex imaging showing patent distal anastomosis of the left femoral–popliteal bypass with translocated non-reversed GSV

index on the right (0.89), with toe-brachial index (0.64) on the left side, ABI (0.84), and toe-brachial index (0.74).

Discussion

In the absence of a suitable ipsilateral greater saphenous vein (GSV), contralateral GSV is a better option as a conduit for femoral–popliteal bypass. In this patient, the adequate length of the contralateral GSV did not permit its use as a sole conduit for the entire length of the femoral–popliteal bypass. Therefore, a long proximal SFA endarterectomy was performed.

Klinkert et al., conducted a prospective randomized trial of above-knee femoral–popliteal bypass with (75 reversed saphenous vein bypass versus 76 PTFE bypasses) with a minimum follow-up of 5 years. They concluded that GSV had a better patency rate at all intervals and needed fewer reinterventions. If the saphenous vein is absent or not suitable for bypass, PTFE is an acceptable alternative conduit for above-knee femoral–popliteal bypass graft [1].

Madabhushi et al. reported 1051 patients (2003–2019). Of these, 328 had at least one revascularization procedure, and 723 died during their follow-up. They demonstrated that revascularization in patients with intermittent claudication is associated with an increased rate of progression to chronic limb-threatening ischemia and increased amputation rates. The study did not differentiate symptoms of intermittent claudication caused by aortoiliac occlusive disease from femoral–popliteal disease. The patient described in this presentation had a failed left SFA artery stenting performed for the symptoms of intermittent claudication. Thrombosis of the left SFA stent resulted in progression of lower extremity ischemic symptoms. The results of iliac stenting are generally more favorable as compared to interventions for femoral/popliteal disease [2].

Joels et al., reported 276 patients who underwent endovascular interventions for the SFA occlusive disease. Early failure (< 200 days) was noted in 24 limbs in 23 patients, resulting in only one major amputation (0.4%). Early failure altered the distal target in 30% of patients if open bypass is subsequently planned [3].

The incidence of wound complications (wound dehiscence, superficial/deep SSI) following lower extremity revascularization in the Veterans Affairs Surgical Quality Improvement Program national dataset from 2005 to 2021 identified 22,114 patients. The wound complication occurred in 1425 patients (9.7%). Predictors

Table 44.2 Wound risks for each risk class in the derivation and validation data sets [4]

Risk groups	Derivation set %	OR	Validation set %	OR
Low risk (0–3)	4.5	Ref	4.5	Ref
Moderate risk (4–7)	8.5	1.9	8.4	1.5
High risk (8–11)	13.8	3.0	13.9	2.5
Very high risk (>12)	23.8	5.2	24.3	4.4

OR Odds ratio. (Permission to use Table granted from Elsevier publishing, license 6170270080459)

Table 44.1 Multivariable predictor of wound complications and risk score calculation in the derivation data set [4]

	B coefficient	Integer score	OR	95%	CI
BMI (>35 kg/m^2)	0.69	4	1.99	1.68	2.36
Non-Hispanic white (vs others)	0.39	2	1.48	1.30	1.69
Endarterectomy with bypass	0.29	2	1.34	1.14	1.57
Absence of CAD	0.24	1	1.27	1.03	1.57
Age (≤73 years)	0.23	1	1.25	1.08	1.46
Diabetes	0.21	1	1.23	1.10	1.37
Operation length (≥6 h)	0.18	1	1.20	1.05	1.37
WBC (>9900/mm^3)	0.17	1	1.18	1.03	1.35

BMI Body mass index, *CAD* coronary artery disease, *CI* confidence interval, *OR* odds ratio, *WBC* white blood cells. (Permission to use Table granted from Elsevier publishing, license 6,170,270,080,459)

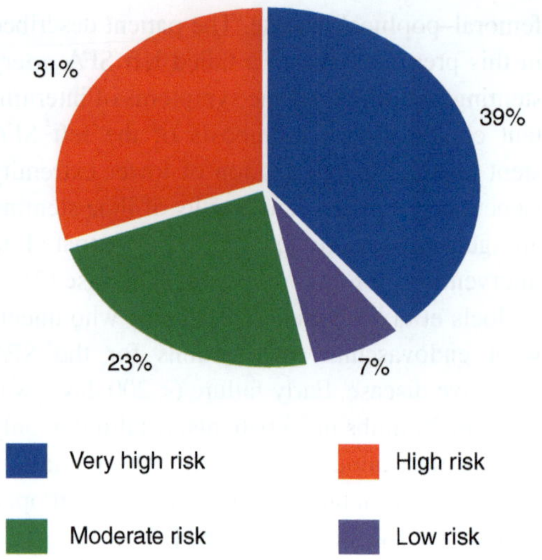

Fig. 44.11 Wound complication rates

of wound complications are recorded in Tables 44.1, 44.2 and (Fig. 44.11).

Among the defined categories in the derivation set, wound complications 4.5% for low risk patients, 8.5% for moderate risk patients, 13.8% for high risk patients, with similar results for the internal validation data set.

Operative indication did not independently predict wound complication. Patients with wound complications had higher rates of reoperation and graft failure [4]. In the patient described in this chapter, the combined procedure of SFA endarterectomy and bypass increased the risk of wound complications.

Multiple Choice Questions

1. A 70-year-old woman, obese, and with type II DM, had a non-healing ulcer on the left leg. She had failed left SFA stent performed for a 16 cm long occlusion of the left SFA a few months earlier. She has diffuse SFA stenosis in the proximal 10 cm segment, occlusion of the distal SFA, with reconstruction of the popliteal artery above the knee with runoff via the peroneal artery and arterial tibial artery with mid-segment stenosis. Duplex arterial imaging showed an incomplete plantar arch. The next best option is:
   A. Left femoral–popliteal endarterectomy
   B. Left femoral–above-knee popliteal bypass using PTFE graft
   C. Left femoral–above-knee popliteal bypass using GSV
   D. Left femoral–infra popliteal bypass using PTFE graft
2. The incidence of wound complications following femoral–popliteal bypass is:
   A. 9–10%
   B. 10–11%
   C. 11–12%
   D. 12–14%
3. The wound complications in patients following femoral–popliteal bypass is associated with:
   A. Higher rates of reoperation
   B. Higher rates of graft failure
   C. Higher rates of reoperation and graft failure
   D. Wound complications have no relationship to graft failure or reoperation

Answers: 1(C), 2(A), 3(C)

References

1. Klinkert P, Schepers A, Burger DH, van Bockel JH, Breslau PJ. Vein versus polytetrafluoroethylene in above-knee femoropopliteal bypass grafting: five-year results of a randomized controlled trial. J Vasc Surg. 2003;37(1):149–55. PMID:12514593
2. Madabhushi V, Davenport D, Jones S, Khoudoud SA, Orr N, et al. Revascularization of intermittent claudicants leads to more chronic limb-threatening ischemia and higher amputation rates. J Vasc Surg. 2021;74(3):771–9. PMID:33775749
3. Joels CS, York JW, Kalbaugh CA, Cull DL, Langan EM 3rd, Taylor SM. Surgical implications of early failed endovascular intervention of the superficial femoral artery. J Vasc Surg. 2008;47(3):562–5. PMID:18295107
4. Xu K, Lin B, Collado L, Martin MC, Carlson SJ, et al. Predicting wound complications following lower extremity revascularization. J Vasc Surg. 2024;79(3):642–650.e642. PMID:37984755

45 Exposed Autologous Femoral–Popliteal Vein Bypass Graft in a Patient with Intraoperative Coagulopathy

Presentation

An 80-year-old woman was admitted to the hospital with severe ischemic rest pain in the right foot with gangrenous skin necrosis on the medial side of the ankle just below the medial malleolus, extending to the heel area (3 × 3 cm) in Dec 2024 (Fig. 45.1). She had a history of hypertension and hyperlipidemia. She was a current smoker with a history of smoking 70 pack years. A doppler arterial evaluation showed an ABI: (0.31 right) and the toe brachial index (0), ABI (0.40 left) and the toe brachial index 0. She had undergone a crossover femoral–femoral graft using an 8-mm Fusion Bioline vascular graft in April 2023 at an outside hospital for left common and external iliac artery occlusion, and bilateral common femoral, superficial femoral, and infrapopliteal arteries showed multifocal stenotic disease. CT angiography and runoff at this admission showed a patent crossover femoral–femoral graft with stenosis of the left common femoral and left superficial femoral artery, and diffuse disease in the infrapopliteal arteries. There was extensive multifocal high-grade stenosis involving the right superficial femoral artery with occlusion of the proximal popliteal artery. Runoff was primarily via the peroneal artery on the right. Lab data—hemoglobin 11.2, hematocrit 35.9, white blood cell count 6200/ml, BUN 14, and creatinine 0.8 mg/dL. Venous mapping showed an adequate

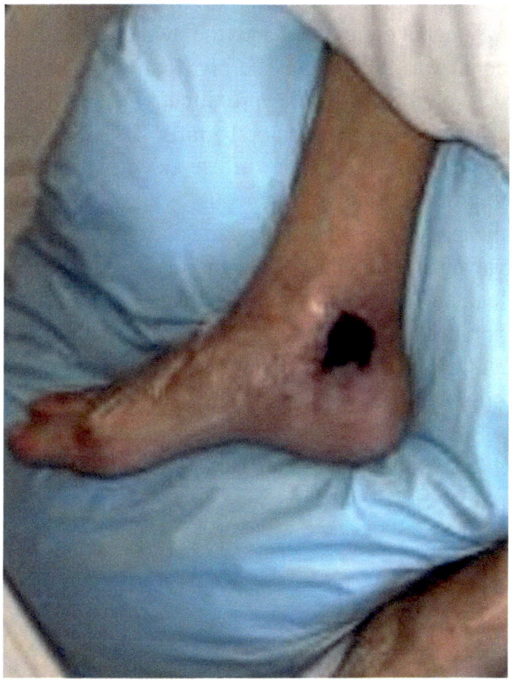

Fig. 45.1 Gangrenous necrosis of the right medial heel area

great saphenous vein (GSV) in the right lower extremity. Triple-phase bone scan showed cellulitis with no evidence of osteomyelitis in the right heel area.

In Dec 2024, the patient underwent abdominal and lower extremity arteriography using a left

S. S. Hans, *Secondary and Tertiary Arterial Reconstructions*,
https://doi.org/10.1007/978-3-032-21214-6_45

brachial artery ultrasound-guided access, which showed a patent crossover femoral–femoral graft. Right superficial femoral artery occlusion at its origin, reconstitution of the popliteal artery above the knee, and runoff primarily with the peroneal artery with a patent tibioperoneal trunk and reconstitution of the distal anterior tibial artery proximal to the ankle via collaterals. There was evidence of left superficial femoral artery occlusion (Figs. 45.2, 45.3, and 45.4).

Following cardiac risk assessment, she underwent right femoral–popliteal artery below-knee bypass in January 2025, using translocated non-reversed GSV. Her preoperative hemoglobin was 8.8, hematocrit 25.3, and the white blood cell count was 9800/mL^3. The proximal anastomosis was performed to the proximal portion of the crossover femoral–femoral graft. The GSV was friable, and there was diffuse oozing from the thigh edges and subcutaneous tissues. Following the passage of the retrograde valvulotome, the valve leaflets in the GSV were rendered incompetent, and a pulsatile flow was obtained. The distal popliteal artery was exposed after dividing the tendons of the pes anserinus and taking down the origin of the soleus muscle from the soleal line.

During the arterial reconstruction, the patient was hypotensive (mean BP 50–55 mmHg) and was treated with vasopressors and fluid resuscitation in the operating room. Two units of packed red cells were given intraoperatively.

In the Intensive Care Unit, the patient developed non-pulsatile swelling of the right upper thigh due to the hematoma. Coagulation profile revealed INR 1.8 and PTT > 100 s; two units of fresh frozen plasma were administered. There was no evidence of active bleeding. The antibiotics were changed from preoperative Ampicillin sodium/Sulbactam sodium to Vancomycin and Zosyn. The patient had spontaneous drainage of the hematoma, with drainage of the old blood. On January 24, 2025, her incision spontaneously opened for a dehiscence of

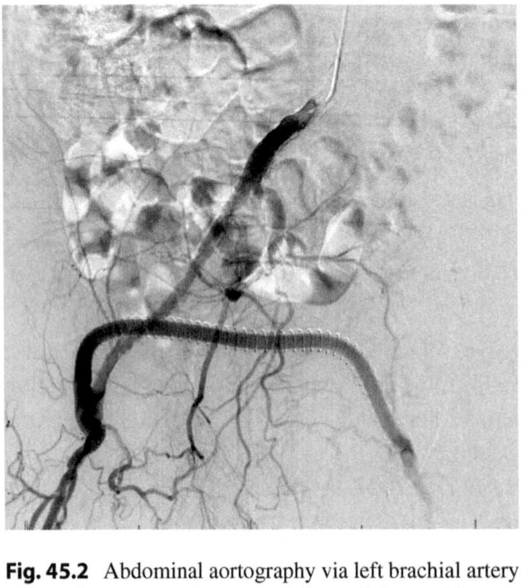

Fig. 45.2 Abdominal aortography via left brachial artery access shows a patent crossover femoral–femoral bypass graft

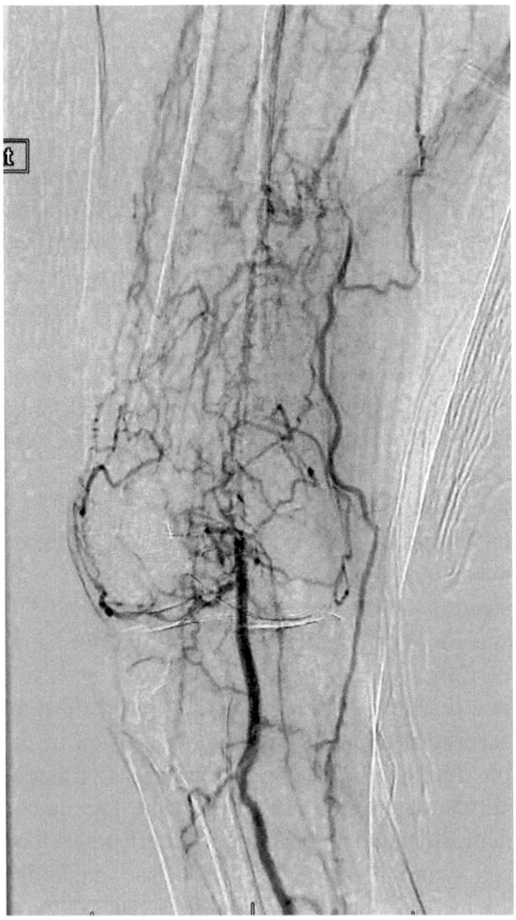

Fig. 45.3 Occlusion of the right superficial femoral artery and reconstitution of the popliteal artery just above the knee

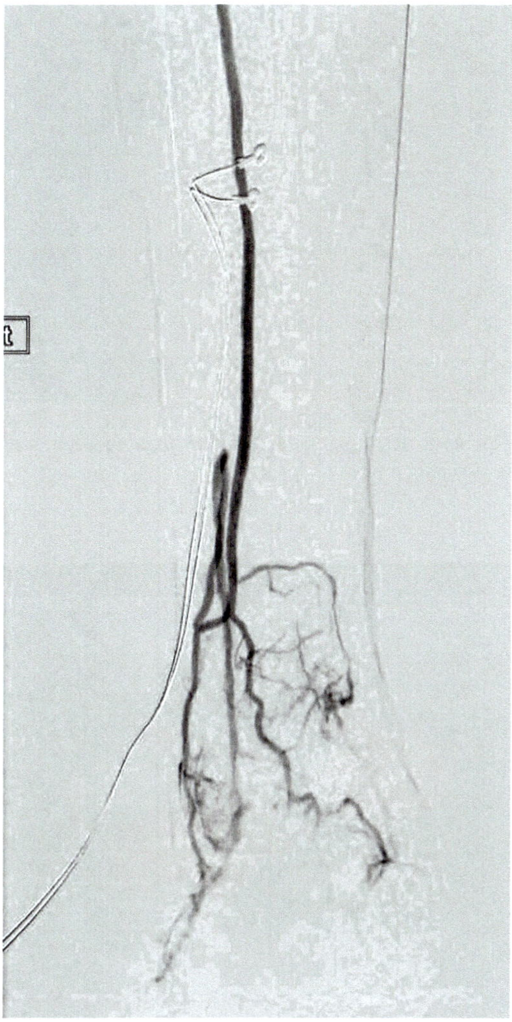

Fig. 45.4 Runoff with the peroneal artery

2.5 cm with drainage of old blood and exposed vein bypass graft (Figs. 45.5, 45.6, and 45.7). The wound culture of the upper thigh was positive for Staphylococcus coagulase, rare Streptococcus, moderate Candida albicans, and a few Klebsiella pneumoniae. She had diarrhea caused by C. difficile infection and started on oral vancomycin and IV cefepime. The thigh incision started to show healing with local wound care and eventually healed by secondary intention (Fig. 45.8). A follow-up of noninvasive arterial testing in April 2025 showed an ABI of 1.0 (right) and the brachial index 0.70 (right), ABI 0.69 (left), and toe brachial index 0.41 (left).

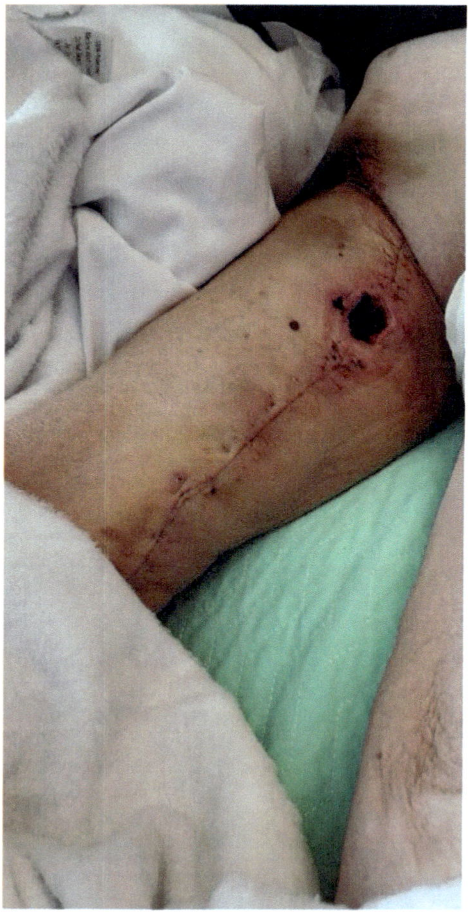

Fig. 45.5 Four weeks following right femoral popliteal bypass, with breakdown of the skin in the upper thigh, with an old blood clot at the base of the ulcer

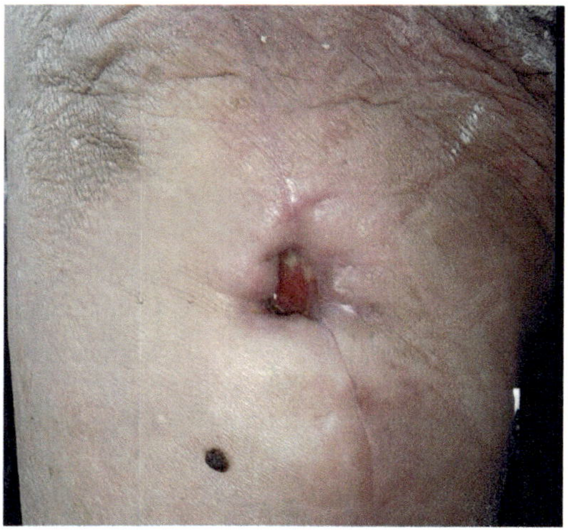

Fig. 45.6 Granulating wound right upper thigh

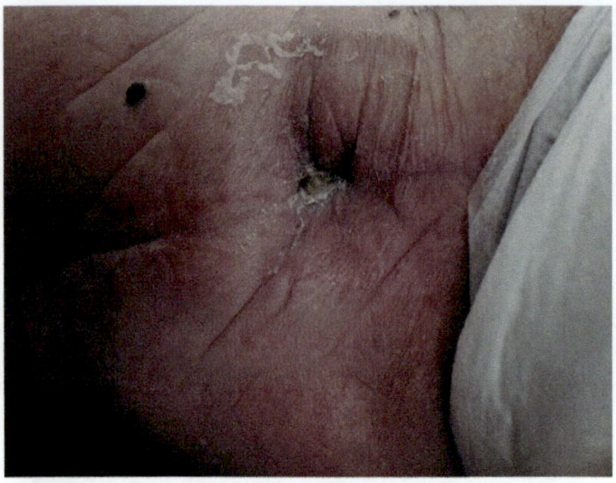

Fig. 45.7 Healing with secondary intention

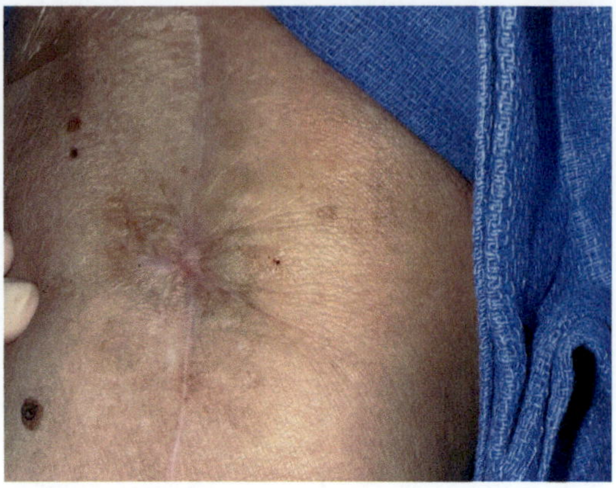

Fig. 45.8 Right groin and upper thigh incision well healed after 8 weeks

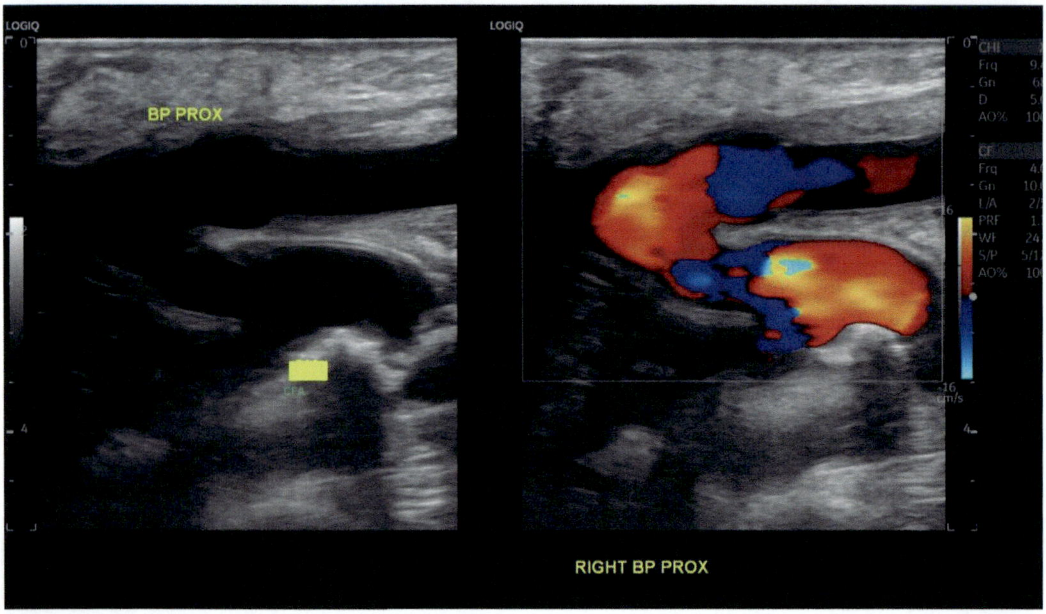

Fig. 45.9 Duplex imaging showing proximal anastomosis and a 4–5 cm segment of popliteal bypass

The skin necrosis in the right heel healed, and her ischemic rest pain resolved. Eight months after the bypass, follow-up duplex mapping showed increased velocity and probable stenosis in the femoral–popliteal bypass just above the knee area (Figs. 45.9 and 45.10). The patient underwent a right femoral arteriogram using antegrade access. Arteriogram showed approximately 20–30% stenosis in the distal portion of the graft with peroneal artery runoff (Figs. 45.11, 45.12, 45.13, and 45.14). The patient did not undergo any intervention and will be followed

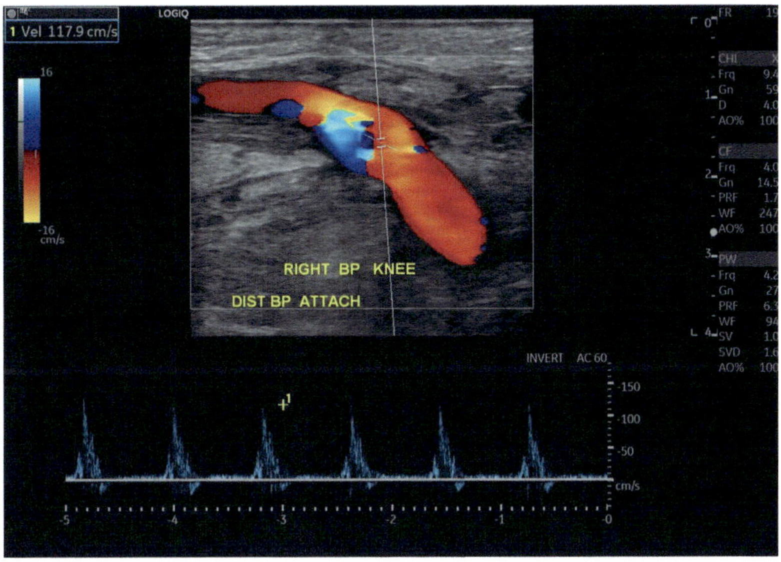

Fig. 45.10 Duplex imaging showing increased velocities in the bypass at the level of the knee

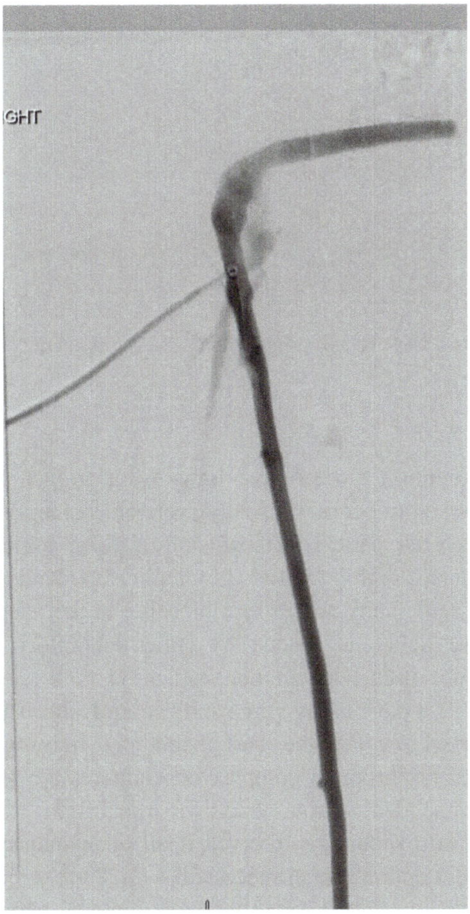

Fig. 45.11 Antegrade right femoral arteriogram shows a patent proximal segment of the crossover femoral–femoral graft and proximal and mid right femoral arterial bypass

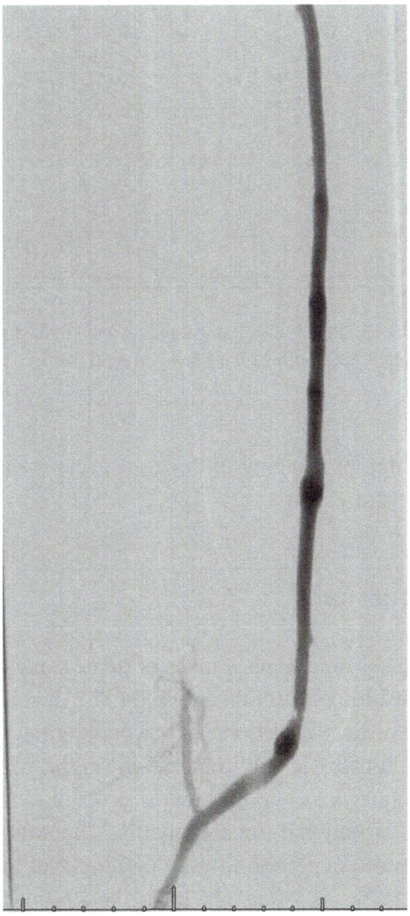

Fig. 45.12 Showing approximately 20–30% stenosis in the distal portion of the femoral–popliteal bypass

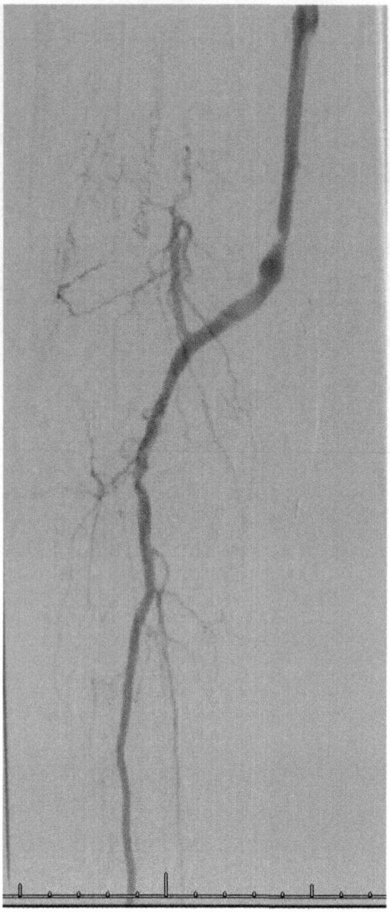

Fig. 45.13 Patent distal anastomosis and small diameter popliteal artery with patent tibio-peroneal trunk

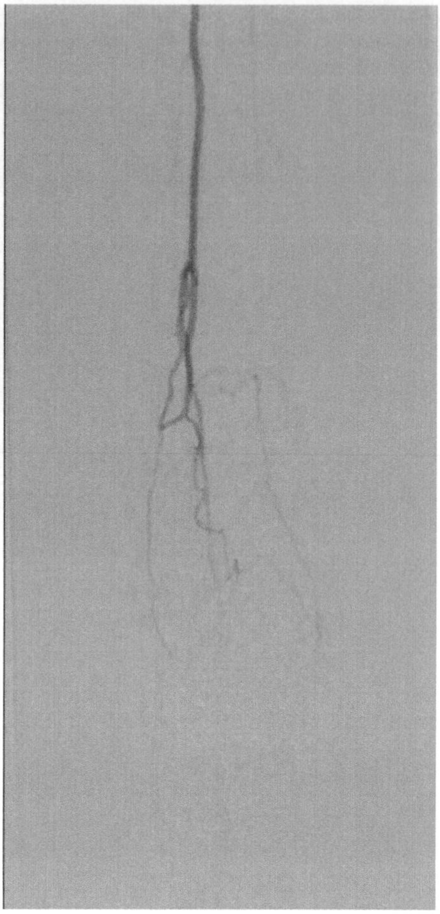

Fig. 45.14 Runoff primarily with the peroneal artery

with duplex imaging of the graft every 3 months for 1 year.

Discussion

Diagnosis and management of acute coagulopathy resulting in significant blood loss during vascular revascularization can be challenging. Acute coagulopathy is multifactorial in origin, with tissue injury and hypotension as precipitating factors. Dilutional coagulopathy, hypothermia, acidemia, hyperfibrinolysis, systemic inflammatory response often results in self-propagating chain of events. The problem is compounded by heparin administration during vascular reconstruction. A restrictive transfusion trigger for packed red cells is usually preferable except for high-risk patients. Transfusion of blood components should be initiated by clinical evidence of coagulopathy and diffuse bleeding in the operative field and guided by either laboratory or point-of-care coagulation studies [1].

If a patient has massive bleeding from major vessel trauma in the chest or abdomen, fibrinogen and prothrombin complex concentrates are recommended during massive transfusion, and rFVIIa should be reserved if all other management options are unsuccessful.

Kim et al. reported femoral–popliteal bypass graft infection (BGI) in 34 patients (2.6%) out of 1315 femoral–popliteal bypasses from 1995 to

2000 [2]. More commonly isolated pathogens were Staphylococcus aureus (55.9%) and polymicrobial cultures (14.7%). Patients with BGI were more frequently complicated by postoperative hematoma, superficial wound infection, lymphocele/lymphorrhea, and use of prosthetic grafts (76.5%) of all graft infections (26/34). Reoperation for BGI involved incision and drainage (n7; 20.6%), graft excision without reconstruction (n12; 35.3%), graft excision with in-line reconstruction (n11; 32.4%), and graft excision with extra-anatomic reconstruction (n2; 5.9%). Nine patients with BGI (26.5%) ultimately required major amputation. Postoperative hematoma and 30-day readmission were independent risk factors associated with BGI. One-year amputation-free survival was 50% (95% CI: 31.9–65.7%) after BGI.

For arteriography in the presence of a cross-over femoral-femoral graft, antegrade femoral artery access via the ipsilateral limb enables intervention of more distal occlusive lesions. This approach is best indicated for use in patients with iliac artery tortuosity, severely diseased aortic bifurcation, prior aorto-femoral graft, or endograft [3]. The safety of antegrade femoral access has been well demonstrated from a large vascular quality initiative study. Results show that the incidence of overall hematoma requiring intervention for arterial occlusive disease was similar with both retrograde and antegrade femoral access [4].

Multiple Choice Questions

1. The best management option for patients with suspected coagulopathy before the results of the coagulation study are available is.
   A. Administration of rFVIIa
   B. Administration of packed cells
   C. Administration of fibrinogen and platelets
   D. Administration of packed red cells and FF plasma
2. The incidence of graft infection following femoral-popliteal bypass is:
   A. 5%
   B. 4.6%
   C. 3.6%
   D. 2.6%.
3. The important factors associated with bypass graft infection are:
   A. Prolonged operation (>6 h)
   B. Postoperative hematoma
   C. 30-day readmission
   D. Postoperative hematoma and 30-day readmission

Answers: 1(D), 2(D), 3(D)

References

1. Chee YE, Liu SE, Irwin MG. Management of bleeding in vascular surgery. Br J Anaesth. 2016;117 Suppl 2:ii85-ii94. PMID:27566811
2. Kim Y, DeCarlo C, Jessula S, Latz CA, Chou EL, et al. Risk factors and consequences of graft infection after femoropopliteal bypass: a 25-year experience. J Vasc Surg. 2022;76(1):248–54. PMID:35276264
3. Wheatley BJ, Mansour MA, Grossman PM, Munir K, Cali RF, et al. Complication rates for percutaneous lower extremity arterial antegrade access. Arch Surg. 2011;146(4):432–5. PMID:21502451
4. Siracuse JJ, Farber A, Cheng TW, Raulli SJ, Jones, et al. Common femoral artery antegrade and retrograde approaches have similar access site complications. J Vasc Surg. 2019;69(4):1160–1166.e1162. PMID:30527937

46 Coil Embolization of a Side Branch Fistula Following Femoral Dorsalis Pedis In Situ Bypass

Presentation

A 71-year-old man was seen in the vascular clinic with dry gangrene of the left big toe of 3 weeks' duration (Fig. 46.1). Medical comorbidities included type II diabetes mellitus, hypertension, hyperlipidemia, and peripheral neuropathy. He is a current smoker with a history of about 60 pack years. Doppler arterial evaluation of the lower extremities showed severe left lower extremity disease at the iliac, left superficial femoral, and infra-popliteal level. Superficial femoral and infra-popliteal level with ABI on right (0.67) and left (0.24) with toe brachial index on right (0.97) and left (0).

He underwent abdominal aortogram and pelvic arteriogram with study of lower extremities in July 2024 using ultrasound-guided right femoral access. The findings were slight aneurysmal dilatation of the common iliac artery (CIA) with severe stenosis in the distal-most segment of the CIA, just proximal to the origin of the hypogastric artery, which was occluded, and stenosis extended into the proximal left external iliac artery. There were 70% stenosis of the common iliac artery and 60% stenosis of the right external iliac artery. Left common femoral artery showed 50% stenosis, left superficial mid-segment occlusion with reconstitution of a diseased popliteal artery above the knee (Fig. 46.2). Distal popliteal artery showed multiple areas of stenosis with atherosclerotic plaque and irregularities of the tibioperoneal trunk and run off primarily with the peroneal artery and reconstitution of distal anterior tibial and dorsalis pedis artery with incomplete plantar arch. Using a 6F Pinnacle sheath from the right femoral access, advanced into the mid left common iliac artery. An 8 mm × 59 mm VBX stent was deployed in the left distal common and proximal external iliac artery, followed by deployment of an 8 × 39 VBX stent for the right common iliac stenosis and a self-expanding 8 × 10 mm smart stent in the right external iliac artery (Figs. 46.3, 46.4, 46.5, and 46.6).

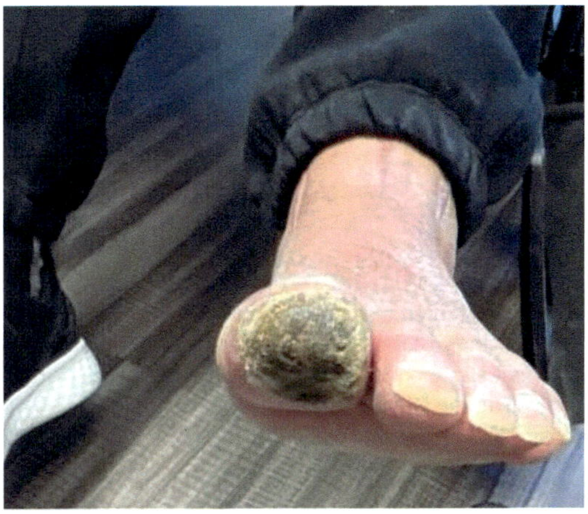

Fig. 46.1 Gangrene of left big toe

S. S. Hans, *Secondary and Tertiary Arterial Reconstructions*,
https://doi.org/10.1007/978-3-032-21214-6_46

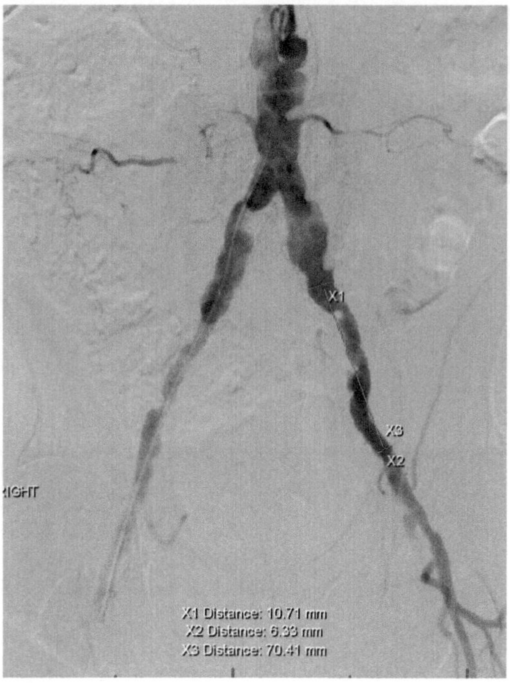

Fig. 46.2 Abdominal aortogram showing marked irregularity of the distal abdominal aorta and 50% stenosis of the right common iliac artery and multiple areas of mild stenosis in the left common iliac artery

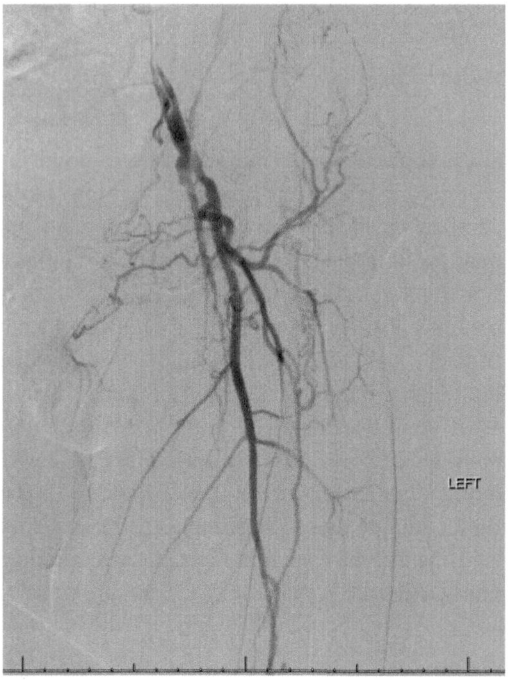

Fig. 46.3 Arteriography showing left superficial artery occlusion

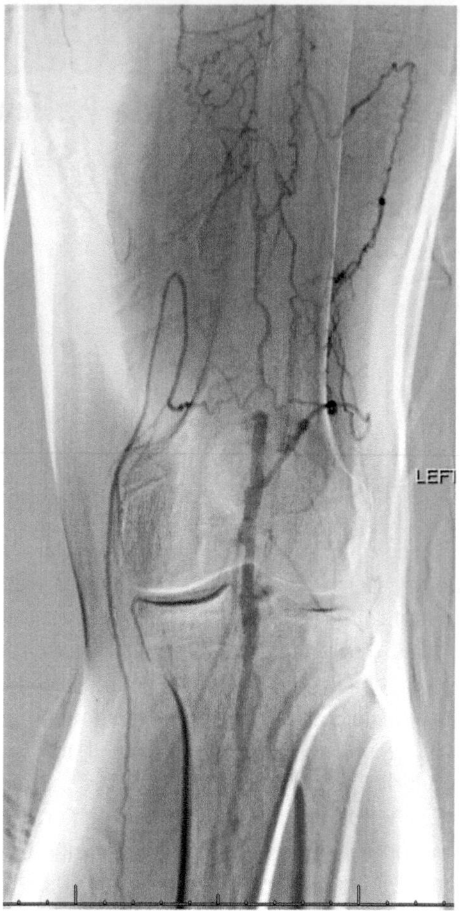

Fig. 46.4 Reconstitution of a severe diseased left popliteal artery with near occlusion of the tibio-peroneal trunk

In August 2024, the patient underwent distal common and proximal superficial femoral endarterectomy and left femoral to dorsalis pedis bypass using skip incisions with exposure of the entire GSV. A retrograde valvulotome was advanced proximally to lyse the valve leaflets to obtain pulsatile flow and route the bypass in the subcutaneous tunnel just above the medial malleolus and anastomosed to the dorsalis pedis artery with 7″ 0″ cardiovascular polypropylene suture. On attempted closure of the dorsal skin, there was tension; therefore, a 4-cm long relaxing incision was made longitudinally anterior and medial to the lateral malleolus.

He had a satisfactory revascularization with significantly improved vascularity to the left big toe. At follow-up, duplex imaging of the graft

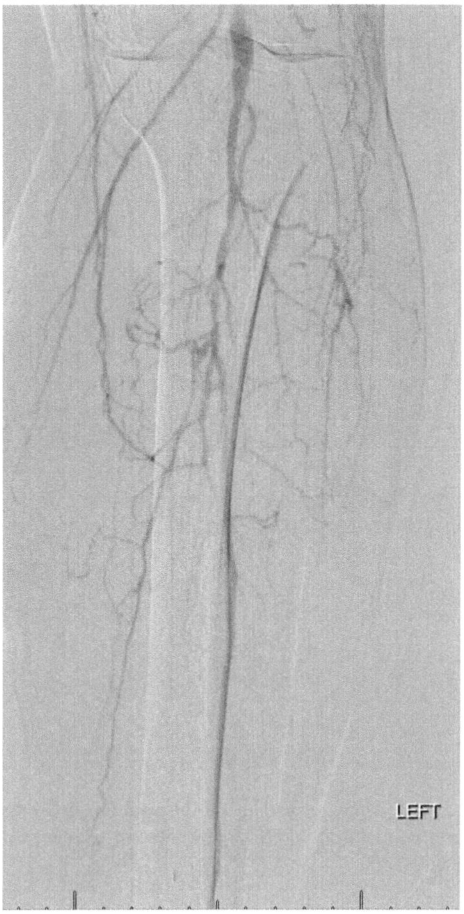

Fig. 46.5 Arteriography showing severe infrapopliteal artery disease

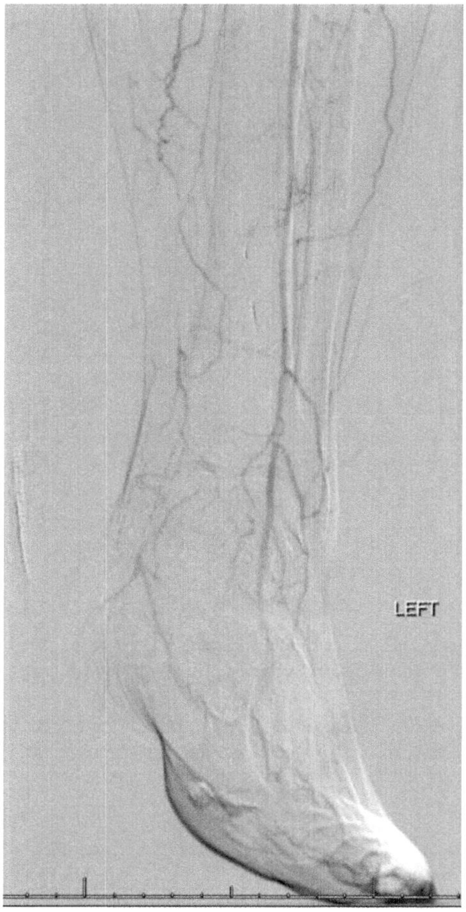

Fig. 46.6 Runoff primarily with diseased anterior tibial artery and Dorsalis pedis artery with incomplete plantar arch

showed increased peak systolic velocity, indicating 70% stenosis at the junction in the mid third of the in situ bypass. Sequential pressures and ABI showed ABI 0.60 (right) and 0.65 (left). The patient was taken to the interventional radiology suite on December 4, 2024, for arteriography. Using ultrasound-guided right femoral artery access and placing the catheter in the proximal left common femoral artery showed 30% stenosis in the proximal segment of the in situ graft and a large AV fistula from the side branch with early filling of the femoral vein (Figs. 46.7, 46.8, 46.9, 46.10, and 46.11). Using a 2.4F microcatheter, via a 5F Kumpe catheter advanced through a 6F, 45 cm Pinnacle sheath with its tip in the distal left external iliac artery, a side branch from the in situ bypass was filling the deep vein (measuring 3 mm in diameter) contributing to significant fistula flow was detected, and micro coil embolization was performed. Another descending branch was cannulated by a microcatheter, and coil embolization was performed, leading to the absence of flow in the fistula (Fig. 46.12). A follow-up duplex imaging of the graft in April 2025 showed 50% stenosis of the proximal segment of the in situ bypass. Ankle brachial index (right) 0.60 (left) 0.65. The gangrenous skin of the left big toe healed by June 2025 (Fig. 46.13).

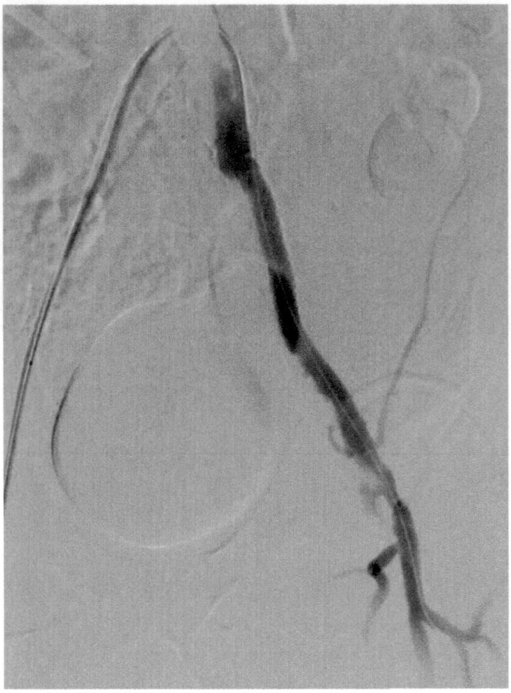

Fig. 46.7 Follow-up aortogram and left lower extremity arteriogram with catheter tip in the left external iliac artery

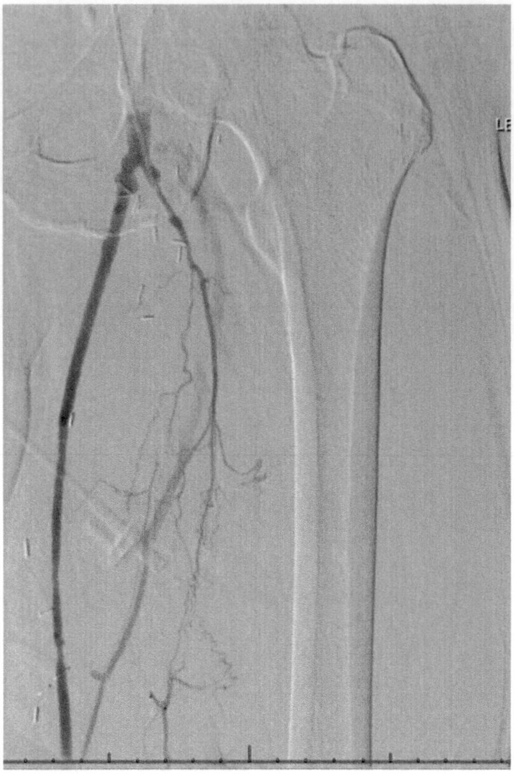

Fig. 46.8 Showing patent left femoral dorsalis pedis in situ bypass with mild stenosis at the mid segment of the bypass

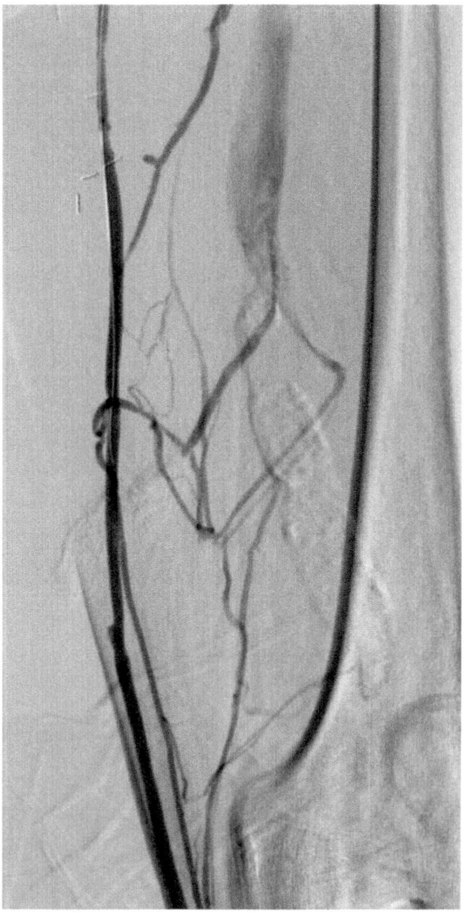

Fig. 46.9 Side branch fistula from the midsegment of the in situ bypass with early filling of the femoral vein

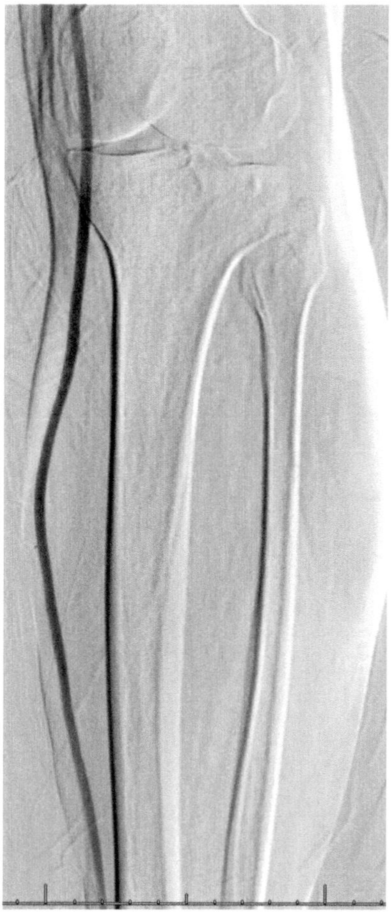

Fig. 46.10 Patent in situ bypass at the level of the knee and upper and mid calf

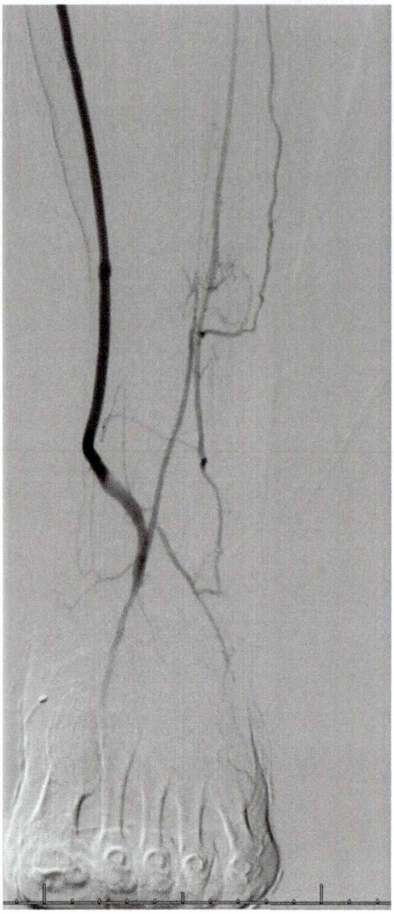

Fig. 46.11 Patent distal bypass to the dorsalis pedis artery

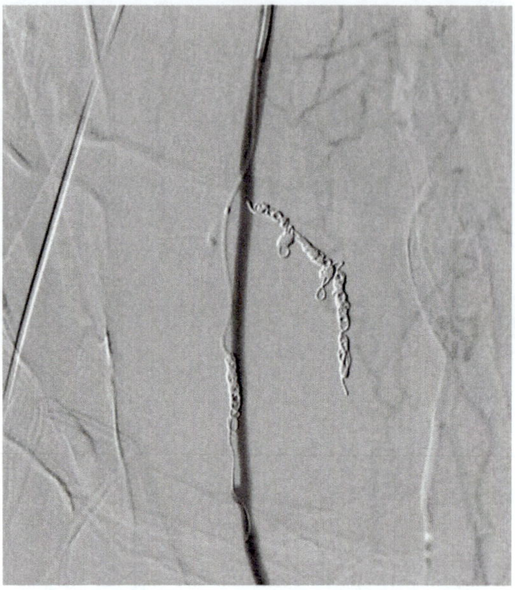

Fig. 46.12 Successful coil embolization of the side-branch fistula using a microcatheter

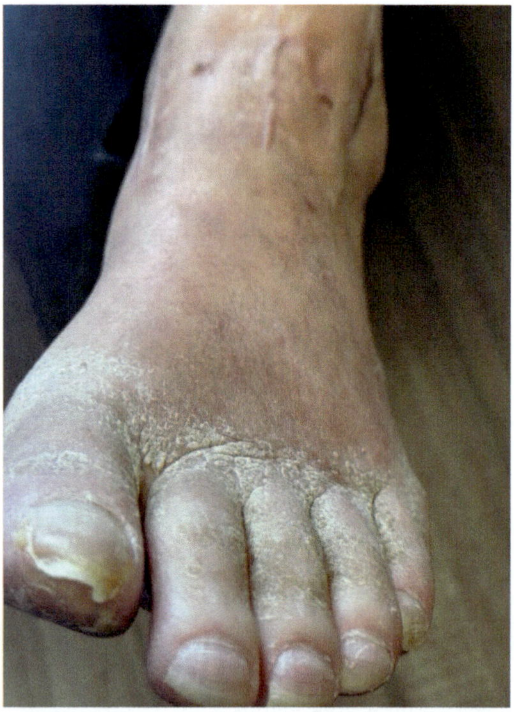

Fig. 46.13 Healing of the gangrene of the left big toe. Two healed scars—one at the dorsum of the left ankle, at the distal anastomotic site and second at the site of the relaxation incision in front of the lateral malleolous

Discussion

Missed saphenous vein tributaries function as arteriovenous fistula following in situ arterial reconstruction of the lower extremity. Many small side branch fistulas that are not filling the deep veins will spontaneously close. Localized edema, cellulitis, skin necrosis, diminished distal arterial flow resulting in graft thrombosis are known complications of retained side branch fistula following in situ bypass. Donaldson et al. reported 455 in situ saphenous vein grafts and reported primary failure in 92 (20%) of the grafts, with perianastomotic stenosis, vein stricture, vein stenosis, and valvulotome injury being the predominant causes. Side-branch fistula was the cause of primary failure in two patients (2.3%) [1]. Rupture of an arterio-venous fistula after in situ has also been reported in the literature [2].

Adjunctive Doppler insonation and intraoperative arteriography are helpful in diagnosing retained side-branch fistulas during in situ bypass reconstruction. O'Donnell et al. have reported on a simplified technique for saphenous vein side branch occlusion during 12 bypass procedures with insertion of a 5F sheath passed into the proximal side branch of the GSV after completing the proximal anastomosis [3]. Prograde flow is established into the bypass, and retrograde valvulotomy is performed. An initial angiogram is obtained. The branches of the GSV are coiled through the proximal sheath, and the distal vein is clamped with a micro bulldog clamp, and flow continues through the fistula. The side branches are identified and selected with a 0.035 angled hydrophilic wire, followed by a hydrophilic angled catheter. A 3 mm, 4 mm, or 5 mm stainless steel Gianturco coil is loaded into the side branch. Coiling was done for side branches larger than 1–2 mm. At follow-up, side-branch fistulas with filling of the deep venous system should be occluded by coil embolization. Successful angioplasty with a drug-eluting balloon for a significant stenosis inferior to an arteriovenous fistula (AVF) connected to a deep venous system has been reported [4]. An ultrasound-guided fistula embolization with cyanoacrylate Glubran has also been reported [2, 4]. Smaller side branch fistulas without filling of the deep venous system usually do not pose a threat to the patency of the bypass and may spontaneously thrombose.

Open ligation of a side-branch AV fistula following in situ bypass is rarely necessary in contemporary vascular practice.

Multiple Choice Questions

1. Retained AV fistula resulting in primary failure of lower extremity in situ bypass occurs in:
   A. 1% of patients
   B. 2–2.5% of patients
   C. 3% of patients
   D. 31–35% of patients
2. The filling deep venous system following a side branch in situ bypass in the lower extremity should be treated to prevent:
   A. Rupture
   B. Thrombosis of the graft
   C. Congestive heart failure
   D. Cellulitis
3. Optimal management of retained fistula following in situ bypass with filling of the deep veins is:
   A. Surgical ligation
   B. Glue injection into the fistula
   C. Coil embolization by femoral artery access
   D. Coil embolization using brachial artery access

Answers 1(A), 2(B), 3(C)

References

1. Donaldson MC, Mannick JA, Whittemore AD. Causes of primary graft failure after in situ saphenous vein bypass grafting. J Vasc Surg. 1992;15(1):113–8. discussion 118-120. PMID:1728669

2. Wolodiger F, Dardik H, Johnson F, Ibrahim IM. Rupture of arteriovenous fistula after in situ saphenous vein bypass. J Vasc Surg. 1991;13(4):503–5. PMID:2010924
3. O'Donnell SD, Gillespie DL, Starnes BW, Parker MV, Johnson CA, et al. Endovascular assisted in situ bypass grafting: a simplified technique for saphenous vein side branch occlusion. J Vasc Surg. 2003;38(4):856–8. PMID:14560245
4. Bertagna G, Adami D, Del Corso A. Percutaneous glue embolization of arteriovenous fistula of in situ saphenous vein bypass graft: case report and literature review. Vascular. 2022;30(4):759–63. PMID: 34233127

Superficial Femoral Artery–Posterior Tibial Artery Bypass for Popliteal Artery Stent Thrombosis

47

Presentation

A 67-year-old man was seen in the emergency room for evaluation of a painful left foot and paresthesia in the left foot for the past 48 h. In June 2025, Doppler arterial evaluation revealed an ABI on the right (1.0), left (0.67); toe brachial index (right 0.90), left (0.36). Medical comorbidities included hypertension, hyperlipidemia, gout, and chronic obstructive pulmonary disease (COPD). Past surgical history included craniotomy (2003) and removal of metastatic lung cancer of the brain, right upper lobectomy (2024). The patient was currently on chemotherapy and immunotherapy. He had a history of a popliteal artery stent performed in 2018 for an ischemic ulcer of the left big toe at an outside ambulatory vascular center. He was a former smoker with a history of smoking cigarettes for 60 pack years.

CT angiography of the left lower extremity showed complete occlusion of the left popliteal artery with patent trifurcation of the popliteal artery and occlusion of the popliteal stent. There was occlusion of the mid-anterior tibial artery. The peroneal artery was small in caliber, and the runoff was primarily with the posterior tibial artery.

Abdominal aortography and run-off study using right femoral artery access revealed a pararenal abdominal aortic aneurysm. The left popliteal artery was occluded at its junction with the superficial femoral artery, with reconstitution of the distal-most position of a small-diameter popliteal artery. The runoff was primarily with the posterior tibial artery and the anterior tibial artery (Figs. 47.1, 47.2, 47.3, 47.4, and 47.5). The plantar arch was incomplete.

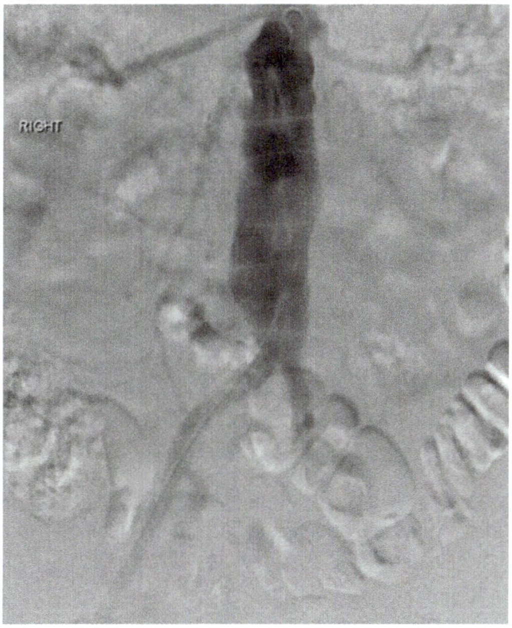

Fig. 47.1 Abdominal aortogram showing abdominal aortic aneurysm on CTA, 5.5 cm pararenal AAA

After cardiac assessment, the patient underwent left mid superficial to mid posterior tibial

S. S. Hans, *Secondary and Tertiary Arterial Reconstructions*,
https://doi.org/10.1007/978-3-032-21214-6_47

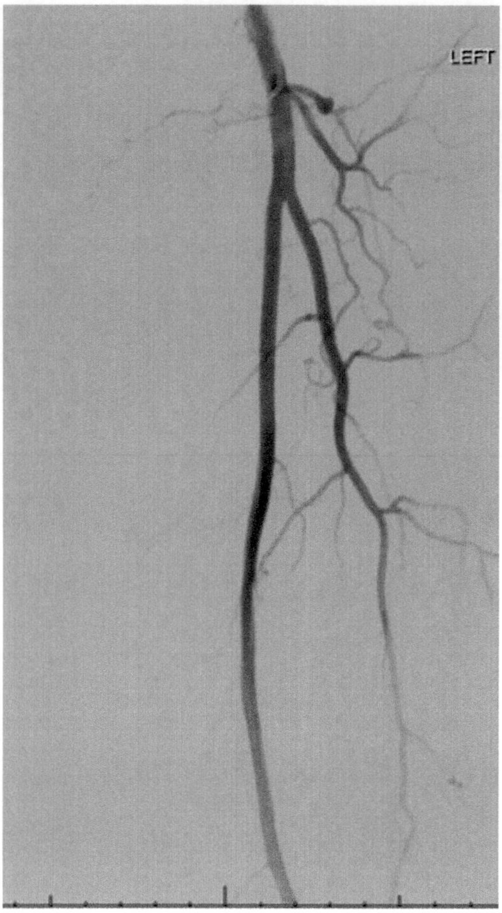

Fig. 47.2 Selective left lower extremity arteriogram showing patent common femoral, Profunda femoris, proximal, and distal superficial femoral artery

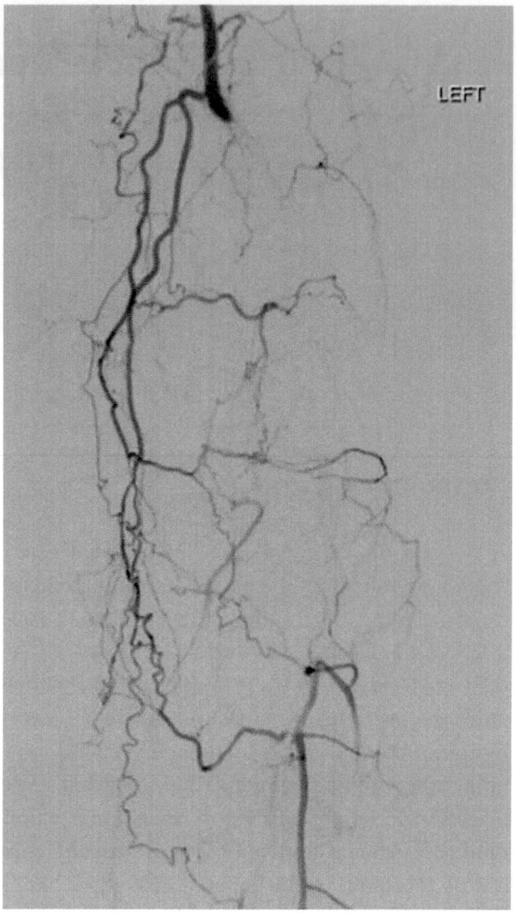

Fig. 47.3 Arteriography showing left popliteal artery occlusion with numerous collaterals

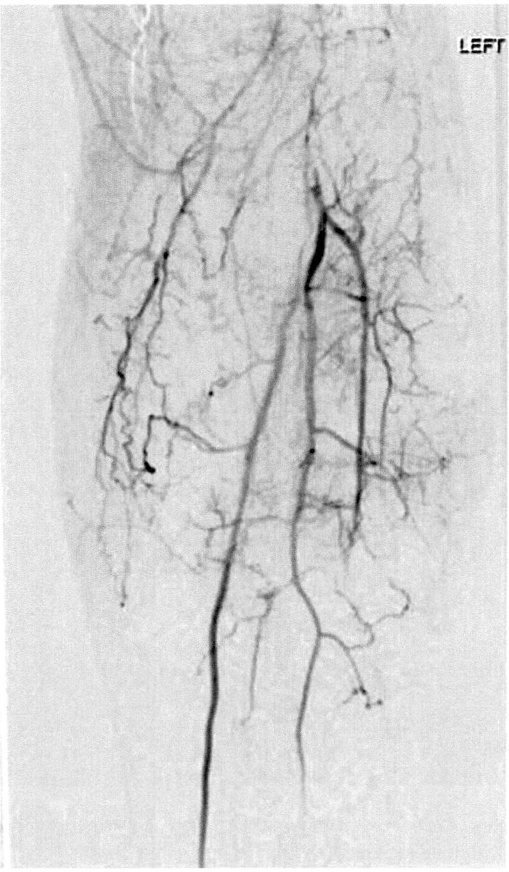

Fig. 47.4 Arteriogram shows distal popliteal artery occlusion with run off via the posterior tibial artery, anterior tibial, and peroneal artery are occluded distally

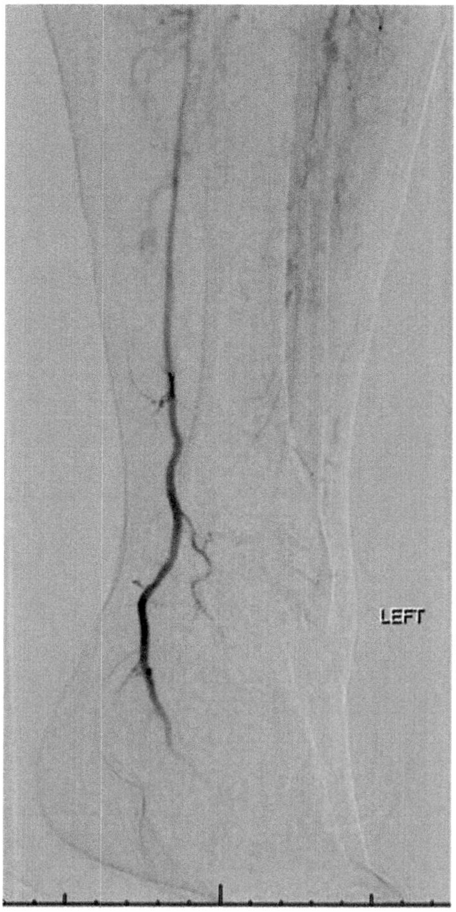

Fig. 47.5 Arteriography showing run off with the posterior tibial artery in its entire length, with an incomplete plantar arch

artery bypass using a non-reversed translocated GSV following vein mapping. The GSV was only 2.5 mm in diameter below the knee. He was discharged on the fifth postoperative day. The patient was seen in the clinic, two weeks following discharge, with cellulitis of the left leg at the incision site with a small amount of serosanguinous drainage. The culture of the groin revealed methicillin-resistant Staphylococcus aureus, which responded to clindamycin. The patient had a follow-up with a non-invasive Doppler arterial study showing patent left femoral–popliteal bypass with ankle-brachial index 1.0 (right) 1.0 (left) and duplex imaging of the graft showing normal flow in the graft. Postoperative CTA showing patent left mid superficial femoral artery to mid posterior tibial bypass (Figs. 47.6, 47.7, and 47.8). Patient had satisfactory healing at the site of incisions (Fig. 47.9). Three months later, the patient under-

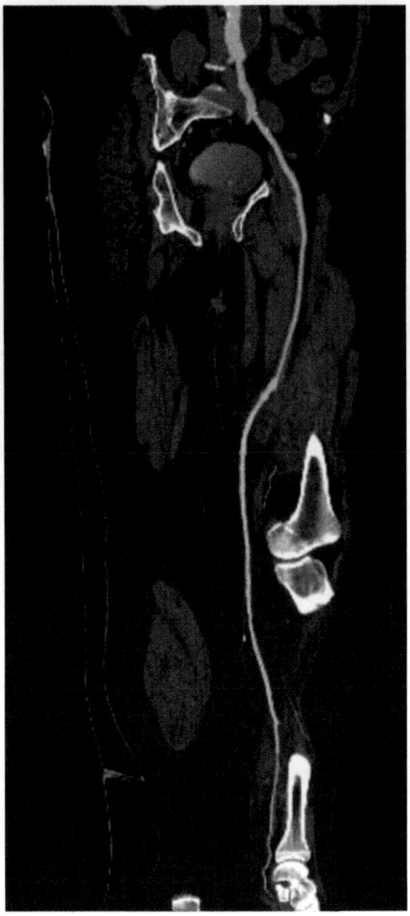

Fig. 47.6 Postoperative CTA showing patent left mid superficial femoral artery-posterior tibial artery bypass with translocated non-reversed GSV

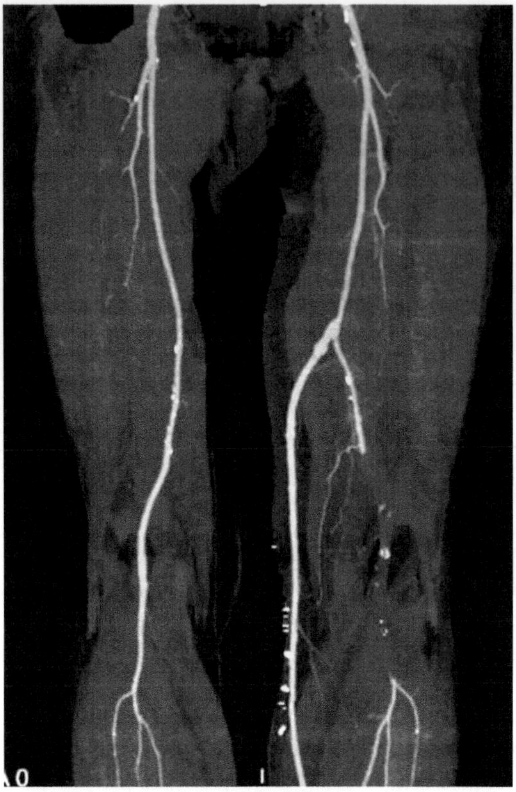

Fig. 47.7 Postoperative CTA showing patent bypass with long-standing popliteal artery occlusion

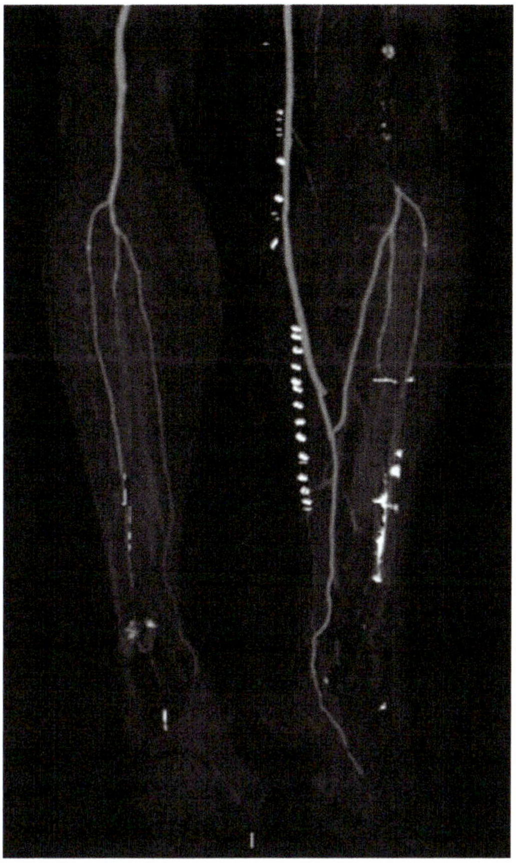

Fig. 47.8 Postoperative CTA showing satisfactory distal anastomosis to mid-posterior tibial artery with satisfactory follow-up of infrapopliteal arteries

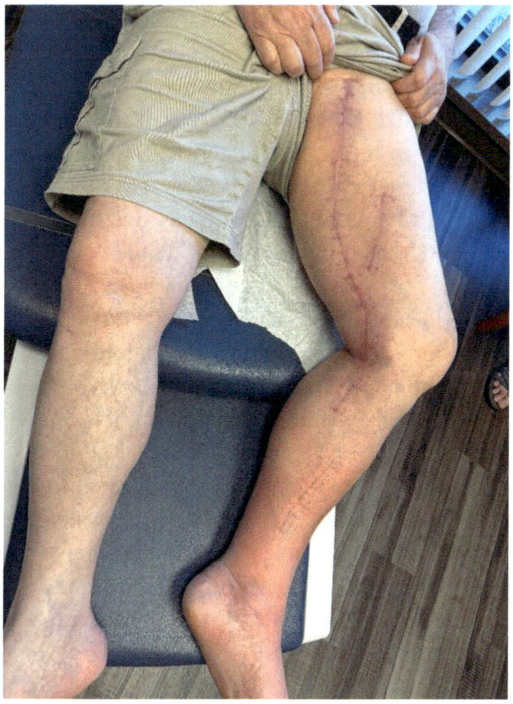

Fig. 47.9 Photograph showing satisfactory healing (scars) from superficial femoral artery to posterior tibial artery bypass graft

went successful Physician Modified Endograft (PMEG) for a 5.5 cm pararenal saccular aortic aneurysm diagnosed by CTA of the abdomen and pelvis.

Discussion

From a systemic review and meta-analysis of MEDLINE, EMBASE, and CENTRAL databases for studies comparing outcomes of primary infrainguinal bypass after a prior failed endovascular intervention for peripheral arterial disease involving 11,886 patients showed no significant difference in 30-day mortality (OR 1.00; 95% CI 0.65–1.54) or 30-day amputation rates (OR 1.26; 95% CI 0.95–1.65), 1 year amputation free survival was higher in the patients who had primary bypass (OR 1.30; 95% CI 1.10–1.52) compared with patients who had bypass after failed endovascular therapy [1]. There was also a worse one-year primary patency (OR 1.65; 95% CI 1.04–2.62) for patients with failed endovascular intervention. The authors noted that because of the observational design of the study, non--uniform patient details and heterogeneity between the studies, the conclusions are somewhat limited [1].

The results of the BASIL-2 trial in 345 patients with critical limb ischemia requiring infrapopliteal revascularization showed that the best endovascular therapy was first associated with a better amputation-free survival strategy (HR = 1.35; 95% CI 1.02–1.80; $p = 0.037$) [2]. This finding is contrary to the results of the BEST-CLI study. The difference in primary outcomes between BEST-CLI and BASIL-2 is likely due to significant differences in the patients' clinical and procedural characteristics [2]. From the Excellence in Peripheral Artery Disease (XLPAD) registry, index procedures resulting in femoropopliteal stent thrombosis were compared to stent procedures. Femoropopliteal stent thrombosis occurred in 26 of 604 patients (4.3%) over a median follow-up of 6 months post-procedure. Stent thrombosis was more likely to occur in men and in patients with chronic significant differences in stent thrombosis between drug-coated and bare metal stents, but the rate of stent thrombosis was significantly higher with self-expanding covered stent grafts compared to bare metal stents. Stent thrombosis was significantly associated with an increased risk of 12-month major adverse limb events [3].

The patient described in this chapter presented with a thrombosed popliteal artery stent with occlusion of a long segment of the popliteal artery, resulting in critical limb ischemia. An open reconstruction with bypass using an autologous GSV was preferred to a repeat endovascular intervention.

Multiple Choice Questions

1. The 30-day mortality and 30-day amputation rates comparing primary bypass with bypass after failed endovascular intervention are:
   A. Similar in both groups.
   B. 30-day amputation rate is higher in the group undergoing bypass after failed endovascular intervention, as compared to the primary bypass group
   C. 30-day mortality is similar in both groups, but the 30-day amputation rate is higher in patients undergoing bypass after failed endovascular intervention, as compared to the primary bypass group
   D. 30-day mortality is higher, but the 30-day amputation rate is similar in patients undergoing bypass after failed endovascular intervention as compared to the primary bypass group.
2. After a median follow-up of 6 months, the incidence of stent thrombosis in the femoral-popliteal segment is:
   A. 4.3%
   B. 5.3%
   C. 6.3%
   D. 8.3%
3. The predictors of early stent thrombosis in the femoral–popliteal segment are:
   A. Diabetes mellitus
   B. Critical leg ischemia
   C. Long segment bare nitinol stents
   D. Critical leg ischemia and covered nitinol stents

Answers: 1(A), 2(A), 3(D)

References

1. Hossain S, Leblanc D, Farber A, Power AH, De Rose, et al. Editor's choice – infrainguinal bypass following failed endovascular intervention compared with primary bypass: a systematic review and meta-analysis. Eur J Vasc Endovasc Surg. 2019;57(3):382–91. PMID:30393063
2. Bradbury AW, Moakes CA, Popplewell M, Meecham L, Bate GR, et al. A vein bypass first versus a best endovascular treatment first revascularisation strategy for patients with chronic limb threatening ischaemia who required an infra-popliteal, with or without an additional more proximal infra-inguinal revascularisation procedure to restore limb perfusion (BASIL-2): an open-label, randomised, multicentre, phase 3 trial. Lancet. 2023;401(10390):1798–809. PMID:37116524
3. Banerjee S, Sarode K, Mohammad A, Gigliotti O, Baig MS, et al. Femoropopliteal artery stent thrombosis: report from the excellence in peripheral artery disease registry. Circ Cardiovasc Interv. 2016;9(2):e002730. PMID:26839391

48 Brachial Artery Bypass Following Failed Thrombectomy

Presentation

A 55-year-old woman was seen in the emergency room in April 2025 with complaints of pain, numbness, and discoloration of the left index and fourth finger of 5 weeks duration. She had a history of well controlled hypertension and was a non-smoker. She had purplish discoloration in the left index and ring finger. Arterial duplex study showed severely diminished perfusion of the left index finger. She underwent extensive Rheumatology work-up including Factor V DNA (Leiden), DNA antibody, JAK-2 mutation, ANA, Scl-70 antibody, Centromere antibody, cytoplasmic antibody, cryoglobulin, neutrophil antibody—all tests were negative. 2D Echocardiogram showed a small PFO, an ejection fraction of 50-50% with a right-to-left shunt. Her symptoms progressively worsened. She underwent CTA angiography on May 3, 2025, which showed an abrupt occlusion of the distal left brachial artery extending to the bifurcation of the brachial artery to the radial and ulnar artery. There was segmental reconstitution of the left proximal radial artery which was of small caliber and hypoattenuating. There was a segmental reconstitution of the distal left radial artery with suspected filling defect at the level of the wrist. The proximal ulnar and radial arteries reconstituted via the deep brachial artery with abrupt occlusion of the distal ulnar artery (Figs. 48.1, 48.2, and 48.3). There was also evidence of remote splenic infarcts.

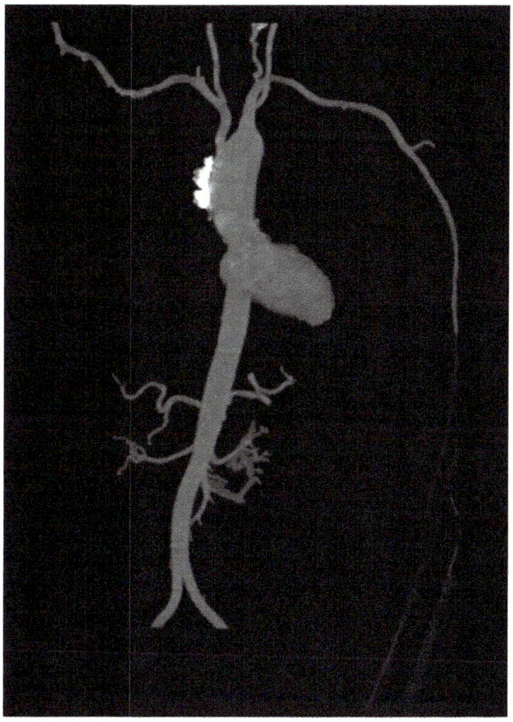

Fig. 48.1 CTA Normal Arch vessels, Abdominal aota, normal left subclavian, axillary and proximal brachial artery

She underwent a selective left subclavian--axillary-brachial arteriogram using an ultrasound-guided right femoral artery access.

S. S. Hans, *Secondary and Tertiary Arterial Reconstructions*,
https://doi.org/10.1007/978-3-032-21214-6_48

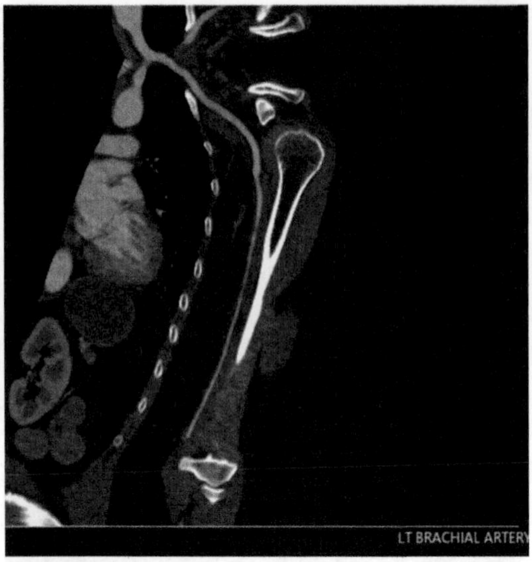

Fig. 48.2 CTA left upper extremity shows left brachial artery occlusion just proximal to the elbow joint

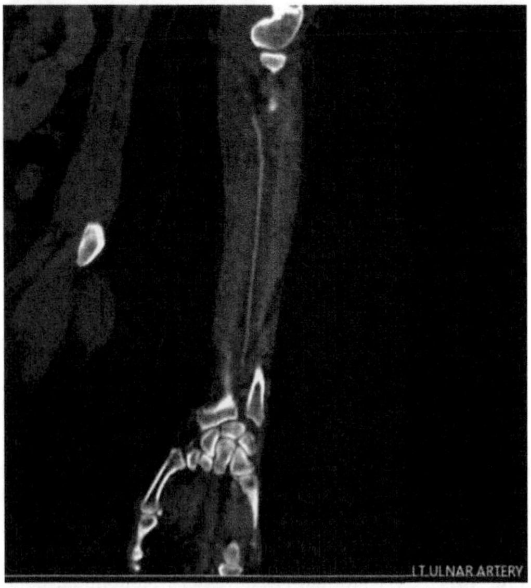

Fig. 48.3 CTA showing patency of the left radial artery with occlusion just proximal to the wrist joint

There was evidence of a left brachial artery occlusion likely thrombotic in nature with filling of the distal most portion of the left brachial artery just proximal to its bifurcation. There was an associated thrombotic radial artery occlusion at the wrist. There were a significant number of collaterals around the elbow area. There was diminished filling of the digital arteries in the left hand (Figs. 48.4, 48.5, 48.6, 48.7, and 48.8). On May 8, 2025, she underwent left brachial artery exploration and thrombectomy, with passage of a number 3 Fogarty balloon catheter into the radial and ulnar arteries. The clot appeared to be subacute on visual inspection of the thrombectomy specimen from the radial and ulnar arteries. A significant amount of thrombus was retrieved from the forearm arteries. Following thrombectomy, a patch angioplasty with a basilic

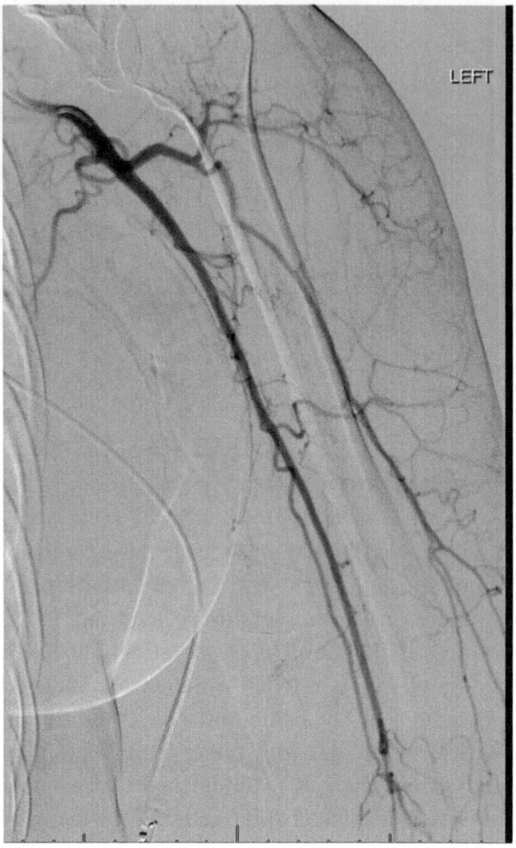

Fig. 48.4 Left proximal brachial arteriogram-(catheter tip) showing small caliber left brachial artery with occlusion just proximal to the elbow joint

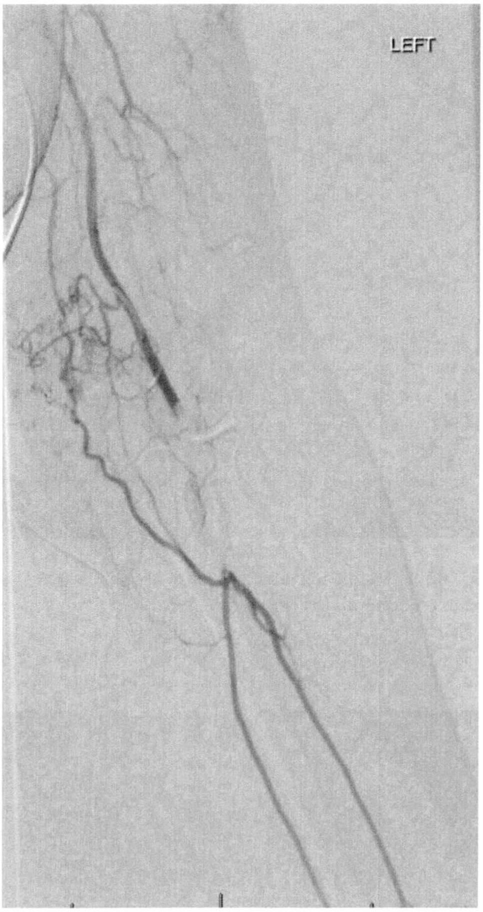

Fig. 48.5 Left upper extremity arteriogram showing distal left brachial artery occlusion with reconstitution just proximal to the brachial artery bifurcation via collaterals

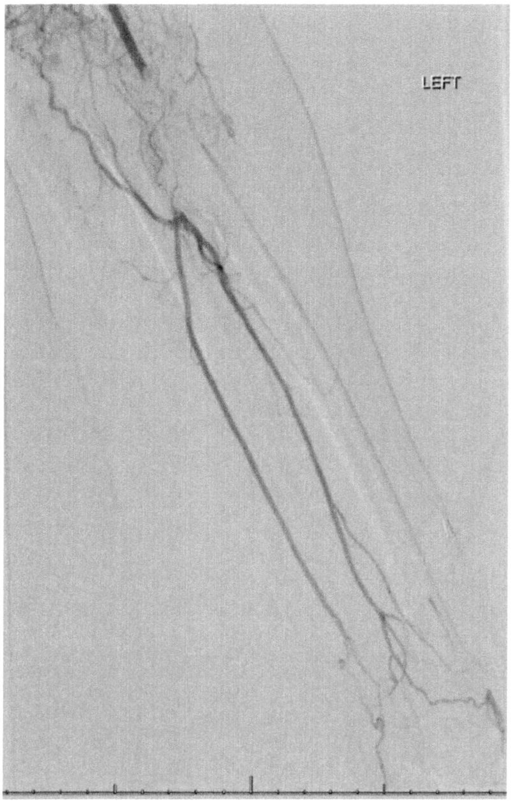

Fig. 48.6 Arteriogram showing left brachial artery occlusion with filling of radial and ulnar arteries with distal occlusion and collaterals at the wrist

vein harvested from the left upper arm was performed. Completion arteriogram showed a satisfactory flow at the thrombectomy site with minimal residual thrombus in the distal radial and ulnar arteries at the level of the wrist. However, 5 days later she developed rethrombosis of the brachial artery confirmed with a CTA on May 13, 2025. She underwent re-exploration of the left brachial artery, rethrombectomy through a longitudinal incision in the basilic vein patch over the brachial artery and passage of No. 3 Fogarty catheter proximally and distally into radial and ulnar arteries. A left mid-brachial to distal brachial reversed saphenous vein bypass was performed after harvesting a left GSV from the thigh. A completion angiogram occlusion of a short segment of proximal ulnar bypass artery (Fig. 48.9). Rethrombectomy via an incision in the bypass showed improved caliber of the proximal ulnar artery (Fig. 48.10). There were focal occlusions of radial and ulnar arteries at the level of the wrist with immediate reconstitution not amenable to any direct thrombectomy (Figs. 48.11, 48.12, and 48.13). Following brachial artery bypass her hand vascularity significantly improved, and she was discharged on Abixaban and clopidogrel after a

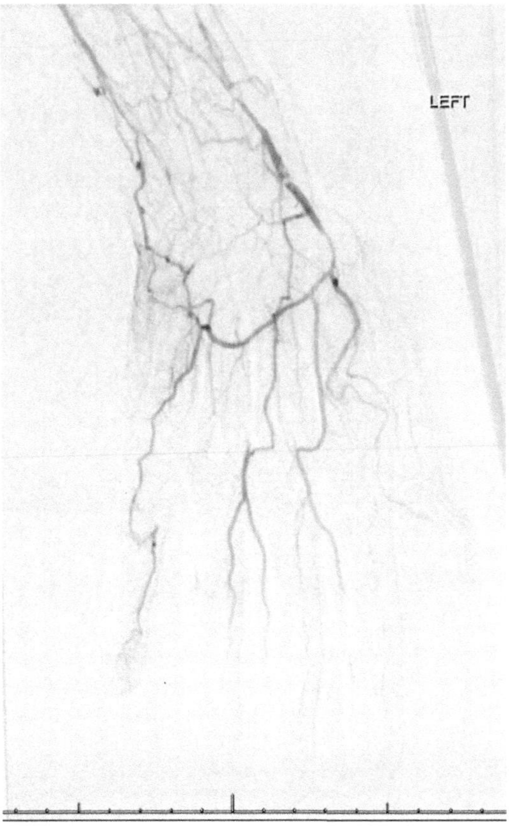

Fig. 48.7 Arteriogram showing filling defect in the left radial artery at the wrist with stenosis proximally. Ulnar artery is occluded at the wrist. Palmer arch is seen

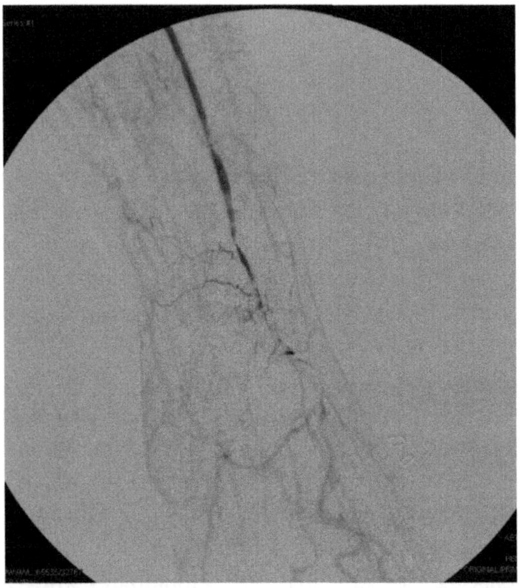

Fig. 48.8 Arteriogram showing areas of stenosis and occlusion of the distal left radial artery at the wrist with incomplete Palmer arch and diminished filling of the digital arteries

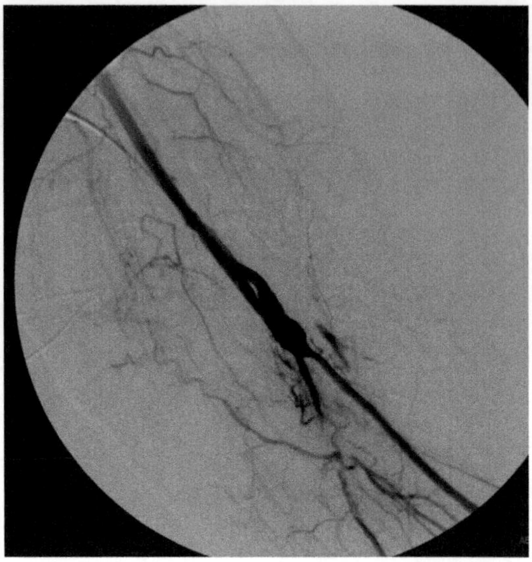

Fig. 48.9 Patent left brachial artery bypass with proximal 3 cm long ulnar artery occlusion

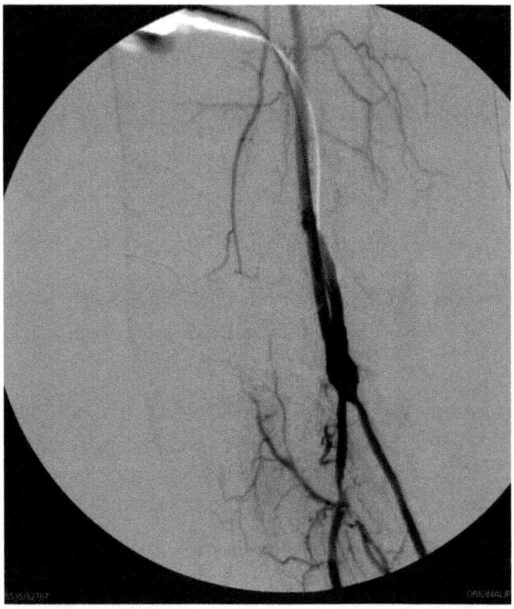

Fig. 48.10 Improved flow following Rethrombectomy of the proximal ulnar artery with 50% residual stenosis

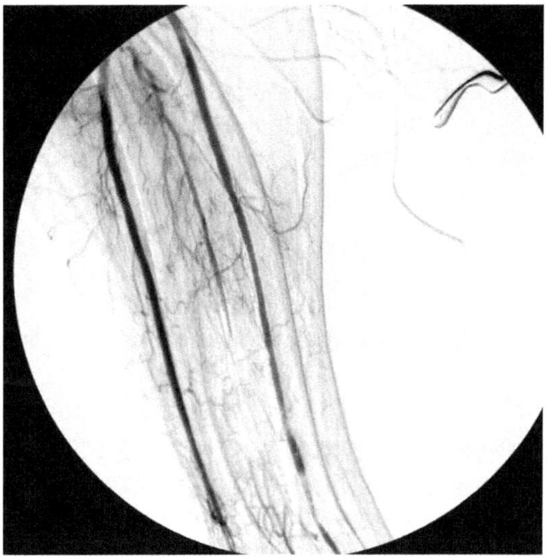

Fig. 48.11 Improved filling of the forearm arteries. Interosseous artery is occluded in its mid-segment

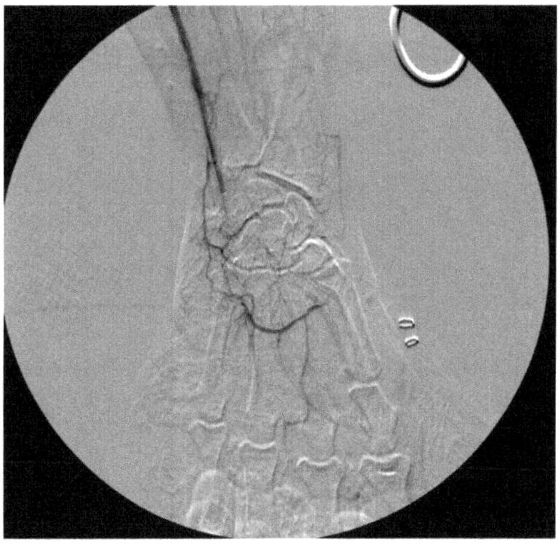

Fig. 48.12 Operative arteriogram shows occlusion of the distal ulnar artery with filling of the Palmer arch via collaterals. There is diminished filling of the digital arteries

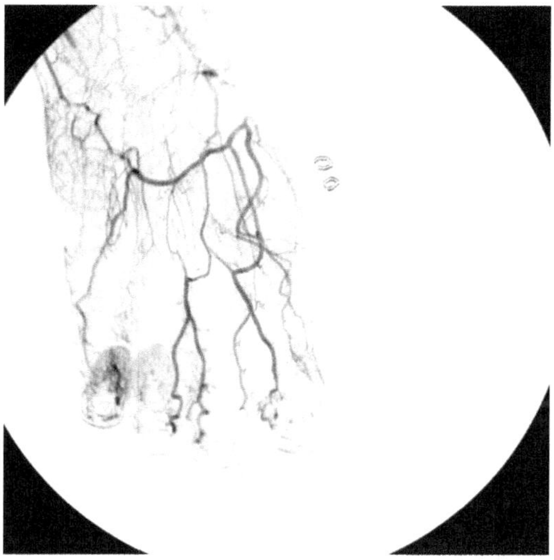

Fig. 48.13 Improved filling of the Palmer Arch

short duration of systemic heparin administration in the perioperative period.

Discussion

The most common cause of an acute brachial artery occlusion is due to an embolus, usually from a cardiac source and rarely from a subclavian/axillary aneurysm caused by a cervical rib [1, 2]. Other causes include trauma such as supracondylar fracture of the humerus, brachial arterial access for cardiac or vascular diagnostic procedures with or without intervention frequently associated with the use of a 6F or a larger sheath. Hypercoagulable states, COVID-19 and HIV infections have also been reported as causes of acute brachial thrombosis [1, 2]. Brachial artery aneurysm and thrombosis secondary to fibromuscular dysplasia in a 29 year-old-man was treated with thromboembolectomy, interposition vein graft and anticoagulation [3]. On histopathology, the residual brachial artery with the aneurysm revealed thickening of the intima, fragmentation of the internal elastic lamina, a thinned and disorganized media, alternating fibrous and loss of smooth muscles. There was absence of inflammatory and fatty infiltrates. Fibromuscular dysplasia affects multiple vascular beds in 28% of cases and screening for the most affected sites such as renal and carotid arteries should be performed. Vasculitis, FMD, and atherosclerosis can also cause both chronic and acute brachial artery occlusion in patients with poor collateral flow.

Brachial artery occlusion occurs in 0.9–4% following cardiac catheterizations using brachial artery access. The brachial artery is also the most common injured artery in civilian trauma (30% of all arterial injuries) [4]. Digital gangrene is a frequent manifestation of connective tissue disease. Thrombangiitis obliterans (Buerger's disease) commonly affects arteries of the lower extremity but may occasionally cause multiple digital artery occlusions and occurs in patients who are current smokers. Upper extremity arterial bypass yields a 52% 5 year patency which is dependent on the underlying condition for which the bypass was performed. For a short-segment bypass as was performed in this patient, long-term results should be much superior.

Multiple Choice Questions

1. The most common cause of brachial artery occlusion is:
   A. Embolic occlusion from a cardiac source
   B. Thrombotic occlusion from brachial artery access
   C. Embolic occlusion from post-procedural aneurysm
   D. Brachial artery aneurysm as a result of FMD
2. Incidence of brachial artery occlusion following brachial artery access for cardiac catheterization is:
   A. 0.5–2%
   B. 0.6–3%
   C. 0.8–3.5%
   D. 0.9–4%
3. A 56-year-ol woman presents to the hospital with ischemic changes in the fingers of the left hand of 4 weeks duration. Arteriogram shows occlusion of brachial artery from just proximal to elbow extending to brachial artery bifurcation with significant collaterals. There is no history of atrial fibrillation or any other cardiac source of embolic occlusion. The best management option is:
   A. Brachial artery thromboembolectomy
   B. Thrombolysis using retrograde femoral artery access
   C. Brachial artery bypass using an autologous vein
   D. Brachial artery bypass using PTFE graft

Answers: 1(A), 2(D), 3(C)

References

1. Eskandari MK: Upper-extremity arterial occlusive disease. eMedicine (7/5/2024). Retrieved from https://emedicine.medscape.com/article/462289-overview?form=fpf
2. Witz M, Lehmann J, Korzets Z. Acute brachial artery thrombosis as the initial manifestation of human immunodeficiency virus infection. Am J Hematol. 2000;64(2):137–9. PMID:10814996
3. Jones JL, de Silva U, Soh HC. Brachial artery aneurysm and thrombosis secondary to fibromuscular dysplasia. J Vasc Surg Cases Innov Tech. 2016;2(3):114–8. PMID:38827196
4. McCollum CH, Mavor E. Brachial artery injury after cardiac catheterization. J Vasc Surg. 1986;4(4):355–9. PMID:3761478

49 Post-radiation Subclavian-Axillary Occlusion with Severe Hand Ischemia

Presentation

In Nov 2007, a 74-year-old woman presented with a painful, cold right upper extremity with paresthesia involving the hand. She had absent right upper extremity pulses (brachial and radial pulse). She was a current smoker with a history of smoking 60 pack-years. Medical comorbidities included hypertension, atrial fibrillation, and chronic obstructive pulmonary disease (COPD). She had a history of carcinoma of the breast with mastectomy followed by radiation nearly 20 years previously, and had bilateral breast implants. She had post-radiation skin changes in the right lower neck and right infraclavicular area. Doppler arterial study showed: wrist-brachial index 0.40 (right) and 1.0 (left). Catheter-based arteriography using femoral artery access showed a 5 cm long right subclavian-axillary artery occlusion (Figs. 49.1 and 49.2). Percutaneous angioplasty using transfemoral artery access followed by an ipsilateral brachial artery access was unsuccessful. She underwent interposition of an 8 mm PTFE interring graft (WL Gore, Newark, DE). Proximal anastomosis was performed end-to-end. The diameter of the distal axillary artery was small with numerous collaterals, which were controlled with silastic vessel loops. The distal anastomosis to the distal segment of the axillary artery was performed in an end-to-side fashion because of the size discrepancy between the graft and the artery (Figs. 49.3 and 49.4).

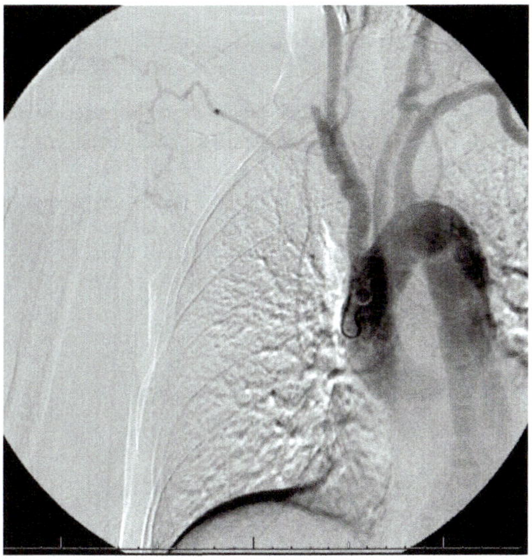

Fig. 49.1 Arteriography showing occlusion of the right subclavian and axillary artery

Two years and four months later, she presented to the ER with acute ischemia of the right upper extremity secondary to thrombosis of the subclavian-axillary artery interposition graft. She

S. S. Hans, *Secondary and Tertiary Arterial Reconstructions*,
https://doi.org/10.1007/978-3-032-21214-6_49

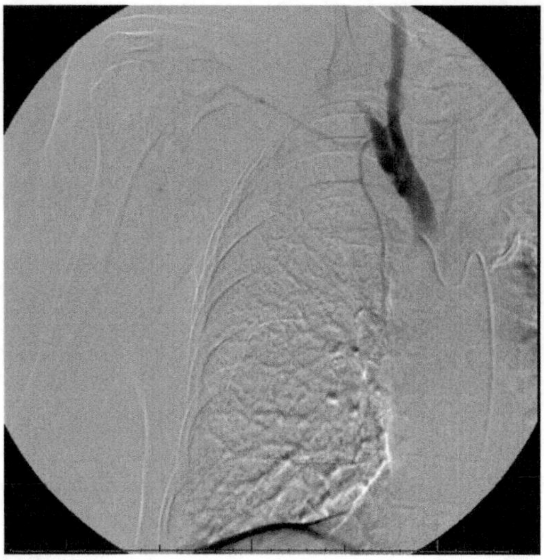

Fig. 49.2 Selective right brachiocephalic arteriogram showing right subclavian and axillary artery occlusion

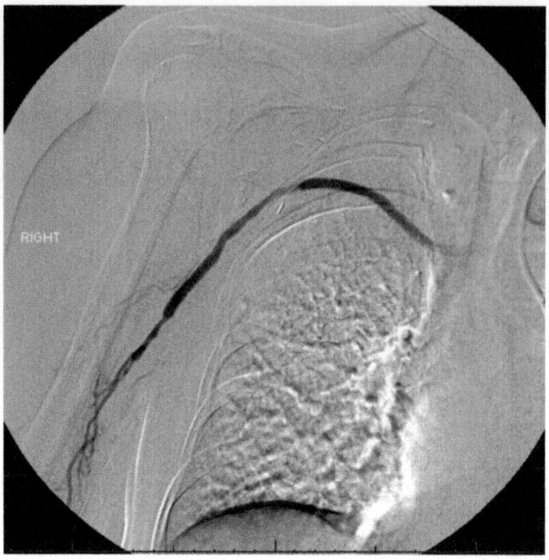

Fig. 49.4 Arteriogram showing diffuse narrowing of the brachial artery in its mid and distal portions

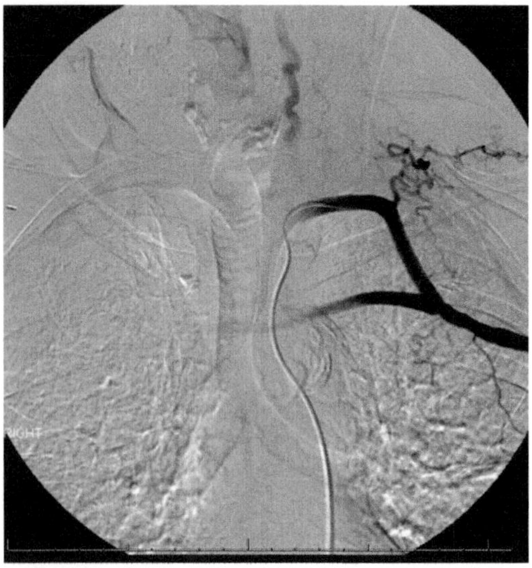

Fig. 49.3 Left subclavian arteriogram showing satisfactory anastomosis of the crossover axillo-axillary artery bypass graft at the donor site

underwent open thrombectomy of the axillo-axillary bypass graft with revision of the graft and distal extension of the graft to the proximal brachial artery using a 6 mm PTFE graft and patch angioplasty (PTFE patch) of the proximal anastomosis after removal of an intimal hyperplastic lesion. The proximal brachial artery measured only 3 mm in diameter.

Three months later, the patient presented with recurrent ischemic symptoms. Catheter-based arteriography using femoral artery access revealed an occluded right axillo-brachial artery with a patent left subclavian and axillary artery. The patient underwent crossover axillo-axillary bypass with graft thrombectomy. Because of the absence of back bleeding after opening of the distal anastomosis with the passage of a No. 3 Fogarty catheter, an incision was made at the elbow, and the brachial artery was exposed. A passage of a Fogarty catheter, proximally, aided in retrieval of an organized thrombus with establishment of a pulsatile antegrade flow.

The patient presented to the ER 9 months later with another episode of recurrent ischemic symptoms of the right hand. The distal anastomosis of the crossover graft (axillo-brachial artery) was thrombosed. Following graft thrombectomy, a translocated non-reversed GSV graft (taken from right thight) was interposed between the distal

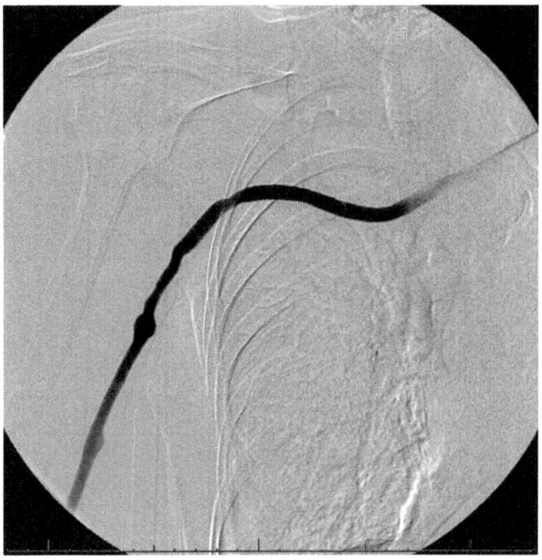

Fig. 49.5 Arteriogram showing proximal segment of a patent brachio-brachial bypass (translocated non-reversed saphenous vein) from right upper arm to lower arm)

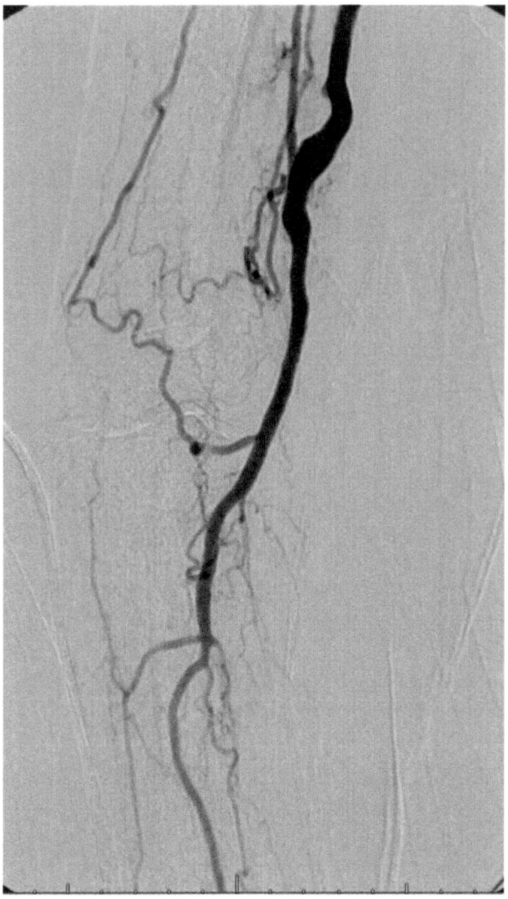

Fig. 49.6 Arteriogram showing the distal segment of the translocated non-reversed GSV graft anastomosed to the distal brachial artery

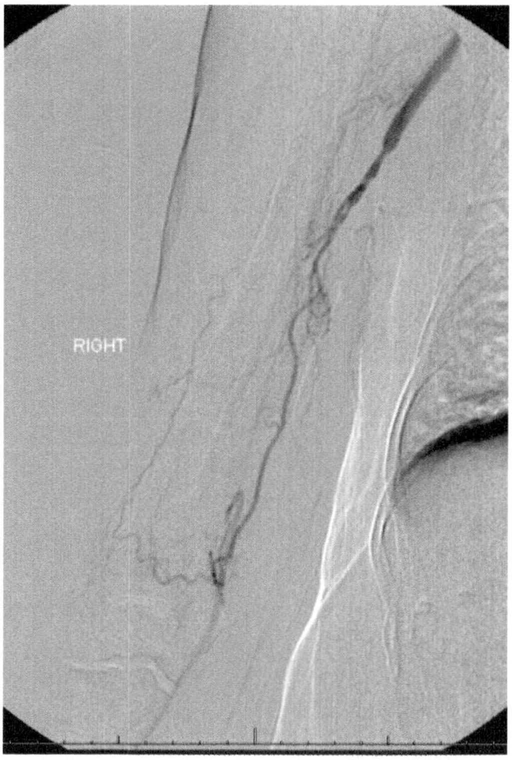

Fig. 49.7 Arteriogram showing occlusion of the brachial artery and stenosis distal to the distal anastomosis of the axillo-brachial bypass

portion of the axillo-brachial graft to the brachial artery at the elbow (Figs. 49.5 and 49.6).

On July 10, 2014 (7 years following her index operation), she underwent thrombectomy via right brachial artery cut down using a Fogarty catheter proximally and distally with reestablishment of diminished blood flow in the hand (Figs. 49.7, 49.8, 49.9, 49.10, and 49.11). The patient had a nearly complete occlusion of the ulnar artery with an incomplete Palmer arch. A follow-up arterial Doppler study (August 2016) showed slightly diminished blood flow in both upper extremities, with wrist brachial index 0.91 (right) and 0.85 (left). Patient died on July 1, 2016, from acute respiratory failure due to advanced COPD.

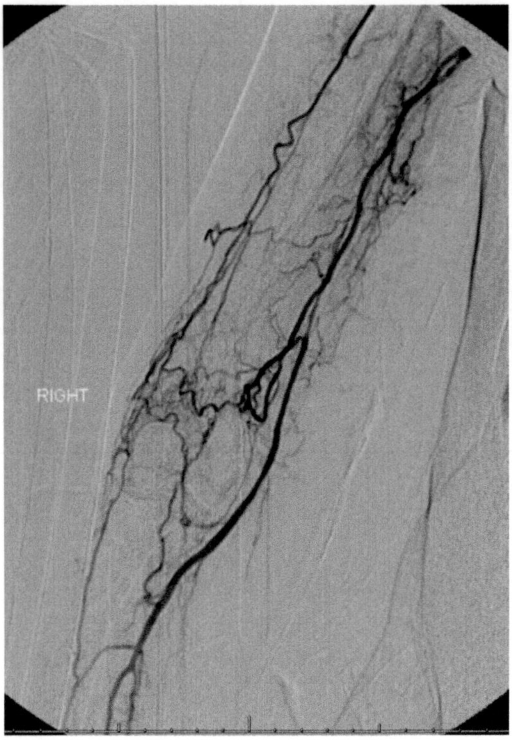

Fig. 49.8 Arteriogram showing occluded right brachial artery with large collaterals

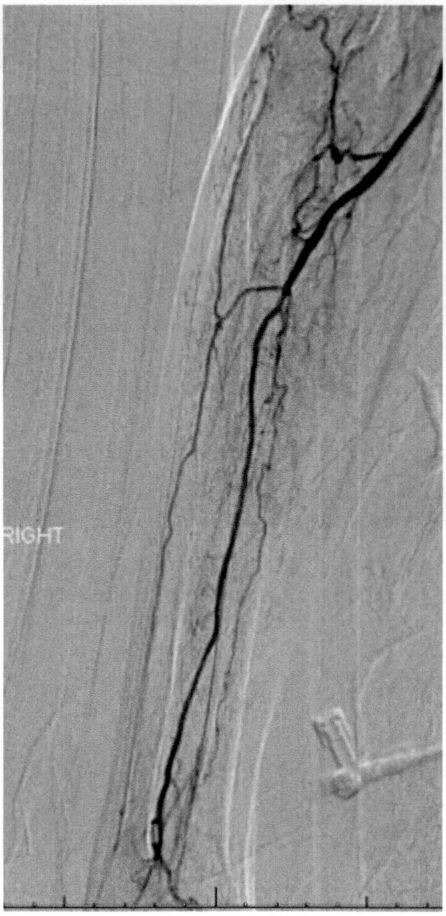

Fig. 49.9 Arteriogram showing a patent right brachial artery but with occlusion of the interosseous and ulnar artery

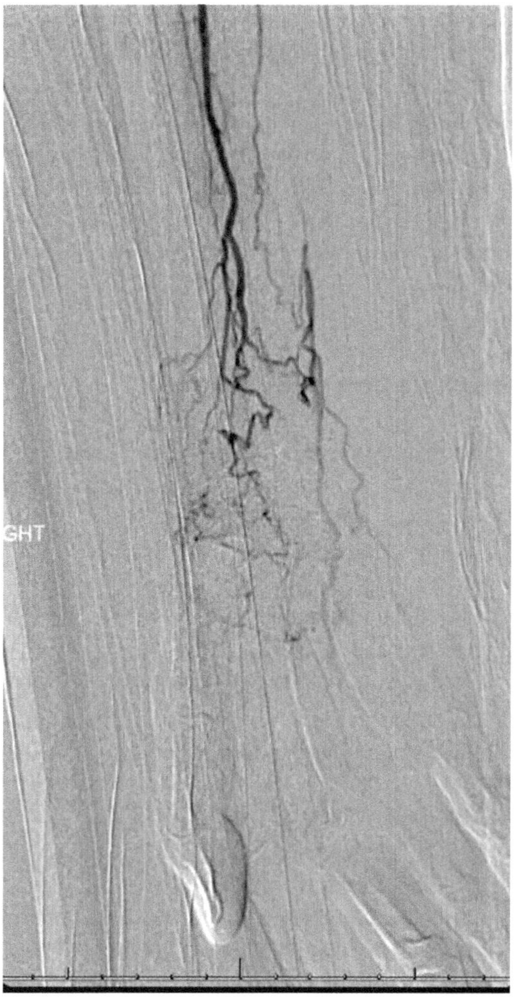

Fig. 49.10 Arteriogram showing patency of the right radial artery with distal occlusion. The faint ulnar artery is reconstituted via collaterals, with diminished flow in the hand vasculature

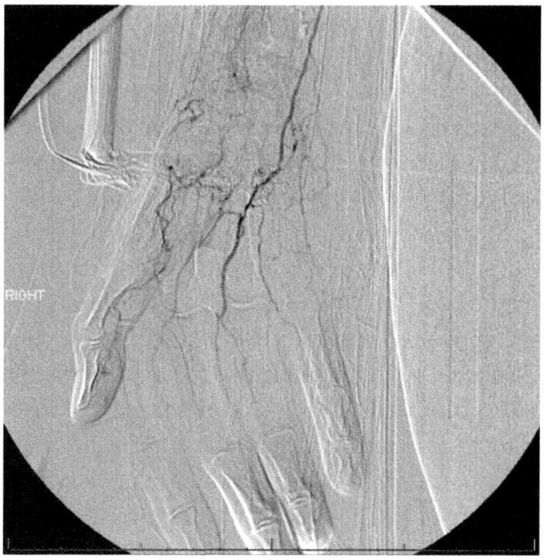

Fig. 49.11 Arteriogram showing diminished filling of the hand vasculature and incomplete Palmer arch vessels

Discussion

Multimodality treatment of breast cancer with surgery, systemic chemotherapy, and radiation therapy has resulted in long-term survival beyond 10 years among half of the treated patients [1]. Recent epidemiological studies have revealed an excess of vascular deaths in women with cancer of the breast who underwent adjuvant radiation therapy [1]. Radiation-induced arteriopathy within the radiation field affects small vessels as well as large vascular trunks [1]. Modrall and

Sadjadi classified radiation-induced arteriopathy according to time of onset: early (≤5 years) by wall thrombosis; intermediate (≤10 years) by wall fibrosis; occlusion in the absence of collaterals; and late (mean 26 years) by accelerated atherosclerosis with peri-arterial fibrosis [2].

Radiation-induced arteriopathy (RIA) involving subclavian-axillary arteries is not well documented in the literature. There are only 39 publications between 1973 and 2015 that comprise only 127 patients in case reports and two cohort studies, with a preponderance of cases after breast cancer. Most patients presented with symptoms of ischemia from arterial stenosis/occlusion [1]. The subclavian artery was the most common artery involved, followed by the axillary artery [1]. Two-thirds of cases have associated radiation-induced brachial plexopathy [1]. The mean time from radiation therapy to radiation-induced atherosclerosis was 16.1 ± 10.8 years [1]. Some patients with minor symptoms (claudication) can be managed medically. Angioplasty with or without stenting has been advocated in some cases with severe stenosis of the subclavian-axillary artery [2]. Most patients with occlusion will require arterial bypass [2]. Due to peri-arterial fibrosis, operative dissection can be challenging, and there is an increased incidence of late graft infection [2]. Restenosis rates are higher in these patients, and therefore, frequent graft surveillance is recommended [2].

The primary revascularization with an interposition axillary graft resulted in an occlusion of the graft, most likely due to intimal hyperplasia exacerbated by graft mismatch between a small diameter distal axillary/proximal brachial artery and the presence of microscopic radiation-induced arteriopathy in the proximal and distal anastomotic sites. In retrospect, the first revascularization should have been a crossover axillo--axillary bypass because likely proximal anastomosis of the interposition subclavian-axillary graft was performed to a diseased portion of the subclavian artery with radiation-induced thickening of its wall. In patients with occlusion involving the first or second portion of the subclavian artery, a carotid-subclavian bypass is an alternative option for revascularization.

Because of recurrent episodes of occlusion due to thrombosis of the grafts and the native brachial artery over a long period of time, the forearm and the hand remained viable despite thrombotic occlusion of the forearm and hand arteries because of the formation of numerous collaterals.

Multiple Choice Questions

1. Radiation-induced vasculopathy following radiation for breast cancer most commonly involves.
   A. Axillary artery
   B. Subclavian artery
   C. Subclavian vein
   D. Axillary vein
2. Association of brachial plexopathy with radiation-induced arteriopathy of the subclavian and axillary arteries occurs in
   A. 50% of cases
   B. 55% of cases
   C. 65% of cases
   D. 75% of cases
3. Accelerated atherosclerosis with peri-arterial fibrosis due to radiation occurs after a mean time period of
   A. 5 years
   B. 10 years
   C. 12–15 years
   D. 16–20 years

Answers: 1(B), 2(C), 3(B)

References

1. Delanian S. Is radiation-induced arteriopathy in long-term breast cancer survivors an underdiagnosed situation?: Critical and pragmatic review of available literature. Radiother Oncol. 2021;157:163–74. PMID:33515666
2. Modrall JG, Sadjadi J. Early and late presentations of radiation arteritis. Semin Vasc Surg. 2003;16(3):209–14. PMID:12975760

50 Hybrid Repair of a Large Traumatic Femoral Artery to Femoral Vein Fistula

Presentation

A 60-year-old woman was referred to the vascular clinic on January 25, 2021, for evaluation of heaviness and discomfort in the right lower extremity for the past 6 months. Comorbidities included hypertension, degenerative arthritis of the hips and knees. She gave a history of a stab wound in the right upper thigh 33 years earlier and was treated at an outside hospital. Physical exam revealed diminished right dorsalis pedis and post-tibial (PT) pulse. A pulsatile mass with a strong thrill was palpable in the right upper thigh. Duplex arterial imaging revealed an ankle brachial index (ABI) of 1.0 on both sides and peak systolic velocity as shown in Table 50.1 below.

Table 50.1 Peak systolic velocity

Artery	Right side	LeftsSide
Common femoral artery (CFA)	205 cm/s	157 cm/s
Profunda femoris	202 cm/s	77 cm/s
Proximal SFA	220 cm/s	94 cm/s

Duplex imaging revealed a large arteriovenous fistula (AVF) in the right upper thigh, but the fistula communication could not be localized. Computerized tomographic arteriography (CTA) showed filling of the IVC in the arterial phase (Fig. 50.1) abdominal aortography and run off study using ultrasound based left femoral artery access showed aneurysmal dilation of the right common iliac artery (CIA), external iliac artery (EIA), right CFA, and a fistulous communication between the profunda femoris artery and profunda femoris vein with poor filling of infrapopliteal arteries on the right side due to a steal from the fistulous communication (Figs. 50.2, 50.3, and 50.4). Preoperative 2D echocardiogram showed left ventricular (LV) ejection fraction of 60% with mild diastolic dysfunction.

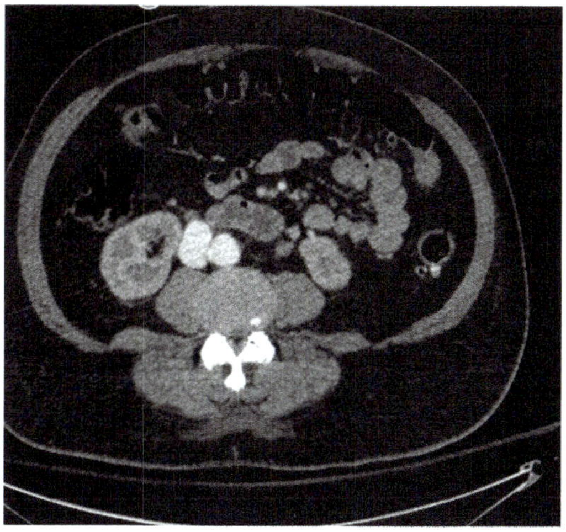

Fig. 50.1 Preoperative CTA showing early filling of the IVC in the arterial phase

Hybrid repair of this very large AV fistula was planned. Under general anesthesia, (February 2021), ultrasound-guided percutaneous puncture of the left common femoral artery and vein was performed. An 8F, 45 cm long Arrow sheath was

S. S. Hans, *Secondary and Tertiary Arterial Reconstructions*,
https://doi.org/10.1007/978-3-032-21214-6_50

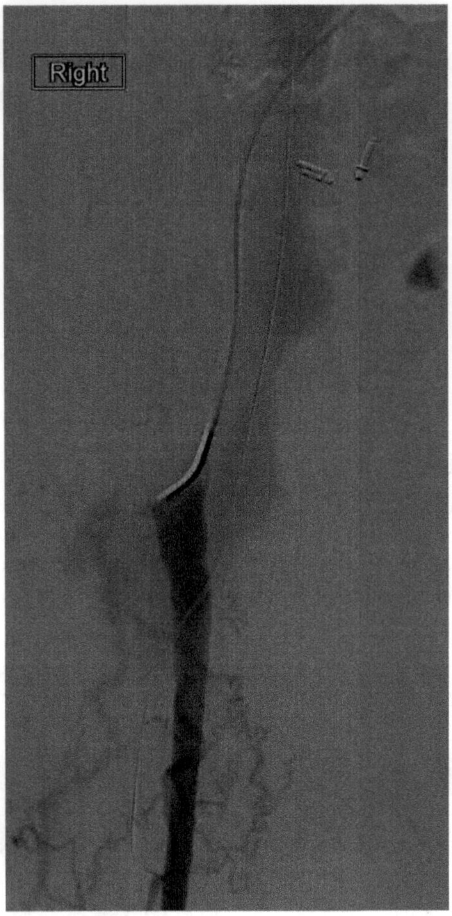

Fig. 50.2 Catheter tip in the proximal SFA, common femoral vein, and external iliac vein filling showing a large fistulous communication

placed in the right external iliac artery, from the left side and a 10F flexor sheath was placed in the distal right external iliac vein following puncture of the left common femoral vein. An 18 mm × 4.0 cm Atlas (Bard, Tempe, AZ) balloon was placed at the junction of the external iliac and common femoral artery. A 20 mm × 4.0 cm Atlas balloon was placed at the site of fistulous communication via a 10F flexor sheath. (The common artery was aneurysmal 22 mm in diameter Tr/AP). Proximal balloon occlusion was positioned for control of bleeding during repair of the large fistula.

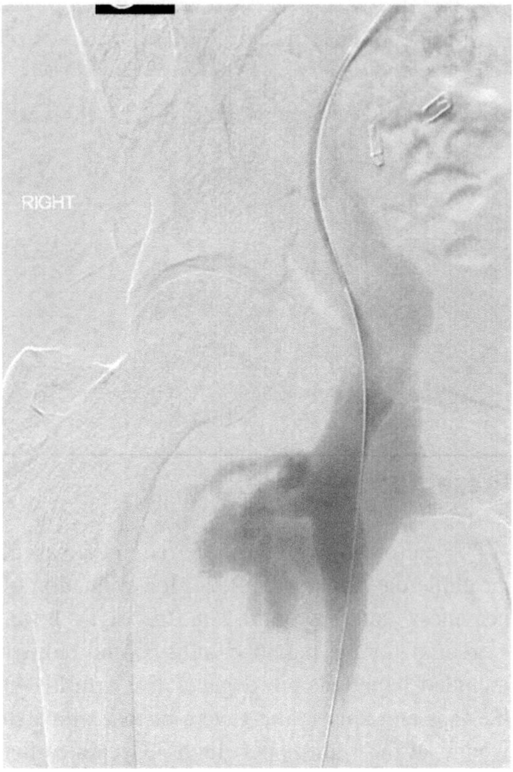

Fig. 50.3 Large AV fistulous communication near the origin of the Profunda Femoris artery

A hockey stick incision was made in the right groin extending to the upper thigh. Intravenous heparin (9000 units/100 mL) was administered during the procedure. The arterial and venous balloons were advanced and inflated in the common femoral artery, proximal superficial femoral artery, and origin of the profunda femoris artery. The common femoral artery was carefully mobilized, and the large venous tributaries were ligated and divided. The common femoral vein was aneurysmal and the silastic vessel loop was not passed around it. At its origin, the superficial femoral artery was thin-walled and had a slight aneurysmal dilatation, resulting in an accidental tear that was repaired. The origin of the profunda femoris artery with fistulous communication was suture ligated. The proximal SFA was mobilized and a silastic vessel loop was passed around the

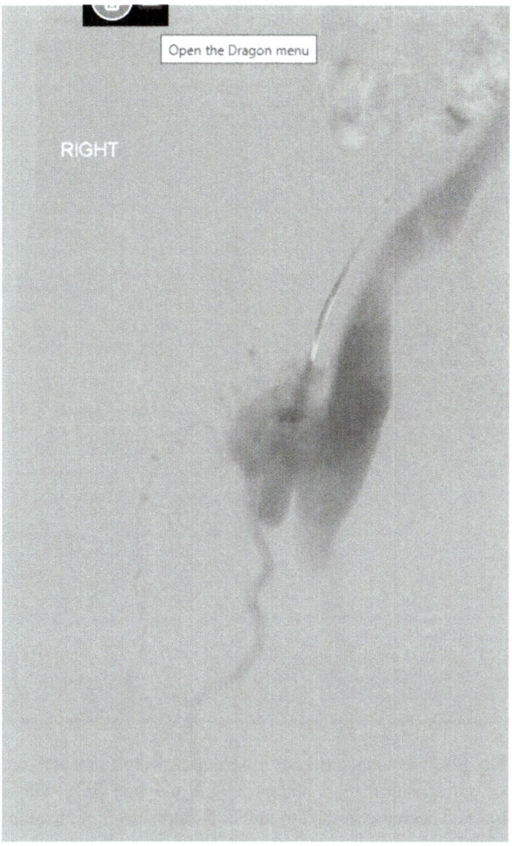

Fig. 50.4 RAO view showing a large fistulous communication with filling of the common femoral vein and the external iliac vein

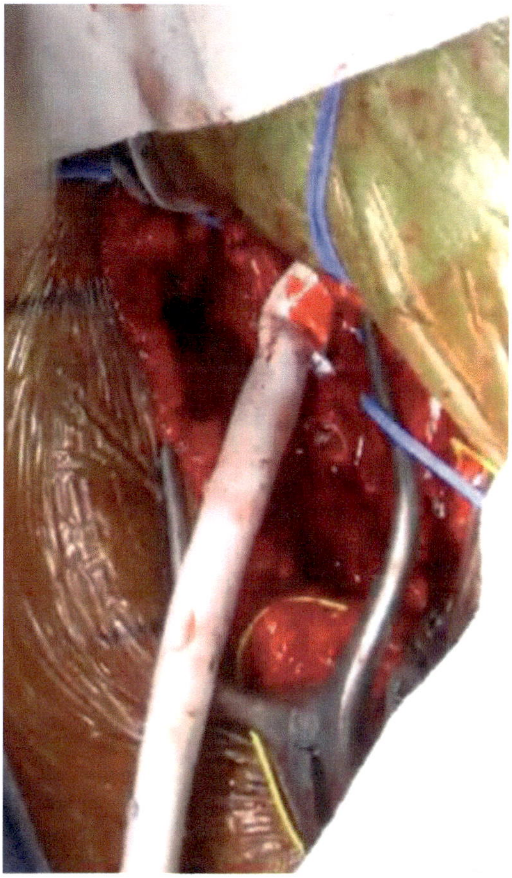

Fig. 50.5 Starting of Proximal Anastomosis of a 10 mm PTFE graft to the proximal CFA

proximal CFA and SFA. The profunda femoris artery and the vein were adherent at one site of the fistulous site. The superficial femoral artery was repaired with a 6′0″ cardiovascular polypropylene suture. A 10 mm PTFE (W.L. Gore—Newark, DE) 5 cm long graft was used as an interpostion graft between the proximal CFA and the proximal SFA (Figs. 50.5 and 50.6). Completion aortogram, pelvic arteriogram, and right lower extremity arteriogram showed a marked decrease in the flow through the fistula with persistent faint filling of the right external iliac vein. One unit of packed cells and 6 liters of isotonic normal saline were administered during four and a half hours of operative time. She was discharged on the fifth postoperative day with ABI of 1.0 on the right and left.

In June 2021, the patient presented with either a residual or a recurrent AV fistula as a result of collateralization or from a missed communication arising from the distal branches of the profunda branches and/or superficial femoral artery. Using ultrasound-guided femoral artery access, right lower extremity arteriogram showed occlusion of the fistula at the proximal SFA and a patent femoral interposition graft (Figs. 50.7 and 50.8). However, there was extensive collateralization throughout the right thigh with retrograde filling of the profunda femoris artery and into the right femoral vein.

Under ultrasound guidance, the right internal jugular vein was punctured using a micropuncture technique, and a 6F, 45 cm long Pinnacle sheath was advanced into the right external iliac

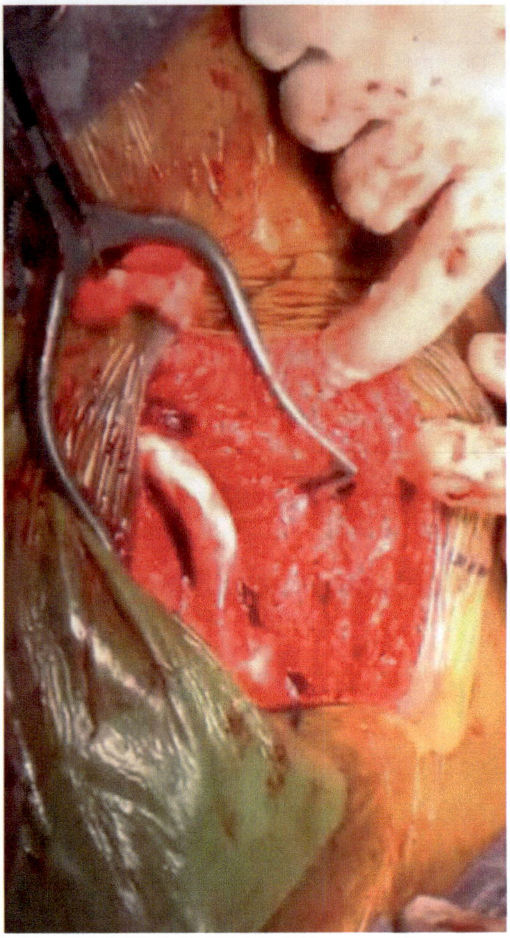

Fig. 50.6 Interposition graft between the CFA and proximal SFA

vein over the guidewire. Common femoral venogram demonstrated a significant enlargement of the right common femoral and external iliac vein. Using a headhunter catheter over-the-wire, the profunda femoris vein was accessed through an AV fistula. There were separate branches arising from the profunda femoris artery contributing to the AV fistula. A 2.6 F Lantern microcatheter (Penumbra Inc., Alameda, CA) was advanced into the circumflex femoral artery, with arteriography demonstrating flow into the fistula. This was selectively embolized using 5 and 6 mm coils. Following this, a medial thigh perforating artery was selectively catheterized and coil embolized. The catheter was retracted into the proximal profunda femoris artery, and another

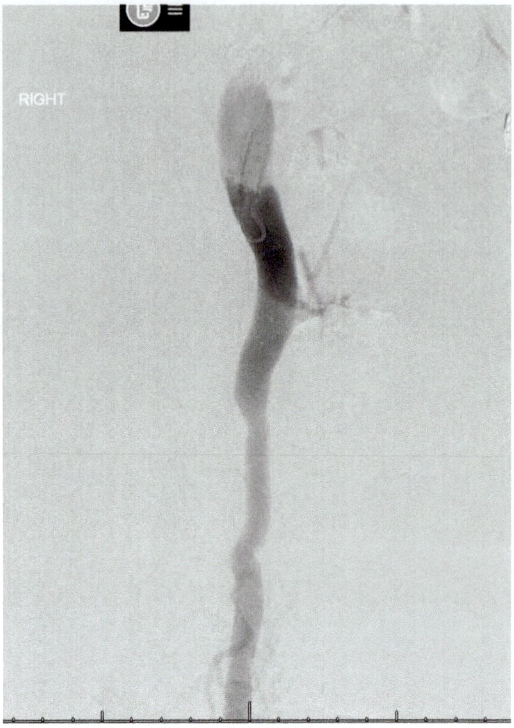

Fig. 50.7 Postoperative arteriogram showing a patent femoral interposition graft and proximal and mid SFA with a marked decrease in-the amount of fistulous communications

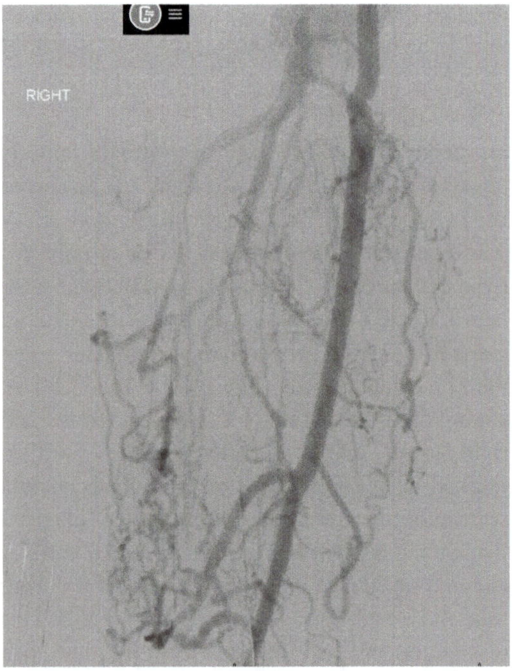

Fig. 50.8 Patent distal SFA with numerous small AV fistula communications arising from the profunda femoris artery and vein branches

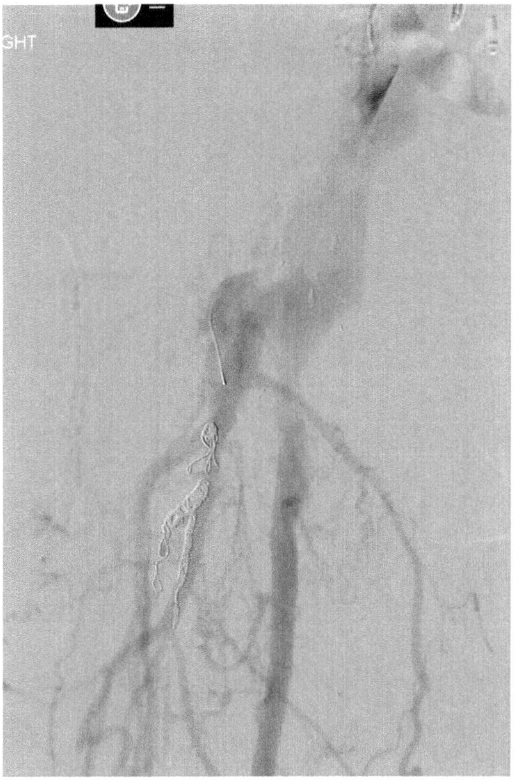

Fig. 50.9 Coil embolization of the branches of the Profunda Femoris vein

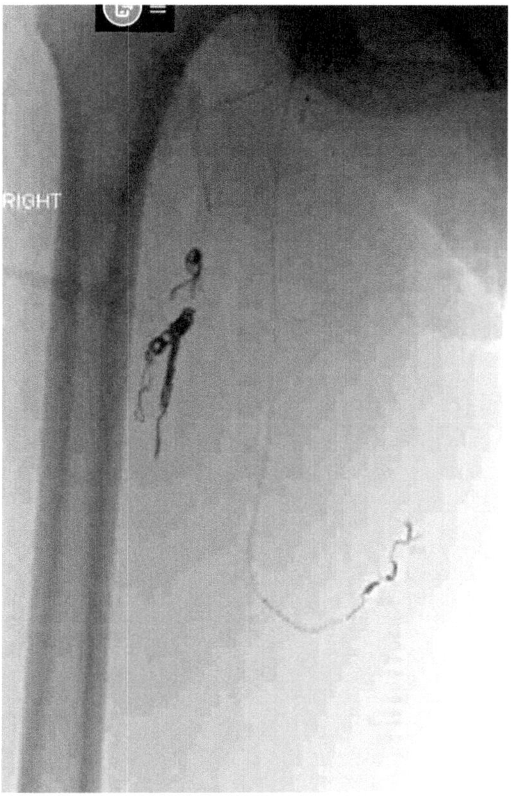

Fig. 50.10 Successful coil embolization of the Profunda Femoris vein and branch of SFA using a microcatheter

fistula communication was selectively embolized with 6 mm coils (Figs. 50.9 and 50.10).

In November 2021, the patient underwent a third intervention for persistent fistulous communication secondary to extensive collateralization between multiple branches of the superficial femoral artery and the profunda femoris artery, with filling of the femoral vein using a left femoral artery access and placement of a 45 cm long 5F Halo sheath that was advanced into the right external iliac artery. Arteriography showed four dominant arteries arising from the SFA with direct communication to the profunda femoris artery, contributing to the persistent/recurrent AV fistula. A 2.6 cm microcatheter was advanced into the ascending segmental branch with coil embolization of this branch and the descending segmental branch. The subsegmental branch was selectively embolized. Another dominant branch of the SFA involving the medial thigh and distal access obtained by a microcatheter and coil embolization was performed with final arteriogram demonstrated absence filling of the AV fistula angiography. Right external iliac artery.

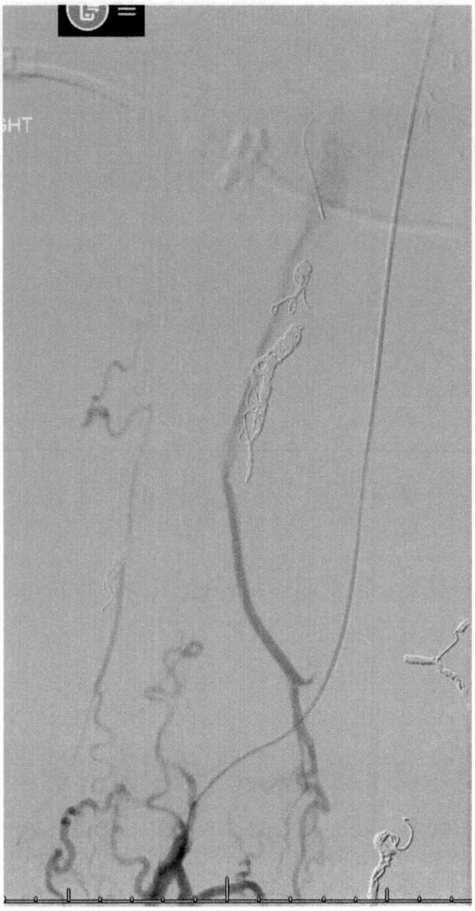

Fig. 50.11 Staged microcoil embolization with the microcatheter tip in the small branches of the distal SFA

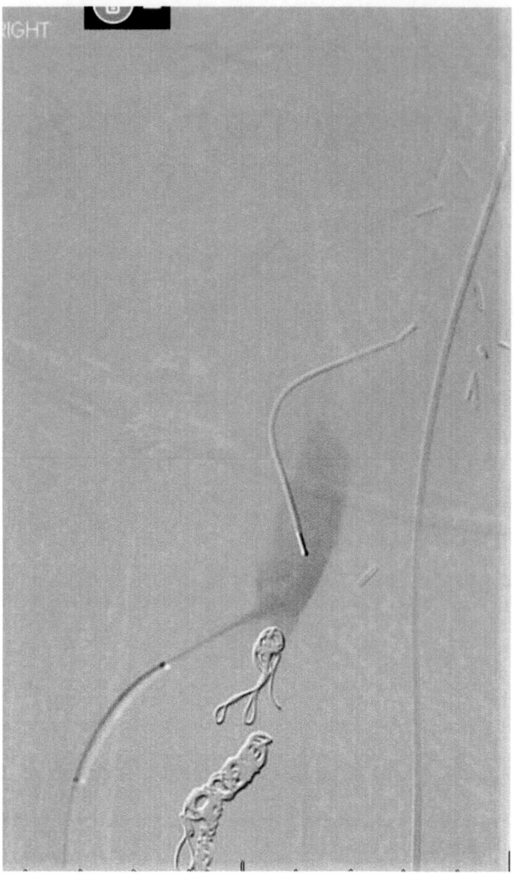

Fig. 50.12 Further coil embolization of the branches of the Profunda Femoris vein

Persistent AV fistula was embolized with coils. Multiple microcatheters were used for selective embolization of profunda and its descending branches (Figs. 50.11 and 50.12).

On June 17, 2024, the patient underwent duplex arterial imaging of the right lower extremity. The patient was uncooperative for completion of the study; there was an elevation of systolic and diastolic velocities suggestive of residual or recurrent femoral AV fistula. There was continuous positive diastolic arterial flow. A follow-up CTA showed a patent femoral interposition graft marked decrease in the fistulous communications in the thigh with filling of the external iliac vein, which appears to have decreased in size (Fig. 50.13).

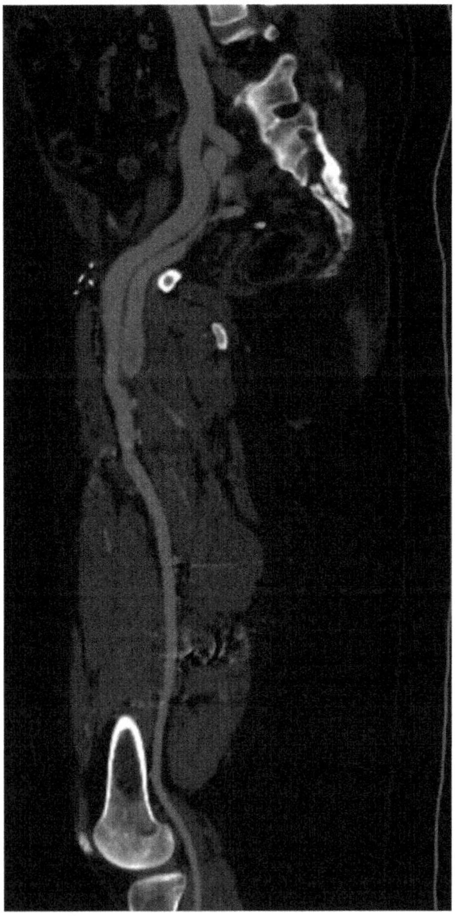

Fig. 50.13 Postoperative CTA showing a patent femoral interposition graft with a marked decrease in the fistulous communication. However, there is persistent filling of the external iliac vein without contrast filling of the IVC

Discussion

Complications of a long-standing acquired femoral arteriovenous fistula of the lower extremity between arterial and venous circulation results in venous hypertension, which in turn causes leg edema and venous ulceration. The patients presenting with a small femoral artery-venous fistula rarely cause any limb symptoms, such as venous hypertension, or systemic symptoms, such as high output congestive heart failure, and can usually be managed conservatively. However, large fistulas like those present in this case usually require repair. Repair isoften challenging and may require open and endovascular techniques (Hybrid repair). Despite all the advances in technology, long-standing fistulas due to a penetrating injury can be difficult to obliterate and frequently recur as closure of a fistulous communication often results in the formation of additional fistulous communications, which continue to enlarge as was demonstrated in this case. Arteriovenous fistulas may occur in the setting of patients with a connective tissue disorder such as Ehlers-Danlos Type IV Syndrome. If fistulous communication is between the SFA and the branch or the main vein, a covered stent can also be considered. A covered stent in the common femoral artery should be avoided.

Rupture of the skin over the fistula, compressive neuropathy, thrombosis, and distal embolization are other rare complications of a large artery-to-vein fistula [1–3]. In patients with a long-standing AV fistula, cardiac overloading may lead to decompensation with heart failure (HF) [1, 3]. From a systematic review and meta-analysis of 274 arteriovenous fistulas by Wenzl et al., the median age was 32 years, and 90% were men. The most frequent mechanism of injury was a stabbing wound (43%) and a gunshot wound (32%). AVF location was the abdomen ($n = 86$; 31%), the lower limb ($n = 79$; 29%), and the neck ($n = 61$; 22%). Risk of heart failure increased with increased feeding artery diameter ($p < 0.001$) [1]. On univariate analysis, HF associated with longer duration from injury to presentation with AVF (11.2 years vs 0.1 years; $p < 0.001$), older median age at presentation (43 years vs 31.1; $p = 0.002$), involvement of large feeding artery (aorta, pulmonary artery, subclavian artery external iliac artery,; 40% vs. 13% $p < 0.001$), shrapnel injuries 11% vs. 2% $p = 0.011$ and injuries to the trunk or lower limb (94% vs. 71% $p = 0.004$) Involvement of a large feeding artery (OR 3.25; 95% CI 1.25–8.42; $p = 0.015$) and every 6 years of delay to presentation (OR 1.30; 95% CI 1.03–1.63; $p = 0.026$) remained independent predictors of heart failure [1]. The AV fistulas distal to the brachial and popliteal artery do not result in heart failure. This case illustrates that because of numerous arteriovenous connections in a long-standing AV fistula, despite satisfactory resolution at the time of the procedure, recurrence is quite common.

Surgical closure of arteriovenous fistula is the mainstay of treatment. Minimally invasive options such as placement of coils and covered stents can be considered depending upon the size and location of the fistula. This option was not considered due to the large size of the fistula and the presence of the aneurysmal femoral artery and vein. A hybrid approach with proximal balloon occlusion and coil embolization helped in reducing blood loss and duration of procedure [1–4]. In this patient, the Profunda Femoris artery had to be sacrificed due to a fistulous communication with an adhered vein. An interposition graft was performed from the proximal CFA to the proximal SFA with ligation of the profunda femoris artery and large fistulous communication with the profunda femoris vein.

Liao et al., described a deep femoral arteriovenous fistula diagnosed over a decade after a small caliber gunshot injury to the groin. The fistula had persisted following two previous attempts. The successful exclusion was achieved via a combination of endovascular techniques. At 4 years of follow-up, the fistula obliteration was durable [4].

Multiple Choice Questions

1. The most frequent mechanism of injury for the formation of AV fistula in the lower extremity is due to:
   A. Iatrogenic vascular access injury during cardiac or vascular intervention
   B. Penetrating stab wounds
   C. Gunshot wound
   D. Vascular injury with femur fracture
2. The risk of heart failure in a patient with an AV fistula is related to:
   A. The size of the feeding artery.
   B. Longer median time from injury to presentation
   C. Size of feeding artery and longer median time from injury to presentation
   D. Presence of AV fistula below the popliteal artery
3. Femoral AV fistula may present years after trauma to the lower extremity with symptoms of:
   A. Pain and discomfort in the lower extremity
   B. Limb edema
   C. Symptoms of intermittent claudication
   D. All of the above

Answers: 1(B), 2(C), 3(D)

References

1. Wenzl FA, Miljkovic SS, Dabestani PJ, Kessler JJ 2nd, Kotaru TR, et al. A systematic review and individual patient data meta-analysis of heart failure as a rare complication of traumatic arteriovenous fistulas. J Vasc Surg. 2021;73(3):1087–1094.e1088. PMID:33002586
2. Nagpal K, Ahmed K, Cuschieri R. Diagnosis and management of acute traumatic arteriovenous fistula. Int J Angiol. 2008;17(4):214–6. PMID:22477453
3. Huang W, Villavicencio JL, Rich NM. Delayed treatment and late complications of a traumatic arteriovenous fistula. J Vasc Surg. 2005;41(4):715–7. PMID:15874939
4. Liao JL, Wang SK, Dalsing MC, Motaganahalli RL. Endovascular treatment of a persistent traumatic deep femoral arteriovenous fistula after gunshot injury. Vasc Endovasc Surg. 2020;54(5):441–4. PMID:32292134

Index

S. S. Hans, *Secondary and Tertiary Arterial Reconstructions*,
https://doi.org/10.1007/978-3-032-21214-6

GPSR Compliance

The European Union's (EU) General Product Safety Regulation (GPSR) is a set of rules that requires consumer products to be safe and our obligations to ensure this.

If you have any concerns about our products, you can contact us on ProductSafety@springernature.com

In case Publisher is established outside the EU, the EU authorized representative is:

Springer Nature Customer Service Center GmbH
Europaplatz 3
69115 Heidelberg, Germany

Batch number: 10732809

Printed by Printforce, the Netherlands